MOLECULAR
BIOLOGY
INTELLIGENCE
UNIT

# Carnitine Today

## Claudio De Simone, M.D.
Università degli Studi di L'Aquila degli Abruzzi
L'Aquila, Italy

## Giuseppe Famularo, M.D.
Università degli Studi di L'Aquila degli Abruzzi
L'Aquila, Italy *and*
Ospedale San Camillo
Rome, Italy

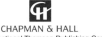

CHAPMAN & HALL
I(T)P An International Thomson Publishing Company

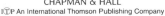

New York • Albany • Bonn • Boston • Cincinnati • Detroit • London • Madrid • Melbourne •
Mexico City • Pacific Grove • Paris • San Francisco • Singapore • Tokyo • Toronto • Washington

LANDES
BIOSCIENCE

AUSTIN, TEXAS
U.S.A.

# MOLECULAR BIOLOGY INTELLIGENCE UNIT
## CARNITINE TODAY
## LANDES BIOSCIENCE
Austin, Texas, U.S.A.

U.S. and Canada Copyright © 1997 Landes Bioscience and Chapman & Hall

Please address all inquiries to the Publishers:
Landes Bioscience, 810 South Church Street, Georgetown, Texas, U.S.A. 78626
Phone: 512/ 863 7762; FAX: 512/ 863 0081

North American distributor:

Chapman & Hall, 115 Fifth Avenue, New York, New York, U.S.A. 10003

CHAPMAN & HALL

U.S. and Canada ISBN: 0-412-13271-0

While the authors, editors and publisher believe that drug selection and dosage and the specifications and usage of equipment and devices, as set forth in this book, are in accord with current recommendations and practice at the time of publication, they make no warranty, expressed or implied, with respect to material described in this book. In view of the ongoing research, equipment development, changes in governmental regulations and the rapid accumulation of information relating to the biomedical sciences, the reader is urged to carefully review and evaluate the information provided herein.

### Library of Congress Cataloging-in-Publication Data
De Simone, Claudio.
   Carnitine today / Claudio De Simone, Giuseppe Famularo.
     p. cm. — (Molecular biology intelligence unit)
   Includes bibliographical references and index.
   ISBN 0-57059-440-6 (alk. paper)
   1. Carnitine—Physiological effect. 2. Carnitine—Metabolism. 3. Carnitine deficiency.
    4. Carnitine—Therapeutic use.
   I. Famularo, Guiseppe. II. Title. III. Series
   [DNLM: 1. Carnitine—metabolism. 2. Carnitine—deficiency. 3. Carnitine—
   therapeutic use. QU 187 D457c 1997]
   QP772.C3D4 1997
   612.3'9—dc21
   DNLM/DLC                                     97-5182
   for Library of Congress                                 CIP

# PUBLISHER'S NOTE

Landes Bioscience produces books in six Intelligence Unit series: *Medical, Molecular Biology, Neuroscience, Tissue Engineering, Biotechnology* and *Environmental.* The authors of our books are acknowledged leaders in their fields. Topics are unique; almost without exception, no similar books exist on these topics.

Our goal is to publish books in important and rapidly changing areas of bioscience for sophisticated researchers and clinicians. To achieve this goal, we have accelerated our publishing program to conform to the fast pace at which information grows in bioscience. Most of our books are published within 90 to 120 days of receipt of the manuscript. We would like to thank our readers for their continuing interest and welcome any comments or suggestions they may have for future books.

Shyamali Ghosh
Publications Director
Landes Bioscience

## DEDICATION

To our good friend Claudio Cavazza, who supported the efforts of two obsessed maniacs in delineating new avenues for carnitine research.

# CONTENTS

# EDITORS

**Claudio De Simone**
Università degli Studi di L'Aquila
degli Abruzzi
L'Aquila, Italy
*chapters 6, 11, 13*

**Giuseppe Famularo**
Università degli Studi di L'Aquila
degli Abruzzi
L'Aquila, Italy *and*
Ospedale San Camillo
Rome, Italy
*chapters 6, 11*

# CONTRIBUTORS

Edoardo Alesse
Department of Experimental
  Medicine
University of L'Aquila
L'Aquila, Italy
chapters 5, 13

Adriano Angelucci
Department of Experimental
  Medicine
University of L'Aquila
L'Aquila, Italy
chapters 5, 13

Roberta Barbato
Universita di Padova
Padova, Italy
chapter 4

Antonio Boschini
Community of San Patrignano
Rome, Italy
chapter 11

Jon Bremer, M.D.
Department of Medical
  Biochemistry
University of Oslo
Oslo, Norway
chapter 1

Michael A. Chirigos, Ph.D.
National Cancer Institute
  (Emeritus)
National Institutes of Health
Bethesda, Maryland, U.S.A.
chapter 8

Grazia Cifone
Department of Experimental
  Medicine
University of L'Aquila
L'Aquila, Italy
chapters 5, 13

Fabio Di Lisa
Universita di Padova
Padova, Italy
chapter 4

Luisa Di Marzio
Department of Experimental
  Medicine
University of L'Aquila
L'Aquila, Italy
chapter 5

Dwayne Ford, M.Sc.
Department of Pathology
Roger Williams Medical Center
Providence, Rhode Island, U.S.A.
chapter 8

Chris Galanos
Max-Planck Institute
for Immunobiology
Stubeweg, Germany
chapter 8

Linda L. Gallo, Ph.D.
Department of Biochemistry
and Molecular Biology
George Washington University
Medical Center
Washington D.C., U.S.A.
chapter 8

W.C. Hülsmann
Thorax Center
Erasmus University
Rotterdam, The Netherlands
chapter 7

Gumilla B. Jacobson, Ph.D.
Uppsala University PET Centre
Uppsala, Sweden
chapter 10

Teruo Kitani, M.D., Ph.D.
Sakai Municipal Hospital
Osaka, Japan
chapter 10

Nicola M. Kouttab, Ph.D.
Department of Pathology
Roger Williams Medical Center
and
Brown University
Providence, Rhode Island, U.S.A.
chapter 8

Hirohiko Kuratsune, M.D., Ph.D.
Hematology and Oncology
Osaka University Medical School
Osaka, Japan
chapter 10

Bengt Långström, Ph.D.
Uppsala University PET Centre
Uppsala, Sweden
chapter 10

Marta E. Leon-Monzon, Ph.D.
Neuromuscular Diseases Section
Medical Neurology Branch
National Institute of Neurological
Disorders and Stroke
National Institutes of Health
Bethesda, Maryland, U.S.A.
chapter 12

Gary D. Lopaschuk
Unversity of Alberta
Edmonton, Alberta, Canada
chapter 3

Takashi Machii, M.D., Ph.D.
Hematology and Oncology
Osaka University Medical School
Osaka, Japan
chapter 10

Sonia Marcellini
Department of Infectious Diseases
University "La Sapienza"
Rome, Italy
chapter 11

Franco Matricardi
Sigma Tau
Pomezia, Italy
chapter 6

Kiyoshi Matsumura, Ph.D.
Subfemtomole Biorecognition
    Project
Japan Science & Technology
    Corporation
Osaka, Japan
chapter 10

Roberta Menabò
Universita di Padova
Padova, Italy
chapter 4

Sonia Moretti
Department of Infectious Diseases
University "La Sapienza"
Rome, Italy
chapter 11

Madiraju S.R. Murthy, Ph.D.
Laboratory of Intermediary
    Metabolism
Clinical Research Institute
    of Montreal
Montreal, Quebec, Canada
chapter 2

Paola Muzi
Department of Experimental
    Medicine
University of L'Aquila
L'Aquila, Italy
chapter 5

Ichiro Nakamoto
Biomedical Laboratories (BML)
Osaka, Japan
chapter 10

Eleonora Nucera
Department of Infectious Diseases
University "La Sapienza"
Rome, Italy
chapter 6

Hirotaka Onoe, Ph.D.
Department of Neuroscience
Osaka Bioscience Institute
Osaka, Japan
chapter 10

Shri V. Pande, Ph.D.
Laboratory of Intermediary
    Metabolism
Clinical Research Institute
    of Montreal
Montreal, Quebec, Canada
chapter 2

Paola Roncaioli
Department of Experimental
    Medicine
University of L'Aquila
L'Aquila, Italy
chapter 5

Barbara Ruggeri
Department of Experimental
    Medicine
University of L'Aquila
L'Aquila, Italy
chapter 5

Gino Santini
Department of Infectious Diseases
University "La Sapienza"
Rome, Italy
chapter 6

Cristina Semino-Mora, M.D.,
    Ph.D.
Neuromuscular Diseases Section
Medical Neurology Branch
National Institute of Neurological
    Disorders and Stroke
National Institutes of Health
Bethesda, Maryland, U.S.A.
chapter 12

Noris Siliprandi
Universita di Padova
Padova, Italy
chapter 4

Maria Teresa Tacconi
Laboratory of Enzyme
  Biochemistry
Istituto di Ricerche Farmacologiche
  "Mario Negri"
Milano, Italy
chapter 9

Mamoru Takahashi, Ph.D.
Diagnosis Division
Asahi Chemical Industry Co., LTD.
Shizupka, Japan
chapter 10

Vito Trinchieri
Department of Infectious Diseases
University "La Sapienza"
Rome, Italy
chapter 11

Italo Trotta
Department of Experimental
  Medicine
University of L'Aquila
L'Aquila, Italy
chapter 5

Sven Valind, M.D., Ph.D.
Uppsala University PET Centre
Uppsala, Sweden
chapter 10

Yasuyoshi Watanabe, M.D., Ph.D.
Department of Neuroscience
Osake Bioscience Institute
Osaka, Japan
chapter 10

Kouzi Yamaguti, M.D., Ph.D.
Hematology and Oncology
Osaka University Medical School
Osaka, Japan
chapter 2

Francesca Zazzeroni
Department of Experimental
  Medicine
University of L'Aquila
L'Aquila, Italy
chapters 5, 13

# PREFACE

The past few years have seen tremendous growth in our understanding of the role of carnitine and its esters in the normal fuel metabolism of cells. Carnitine, indeed, acts as a key factor in the transport of long-chain fatty acids across mitochondrial membranes into the matrix where they undergo β-oxidation and energy production. It is now apparent that a deranged carnitine metabolism resulting in low cellular levels contributes to the pathogenesis of many human diseases. Detailed immunologic, metabolic and biochemical studies have yielded important insights into the reaction mechanisms and molecular interactions, explaining the pathological consequences of carnitine deficiency. These advances are of considerable clinical interest because of their potentially relevant implications for the therapy of diseases with an otherwise poor course, such as the acquired immunodeficiency syndrome (AIDS), septic shock and chronic fatigue syndrome.

The first five chapters of this book address the most recent advances of basic studies investigating the metabolic role of carnitine.

Chapter 1 by Jon Bremer deals with the functions of carnitines in cellular metabolism. The author presents an up-to-date review of the mechanisms of biosynthesis and transport of carnitine and illustrates how carnitine regulates fatty acid oxidation and energy metabolism. The role of carnitine acetyltransferases is also depicted.

Murthy and Pande in chapter 2 focus on the molecular biology of carnitine palmitoyltransferases and discuss the potential role of carnitine in transcriptional gene regulation. They suggest that the metabolic roles of carnitine and carnitine palmitoyltransferases are likely to extend to the nucleus and that the potential of the carnitine system to modulate the intranuclear fatty acyl-CoA levels is one way by which this system may influence the fatty acid-mediated control of gene transcription.

It is now evident that carnitine also has an important role in the regulation of glucose oxidation. In chapter 3 Lopashuk addresses this issue and highlights how carnitine can relieve the inhibition of the pyruvate dehydrogenase complex, the rate-limiting enzyme for glucose oxidation. This role of carnitine may explain some of the beneficial effects associated with carnitine therapy in several human diseases. Furthermore, it is likely that the well-documented beneficial effects of carnitine therapy in ischemic hearts correlates with its ability to overcome fatty acid inhibition of glucose oxidation during reperfusion.

Chapter 4 by Di Lisa and coworkers deals with carnitine and mitochondrial dysfunction. They review how decreased carnitine availability results in decreased mitochondrial energy production because of impaired mitochondrial oxidation of substrates. This mechanism explains both functional (i.e. impairment of muscle contractility) and structural (i.e. lipid storage and steatosis) abnormalities found in several inborn metabolic errors and acquired disorders.

Alesse and coworkers report in chapter 5 exciting data from their laboratory about the ability of carnitine to interfere with Fas-induced apoptosis in human T cell lines. This appears to involve the inhibition of an acidic sphingomyelinase that generates ceramide, an endogenous mediator of apoptosis and human immunodeficiency virus (HIV) replication. These results may have a crucial impact on the design of therapeutic strategies directed at reducing apoptosis and viral replication in subjects infected with HIV.

The next section of the book highlights the impact of recent progress in basic studies of carnitine on clinical medicine.

In chapter 6 Famularo and colleagues review the clinical disorders in which carnitine deficiency may be most frequently encountered. Even though the primary syndromes of carnitine deficiency are rare, prompt recognition is essential because carnitine therapy is very effective and may significantly improve an otherwise fatal course. Additionally, acquired disorders, such as myocardial diseases, diabetes, hemodialysis and sepsis, and iatrogenic factors resulting in secondary syndromes of carnitine deficiency, are discussed in depth. The authors suggest that carnitine supplementation should be considered in the management of these conditions.

Chapters 7 and 8 focus on the role of carnitine administration to protect against tissue injury in models of ischemia and infection. Hülsmann presents an overview of the molecular mechanisms contributing to the protective effects exerted by carnitine administration against tissue injury in experimental models of ischemia followed by reperfusion and of lipopolysaccharide toxicity. Meanwhile, Kouttab and coworkers provide evidence that carnitine can improve the course of sepsis in animal models infected with bacteria or injected with lipopolysaccharide. The main effect observed in these studies is the ability of carnitine to modulate the production of several cytokines, and in particular to significantly decrease the production of tumor necrosis factor-alpha, a cytokine implicated in the pathogenesis of septic shock. In addition, the authors report that at least 30% of animals treated with carnitine showed increased survival. These results highlight a potential new avenue for the treatment of infections, particularly those leading to the syndrome of septic shock, involving the use of carnitine in combination with other agents such as antibiotics and antibodies against certain cytokines or their receptors.

In chapter 9, Tacconi suggests that an involvement of carnitine in the pathogenesis of Reye's and Reye-like syndrome can be envisaged.

These syndromes comprise a class of multifactorial metabolic diseases that have a common marker in the derangement of liver mitochondria and the onset of encephalopathy. Oxidative metabolism is impaired by a subsequent shift toward alternative pathways of oxidation. Altered carnitine metabolism, with low levels in skeletal muscle, high plasma levels, and increased urinary loss during the acute phases of Reye's syndrome, has been reported. Experiments performed in animal models suggest a potential role for carnitine in the therapy of these syndromes.

Kuratsune and colleagues discuss in chapter 10 the finding of serum acylcarnitine deficiency in the face of normal free carnitine levels—a peculiar abnormality of carnitine metabolism—in patients with chronic fatigue syndrome. Since the physiological and biological roles of serum acylcarnitine are still unclear, the authors have investigated the brain uptake and metabolism of acylcarnitine by positron emission tomography. They suggest that serum endogenous acylcarnitine could be an important metabolic substance in mammals. Furthermore, acylcarnitine deficiency in serum and/or cells may be related to the signs and symptoms of patients with chronic fatigue syndrome and it appears that acylcarnitine therapy markedly improves daily activity scores and reduces symptom severity in these subjects.

In chapter 11, De Simone and coworkers review the evidence for carnitine deficiency in patients infected with HIV. Even though studies of carnitine therapy in these subjects are difficult to carry out because of the multifactorial mechanisms implicated in the pathogenesis of carnitine deficiency, preliminary reports have demonstrated that carnitine therapy may significantly improve several metabolic and immunologic parameters of the disease. This impact of carnitine treatment appears to be associated with the downmodulation of cell-associated ceramide, an endogenous mediator of apoptosis and HIV replication. This appears to explain their recent finding of a reduced frequency of apoptotic CD4 and CD8 cells. Interestingly, the decline in CD4 counts observed during the pretreatment follow-up period was reversed and a net gain of CD4 cells per day was obtained.

Semino-Mora and Leon-Monzon in chapter 12 review the role of carnitine deficiency in the pathogenesis of mitochondrial myopathy of zidovudine. They suggest that carnitine therapy can be envisaged in order to prevent or treat this severe dose-limiting toxicity of zidovudine therapy.

Alesse and colleagues discuss in chapter 13 the impact of L-carnitine therapy on liquoral glutamate levels in subjects with AIDS dementia complex. They found that carnitine therapy resulted in a significant reduction in the levels of glutamate, which is believed to act as a pivotal mediator in the pathogenesis of AIDS-dementia complex. These results point to a potential role of carnitine in the treatment of HIV-mediated injury to the central nervous system.

We wish to thank all the contributors for providing such clear and informative chapters, which provide a stimulating overview of the burgeoning field of carnitine metabolism in both basic sciences and clinical medicine. We hope that this book will stimulate in-depth research to clarify the role of carnitine in the pathogenesis and treatment of several human diseases.

*Claudio De Simone*
*Giuseppe Famularo*

# The Role of Carnitine in Cell Metabolism

Jon Bremer

## A CENTURY OF CARNITINE RESEARCH

The sequence of basic detections in carnitine research listed be low represents main events which have led to our present understanding of the
function of carnitine in the oxidation of fatty acids. This research had a
slow start. Carnitine was isolated from meat extracts at the beginning of the
century, but in spite of many studies on its biological effects, (reviewed by
Fraenkel and Friedman)[1] its function remained a riddle for half a century.

| Year | Discovery |
|---|---|
| 1905 | Carnitine (Cn) was isolated from muscle.[2] |
| 1927 | The chemical structure of Cn was estabished.[3] |
| 1952 | Cn was shown to be a vitamin ($B_T$) for a meal worm (*Tenebrio molitor*).[4] |
| 1955 | Cn was shown to stimulate fatty acid oxidation in liver homogenates.[5] |
| | Reversible enzymatic acetylation of Cn in liver was detected.[6] |
| 1961 | Butyrobetaine was shown to be a Cn precursor.[7,8] |
| 1962-63 | Fatty acid esters of Cn were shown to be intermediates in fatty acid oxidation.[9-11] |
| 1965 | High concentrations of Cn were found in epididymis and sperm.[12] |
| 1966 | CPT was localized in the inner mitochondrial membrane and acyl-CoA synthetase in the outer mitochondrial membrane.[13,14] |
| 1970 | Formation of branched chain acylcarnitines from branched chain amino acids was detected.[15] |
| 1971 | Lysine was shown to be a precursor of Cn.[16] |

*Carnitine Today,* edited by Claudio De Simone and Giuseppe Famularo.
© 1997 Landes Bioscience.

1973        Cn acyltransferases were detected in peroxisomes.[17]
            Inborn errors in Cn metabolism were found.[18,19]
1975        Cn translocase was demonstrated in mitochondria[20,21]
1977        Malonyl-CoA was shown to be an inhibitor of CPT-I.[22]
1980-81     Fatty acid oxidation was found to be less inhibited by
            malonyl-CoA in livers of fasted rats.[23,24]
1987        CPT-I was shown to be localized in the outer membrane of
            the mitochondria.[25]
1988-95     Several genes of Cn acyltransferases were cloned and their
            regulation studied (see chapter 2).
1995        Direct evidence was obtained for the function of Cn in the
            transfer of acyl groups from the peroxisomes to the mito-
            chondria. [26]

The first crucial event was the report in 1955 by Fritz,[5] who found
that carnitine stimulates fatty acid oxidation. In the following years this led
to the detection of the carnitine acyltransferases and carnitine esters as
intermediates in the oxidation of fatty acids in mitochondria.

Carnitine became interesting in clinical medicine when lack of carnitine or carnitine palmitoyltransferase was detected in inborn errors in
1973.[18,19]

Interest in carnitine in basic research got a boost in 1978 when
McGarry et al[22] reported that CPT-I is inhibited by malonyl-CoA, thus demonstrating that this enzyme has a critical regulatory function in metabolism.

Medline lists about 2000 articles over the last 10 years dealing with
carnitine. This extended effort has shown how carnitine and the carnitine
acyltransferases function in the regulated transport of fatty acids into mitochondria for oxidation. It is also likely that the carnitine acyltransferases
function in the transport of fatty acids across other cellular membranes.
However, we still have a poor understanding of the significance of these
processes.

This chapter deals with the functions of carnitine in cellular metabolism. With the great number of articles published in recent years it is evident that the references here included must be limited and subjective. Still,
it is hoped that this review will represent a reasonably accurate picture of
our present knowledge.

## BIOSYNTHESIS, UPTAKE AND EXCRETION

### BIOSYNTHESIS AND ABSORBTION

Carnitine turns over relatively slowly in the body. In the rat about 7%
of the body pool is excreted in the urine each day.[27] Both uptake from the
diet and de novo synthesis are relatively slow processes. The pathway of
carnitine synthesis has been reviewed.[28] It is sufficient to recall here that in

animals and man carnitine is formed from trimethyllysine which is liberated from body proteins. Most tissues can convert trimethyllysine to butyrobetaine, although in the rat the kidneys are particularly active.[29] The last step, the hydroxylation of butyrobetaine to carnitine, is limited to liver and a few other tissues, depending on species. In rat the butyrobetaine hydroxylase is found only in liver and testis; in man in liver, kidney and brain. In sheep it is also present in skeletal muscle.[30] Most of the carnitine is found in skeletal muscle (about 1 mM in rat,[31] 3 mM in man[32]), with the highest concentration in epididymis (varying with species, up to 80 mM[33]), yet it is formed mainly in liver. It is evident, therefore, that an extensive transport and redistribution of carnitine takes place. Availability of trimethyllysine seems to regulate the rate of carnitine biosynthesis.[34] No other regulation of its biosynthesis has been found. Its absorption in the gut is slow and is influenced by the carnitine content of the diet.

## EXCRETION

The normal concentration in blood plasma is 25-50 μM. Carnitine is a threshold substance with a rapid turnover in the kidney.[35] It is likely, therefore, that the level of carnitine in the blood is regulated mainly by the kidneys. In perfused rat kidneys more than 95% of the carnitine in the ultrafiltrate is reabsorbed at 30 μM (-)carnitine in the perfusate, and a clearance of about 40 ml rat plasma/day could be calculated. The clearance rose rapidly with higher concentrations, (especially over 100 μM), showing that excess plasma carnitine is rapidly excreted in the urine. Reabsorptions of more than 95% were found also with (+)carnitine, butyrobetaine, and isobutyrylcarnitine, showing that the the reabsorption mechanism has a relatively low specificity.[35] However, acylcarnitines formed in the kidney itself during perfusion "leaked" more readily into the urine than into the perfusate.[36] This may explain the apparently higher fractional excretion of acylcarnitines than of carnitine itself in man.[37]

## UPTAKE AND RELEASE IN TISSUES

Since most tissues have carnitine concentrations 10-100-fold higher than blood plasma, an active uptake of carnitine must take place, but at vastly different rates. Brooks and McIntosh[31] found that the turnover times for carnitine in kidney, liver, heart, skeletal muscle and brain in relation to blood plasma in the rat are 0.4, 1.3, 21, 105 and 220 hours respectively. There is probably more than 1000-fold difference in maximum uptake rates in kidney and liver compared to the maximum rates in skeletal muscle and brain. The $K_m$ of the liver transporter also is at least 100-fold higher than the $K_m$ for the muscle transporter. Early studies on uptake and release in different organs have been reviewed.[28] More recent studies have shown that uptake in kidney and other tissues is sodium dependent,[38-40] suggesting a cotransport with sodium down the extracellular/intracellular sodium gradient. An uptake in muscle by an exchange-diffusion process against butyrobetaine is also suggested.[41] Such an exchange diffusion may be the mechanism by which (+)carnitine provokes (-)carnitine deficiency.[42] It is not known whether this exchange uptake takes place on the same carrier as the sodium-dependent uptake. The carriers in cell membranes have not been isolated and characterized. They show little stereospecificity since the transport of (+)carnitine and butyrobetaine is not very different from the transport of the physiological isomer (-)carnitine.

The uptake and release of carnitine in liver and epididymis are hormone regulated. Liver carnitine is higher in fasted rats, and carnitine uptake is stimulated by glucagon.[43] The most pronounced difference is seen in sheep where liver carnitine concentration in diabetic sheep is increased 6-fold compared to normal animals.[44] Uptake and release take place over different membrane carriers by different mechanisms.[45] Acylcarnitines are released from the liver more rapidly than carnitine itself.[46] In epididymis carnitine uptake is stimulated by testosterone.[47]

INTRACELLULAR MEMBRANE TRANSPORT

Mitochondria contain a carnitine tranlocase in the inner membrane which rapidly exchanges extra- and intramitochondrial carnitine and acylcarnitines.[20,21,48] (Fig 1.1). This carrier also permits a slow net one-way transport. It requires the presence of cardiolipin in the membrane.[49] There seems to be microcompartmentalization of this translocase and the carnitine acyltransferases in the membrane because when incoming carnitine is acetylated in the matrix of the mitochondria, the tranlocase exchanges the acetylcarnitine formed with new extramitochondrial carnitine without equilibration with the whole intramitochondrial carnitine pool.[50] This microcompartmentalization may permit channeling of fatty acids to oxidation without equilibration with the whole matrix pool of (acyl)carnitines. (See also the section on the regulation of fatty acid oxidation in liver.)

# CARNITINE ACYLTRANSFERASES

## CARNITINE ACETYLTRANSFERASE

### Topography

Carnitine acetyltransferase is found in mitochondria, in peroxisomes, and in endoplasmatic reticulum in rat liver.[54,55] The enzymes of mitochondria and peroxisomes are structurally very similar and it has been suggested that they are formed from the same gene by alternative splicing.[56] The acetyltransferase of mitochondria is latent, i.e. the enzyme is localized in the matrix or on the matrix side of the inner mitochondrial membrane. In intact isolated mitochondria, therefore, it cannot use added acetyl-CoA because added CoA and CoA esters cannot penetrate the inner mitochondrial membrane. It reacts only with acetyl-CoA generated intramitochondrially, e.g. from pyruvate, and with carnitine which can exchange with acetylcarnitine via the carnitine translocase.[20,21] Isolated mitochondria, therefore, oxidize added acetylcarnitine,[9] but not added acetyl-CoA in the presence of carnitine.[57] However, acetyl-CoA formed in the peroxisomes may be converted to acetylcarnitine and oxidized in the mitochondria (see below).

## Specificity and properties

The acetyltransferase was the first carnitine acyltransferase to be purified and crystalized.[58] The enzyme in animal tissues has a relatively broad specificity with regard to acyl groups since it reacts with straight chain acyl-CoA esters up to decanoyl-CoA with decreasing rates.[59,60] Fluoroacetylcarnitine is as good a substrate for the enzyme as is acetylcarnitine.[61] In

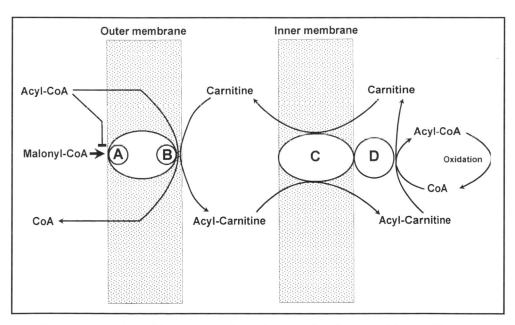

Fig 1.1. The organization of the carnitine-dependent transfer of activated fatty acids into mitochondria. AB: Carnitine palmitoyltranferase I (CPT-I) in the outer mitochondrial membrane with its regulatory malonyl-CoA site (A) on the external surface, and its substrate site (B) on the inner surface. The outer membrane also contains the long-chain acyl-CoA synthetase and the glycerophosphateacyltransferase which competes with CPT-I for the acyl-CoA formed by the synthetase.[144] C: Carnitine/acylcarnitine tranlocase in the inner mitochondrial membrane. D: Carnitine palmitoyltransferase II (CPT-II) on the inner surface of the inner mitochondrial membrane. This is also the localization of the mitochondrial carnitine acetyltranferase.

isolated mitochondria fluoroacetylcarnitine, therefore, leads to fluoroacetyl-CoA and fluorocitrate formation and a complete block in the citric acid cycle.[61] Bromoacetyl-CoA and bromoacetylcarnitine are interesting suicidal substrates for the enzyme.[62,63] They inhibit by two mechanisms. Bromoacetylcarnitine alone leads to an alkylation of a histidine residue at the catalytic site of the enzyme. In the presence of CoASH its SH group is alkylated and a carboxymethyl-CoA carnitine ester is formed. This product is extremely tightly bound to the enzyme (dissociation constant $K_d = 10^{-10}$) because the inhibitor is bound to both the carnitine- and the CoA substrate sites. Thus, these results prove that the enzyme has close, but separate substrate sites for carnitine and CoA with a histidine residue. This is most likely a common feature for all the carnitine acyltransferases. A histidine residue essential for its catalytic activity has been found also in the mitochondrial CPT-II.[64] The acetyltransferase also reacts with branched chain acyl-CoA from the degradation of branched chain amino acids,[15] and with pivaloyl-CoA (trimethylacetyl-CoA) which is formed from pivalic acid used in antibiotics like Pivampicillin.[65]

In *Candida tropicalis* the enzyme has a much narrower chain length specificity.[66] In this organism it is highly specific for acetyl-CoA and shows almost no activity with propionyl-CoA.

In animal tissues the enzyme is inhibited by long-chain acyl-CoA esters. It is a peculiar feature that palmitoyl-CoA acts as a competitive inhibitor toward both carnitine and acetyl-CoA.[59] The enzyme is present in all tissues, but its activity varies. It is high in rat heart and low in rat liver. However, in the liver both the mitochondrial and the peroxisomal activities increase many-fold when clofibrate or other peroxisome proliferators like 3-thia fatty acids are fed.[67,68]

## Functions

Different functions have been suggested for carnitine acetyltransferase and for acetylcarnitine. All of these functions depend also on the simultaneous activity of the carnitine translocase in the inner membrane of the mitochondria (Fig 1.1).[20,21,48] These functions can be grouped under four headings:

a. Transfer of acetyl and other short acyl groups from peroxisomes to mitochondria.

b. Export of excess acetyl and branched chain acyl groups from mitochondria and from the cell. This buffers mitochondrial free CoA.

c. Acetylcarnitine as a temporary energy substrate.

d. Acetylcarnitine as a regulator of fatty acid oxidation (This point will be discussed as part of the regulation of fatty acid oxidation in the heart).

## Transfer of ac(et)yl groups from peroxisomes

Such a function for carnitine and the acetyltransferase has been assumed since the detection of fatty acid β-oxidation and carnitine acyltransferases in peroxisomes.[17] However, this idea has been difficult to prove because alternative mechanisms for transfer of peroxisomal products exist, at least in liver. Peroxisomes and cytosol in liver contain acetyl-CoA and acyl-CoA hydrolases, and in isolated hepatocytes free acetate has been shown to be the main product of peroxisomal β-oxidation.[69] Thus, in rat liver fatty acid oxidation in the peroxisomes does not depend on the normally low activity of carnitine acetyltransferase. In other tissues the situation may be different. Propionyl-CoA produced in the β-oxidation of pristanic acid (an α-methyl fatty acid) in peroxisomes of fibroblasts depends on the carnitine system for transfer to the mitochondria for further oxidation.[26] So far, this is the only direct evidence for such a carrier function of carnitine. Indirect support for this idea was obtained in studies by Skorin et al[70] who found that tetradecylglycidic acid, an inhibitor of peroxisomal carnitine acyltransferase (and of CPT-I), leads to a more extensive oxidation of fatty acids in peroxisomes in the liver, presumably because export of partially oxidized, shortened fatty acids as carnitine esters is prevented.

## Buffering of mitochondrial CoA

Under some conditions acetyl-CoA and other short CoA esters may accumulate in the mitochondria. In liver the acetyl-CoA/CoA and the acetylcarnitine/carnitine ratios increase in starvation (Fig 1.2). In muscle these ratios increase with acute excercise. In normal rat liver there are significant amounts of propionylcarnitine which vary opposite the long-chain acylcarnitines. In some inborn errors propionyl-CoA and other coenzyme A esters may accumulate. In these conditions a parallel accumulation of the corresponding carnitine esters in the cytosol takes place.[71-74] Administration of the xenobiotic acid pivalic acid (trimethylacetate) leads to a similar accumulation of pivaloylcarnitine.[65] Evidently the carnitine acetyltransferase and the carnitine translocase in the mitochondria permit transfer of the excess acyl groups to carnitine in the cytosol.[15,75] This may relieve disturbances of mitochondrial metabolism.[74] It is important that liver carnitine and carnitine esters equilibrate rapidly with the blood plasma. Carnitine esters are released even more rapidly from the liver than carnitine itself,[46] and in kidney they are released to the urine.[36] These reactions represent an export route for "unwanted" acyl groups, and also represent a mechanism for carnitine loss from the body.

Muscle and brain carnitine equilibrate much more slowly with blood plasma.[31] Excretion of acyl groups as carnitine esters from muscle tissues is

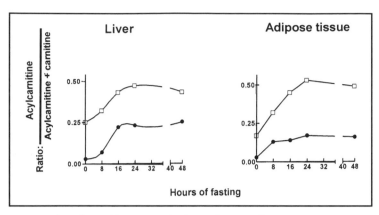

Fig 1.2. The effect of fasting on the long-chain acylcarnitine/carnitine—
and on the acetylcarnitine/carnitine ratios—in liver and adipose tissues in rats. Fasting has a similar effect on these ratios in other tissues.
The figure is a modified reproduction from Bøhmer[132] with permission
from Biochim Biophys Acta and the author.

therefore slow and of more dubious physiological significance. Loss of carnitine from muscle by this mechanism must also be a slow process which
develops over months in man when for example, pivalic acid-containing
drugs are administered.[76]

### Acetylcarnitine as temporary energy substrate

Acetylcarnitine formed in the mitochondria (or in the peroxisomes)
will normally have to be transferred back to the mitochondria for utilization. In liver and muscle this pool will represent very little in relation to the
total energy production and the total turnover of acetyl groups in the citric
acid cycle. However, in some cells acetylcarnitine may be of physiological
significance as a short-lived energy source. Mature sperm have a relatively
high level of acetylcarnitine which can be utilized as an energy source for
their motility.[77] Similarly, mononuclear phagocytes have a high level of
acetylcarnitine which is used as energy source in their immune response
and hydrogen peroxide formation.[78] Acetylcarnitine also seems to function
as an initial energy source in insect flight muscle.[79]

### CARNITINE LONG-CHAIN ACYLTRANSFERASES

The function of carnitine and carnitine acyltransferases can be understood only in relation to the transport of activated fatty acids across
membranes. If membrane transport is disregarded, the carnitine

acyltransferases represent dead-end freely reversible reactions in intermediary metabolism:

carnitine + acyl-CoA ↔ acylcarnitine + CoA

Carnitine esters formed can be metabolized only by reformation of coenzyme A esters by the carnitine acyltransferases. The only exception is hydrolysis to carnitine and free fatty acids by carnitine ester hydrolases.[51,52] These enzymes have no established physiological significance, but it has been speculated that they prevent excessive accumulation of long-chain acylcarnitines. One of these enzymes was found on the luminal side of the endoplasmic reticulum in the liver and it was assumed that it is active in the transport of carnitine out of the cell.[52] However, in the liver acylcarnitines are released to the blood without hydrolysis.[46]

The carnitine acyltransferases are membrane-bound and their long-chain acyl substrates are poorly soluble in water. It has been difficult, therefore, to develop good assay procedures and to purify the different carnitine acyltransferases.[53] Only slowly has it become established that different parts of the cell contain separate transferases with similar chain length specificities. The existence of these different carnitine acyltransferases has also been proven with gene technology methods (see chapter 2).

Table 1.1 shows the different established carnitine acyltransferases in animal tissues and their cellular localization, chain length specificity and sensitivity to malonyl-CoA. There is some confusion in the nomenclature of the carnitine acyltransferases. The short-chain carnitine acyltransferase is usually called "acetyltransferase," but sometimes this enzyme shows higher activity with propionyl-CoA. The long-chain acyltransferases of mitochondria are most often called carnitine palmitoyltransferase I and II (CPT-I and CPT-II), but these enzymes are usually more active with medium chain length acyl-CoAs. The peroxisomal carnitine acyltransferases (beside the acetyltransferase) are often called carnitine octanoyltransferase, but their chain length specificity is probably not very different from the CPT-I and -II of mitochondria, as are the specificities of the carnitine acyltransferases of endoplasmic reticulum. In Table 1.1 the names carnitine acetyltransferase, CPT-I and CPT-II have been used as these are most common in the literature. The others are simply called peroxisomal-, microsomal- and nuclear carnitine acyltranferases.

It is striking that at least three different cell organelles contain two carnitine long-chain acyltransferases, one malonyl-CoA sensitive and one malonyl-CoA insensitive. The general significance of this is still uncertain, but based on the extensively studied mitochondrial system it is reasonable to assume that the systems in peroxisomes and in endoplasmic reticulum also function in regulating the transport of fatty acids across their membranes.

Here we will look at the different carnitine acyltransferases and some of their properties and suggested functions. The roles of the mitochondrial carnitine acyltransferases in the regulation of fatty acid metabolism in different tissues will be discussed later.

MITOCHONDRIAL CPT-I AND CPT-II

Topography

Studies on the carnitine-dependent oxidation of fatty acids in intact mitochondria showed that these particles had to contain an outer and an inner CPT (CPT-I and CPT-II), (Fig. 1.1) or alternatively that the substrates could reach the enzyme from both sides of the membrane.[14] The detection of carnitine translocase[20,21] showed that there had to be two different CPT pools, and this was definitely confirmed when CPT-I was found in the outer membrane of the mitochondria. This permitted its separation from CPT-II by mechanical means in the form of isolated outer mitochondrial membranes.[25] Still, characterization of CPT-I has been difficult because the enzyme is membrane bound and it is labile to the detergents needed to solubilize it. When purified the enzyme loses its activity and its sensitivity to malonyl-CoA.[89-91]

We once suggested that CPT-I might be regulated by a separate malonyl-CoA binding regulatory peptide in the mitochondrial membrane.[92] This idea has died hard because it received experimental support in membrane reconstitution experiments.[93-95] However, there is now compelling evidence that the inhibitory malonyl-CoA site and the catalytic site reside on a single polypeptide.[96] Component(s) in the membrane which influence(s) the activity of CPT-I, therefore, probably do(es) not act by forming complex(es) with malonyl-CoA. The CPT-I peptide is different in liver and other tissues. Both the liver CPT-I isoenzyme (94 kDa) and the muscle CPT-I isoenzyme (86 kDa) are malonyl-CoA sensitive. The CPT-II isoenzyme which is malonyl-CoA insensitive is the same in all tissues (66 kDa).[97-99]

When intact mitochondria are treated with proteases the inhibitory effect of malonyl-CoA decreases with little inactivation of the enzyme. However, when the mitochondria are disrupted the enzyme is rapidly inactivated by proteases.[25] Malonyl-CoA protects the enzyme against proteolysis.[100] These results show that the enzyme most likely spans the outer mitochondrial membrane with the malonyl-CoA inhibitory site facing the cytosol and the substrate sites facing the intermembrane space. Studies with

Table 1.1. Carnitine acyltransferases in animal tissues

| Organelle Enzyme | Specificity | Sensitive to malonyl-CoA | Refs |
|---|---|---|---|
| **Mitochondria** | | | |
| **-inner membrane** | | | |
| Acetyl-transferase | $C_2$-$C_{10}$ | No | 9,80 |
| CPT-II | $C_6$-$C_{18}$ | No | 13,60,81 |
| **-outer membrane** | | | |
| CPT-I | $C_6$-$C_{20}$ (?) | Yes | 22,25 |
| **Peroxisomes** | | | |
| Acetyl-transferase | $C_2$-$C_{10}$ | No | 17,54 |
| P-acyl-transferase I | $C_4$-$C_{16}$ | Yes | 54,82 |
| P-acyl-transferase II (soluble) | $C_4$-$C_{16}$ (?) | No | 53 |
| **Microsomes (ER)** | | | |
| M-acyl-transferase I | $C_6$-$C_{16}$ | Yes | 83,84 |
| M-acyl-transferase II | $C_6$-$C_{16}$ | No | 84 |
| **Sarcoplasmic reticulum** | | | |
| Acyl-transferase | (?) | Yes | 85 |
| **Cytoplasmic membrane** | | | |
| Acyl-transferase | $C_6$-$C_{22}$ | Yes | 86,87 |
| **Nucleus** | | | |
| N-acyltransferase | (?) | (?) | 88 |

inhibitors[101,102] and studies on CPT from patients with mutant CPT[103] have also indicated that CPT-I has different binding sites for malonyl-CoA and for substrate acyl-CoA. Figure 1.1 shows how CPT-I, (acyl)carnitine translocase, and CPT-II take part in the transfer of fatty acids into mitochondria with CPT-I's inhibitory allosteric site for malonyl-CoA on the external surface of the outer membrane.

## Specificity of CPT-I and CPT-II

Both CPT-I and CPT-II have broad chain length specificities. CPT-I reacts with CoA esters at least down to octanoyl-CoA and up to stearoyl-CoA.[104,105] Very long-chain fatty acids ($C_{20-24}$) have not been tested directly as substrates for CPT-I. However it has been shown that oleic acid ($C_{18:1}$) and gondoic acid ($C_{20:1}$) are well oxidized by isolated liver mitochondria, while erucic acid ($C_{22:1}$) is not. With erucic acid erucoyl-CoA accumulated.[106] It is likely therefore that the erucoyl-CoA is a poor substrate for CPT-I. CPT-I also discriminates against branched chain fatty acids,[107] dicarboxylic acids,[52,108] and acids with a double bond in the $\alpha\beta$-position.[109] In comparison, carnitine acetyltransferase does not discriminate against branched chain carboxylic acids formed from branched amino acids.[15] Thus, CPT-I prevents branched chain fatty acids from entering the mitochondria. Carnitine acetyltransferase permits branched chain carboxylic acids to escape if the mitochondria are unable to break them down.

A peculiar feature of CPT-II is a different chain length specificity depending on reaction direction.[110] In the direction of acylcarnitine formation, the optimum chain length of the acyl-CoA substrate was found to be decanoyl-CoA, while in the direction of acyl-CoA formation the optimum chain length of the acylcarnitine was myristoyl- or palmitoylcarnitine. This change in chain length specificity may be connected with a kinetic peculiarity of the enzyme. Long-chain acyl-CoA is, in addition to being a substrate for the enzyme, a competitive inhibitor for the second substrate carnitine. It also inhibits carnitine acetyltransferase competitively to both carnitine and to acetyl-CoA.[59] Therefore, the apparent $K_m$ of CPT-II for carnitine increases with the concentration of long-chain acyl-CoA, thus slowing down the reaction rate. Both CPT-I and CPT-II show this effect of a long chain acyl-CoA substrate.[111,112] The apparent change in $K_m$ is significant in relation to the normal concentration of carnitine in the liver (approximately 0.25 mM in the rat).

In the opposite direction long-chain acyl-CoA gives a strong product inhibition of CPT-II.[113] These features of the CPT enzymes will slow down the transfer of activated fatty acid to the mitochondria when the extramitochondrial acyl-CoA level is high, thus preventing "flooding" of the mitochondria with acyl-CoA. This will save free CoA for other CoA-dependent reactions in the mitochondria.

### Inhibition by malonyl-CoA

The inhibition of CPT-I by malonyl-CoA is very specific in relation to free CoA and other CoA esters. Methylmalonyl-CoA, succinyl-CoA, and other short-chain acyl-CoA esters are less inhibitory, by at least one order of magnitude.[114] It is likely that malonyl-CoA inhibits allosterically at its separate inhibitory site while CoA and other CoA esters inhibit at the substrate site facing the intermembrane space in the mitochondria.[102] In sheep the specificity of the allosteric site is different. In sheep liver methylmalonyl-CoA is as inhibitory as malonyl-CoA.[115] This is probably connected with the importance of propionate and methylmalonyl-CoA as glucose precursors in ruminants in the fed state. In addition the level of malonyl-CoA and its inhibitory effect are similar to those in other species in spite of a very low rate of fatty acid synthesis in sheep liver. Therefore in ruminants CPT-I probably is regulated by malonyl-CoA and methylmalonyl-CoA together.[115]

In spite of the specificity of malonyl-CoA as inhibitor of CPT-I, similar inhibition is found with apparently unrelated compounds, e.g. hydroxyphenylglyoxalic acid.[116] This and other inhibitory compounds have shown that the CoA structure is not required for the allosteric inhibition, which seems to depend on the presence of two carbonyl groups in close juxtaposition.[102]

A series of fatty acid derivatives acts more or less as specific inhibitors of the CPTs and carnitine translocase. Tetradecylglycidic acid (as the coenzyme A ester) inhibits CPT-I irreversibly while CPT-II is not inhibited.[117] This inhibitor has been used in many studies on the function of CPT-I. Another oxirane-2-carboxylic acid derivative inhibits the liver CPT-I isoenzyme while it does not inhibit the heart isoenzyme.[118] Tetradecylthioacrylyl-CoA is a strong inhibitor of CPT-II, while CPT-I is not inhibited.[109] Decanoyl-(+)carnitine and other fatty acid esters of the unphysiological isomer (+)carnitine inhibit mitochondrial carnitine translocase[21] and are used as a specific inhibitor of mitochondrial fatty acid oxidation.[119]

CPT-I is inhibited by malonyl-CoA in all tissues.[120,121] Since the level of malonyl-CoA varies with the nutritional state,[122,123] this inhibition evidently is important in the regulation of fatty acid oxidation. However, this inhibition is very different in liver and other tissues. The regulation of CPT-I and fatty acid oxidation in liver and other tissues will, therefore, be discussed in a separate section.

PEROXISOMAL ACYLTRANSFERASES

Besides the carnitine acetyltransferase which has already been discussed, the peroxisomes contain two carnitine acyltransferases with a broad chain length specificity, one membrane bound and sensitive to malonyl-CoA, and one soluble or easily extractable and insensitive to malonyl-CoA.[53,82] Isolated peroxisomes do not require carnitine for the oxidation of fatty acids, but there is evidence that the carnitine acyltransferases are active in the transfer of acyl groups from the peroxisomes to mitochondria for oxidation.[26] It has been assumed that the peroxisome membrane is freely permeable for CoA and CoA esters, but permeability changes during isolation cannot be excluded. Buechler and Lowenstein[124] have concluded from cell experiments with tetradecyglycidic acid, (+)carnitine esters and α-bromofatty acids that carnitine is needed for transport of fatty acids into peroxisomes. On the other hand, decanoyl-(+)carnitine does not inhibit chain shortening of erucic acid to oleic acid, a process which most likely takes place in peroxisomes,[119] and Skorin et al[70] found that inhibition of the carnitine acyltranferases with tetradelylglycidic acid increased the extent of fatty acid oxidation in the peroxisomes, presumably by preventing acyl-CoA intermediates to "escape" as carnitine esters. Thus, there is no general agreement on the function of the carnitine acyltransferases in peroxisomes.

### Microsomal Carnitine Acyltransferases

Both malonyl-CoA sensitive and malonyl-CoA insensitive carnitine acyltransferases have been found in microsomes (endoplasmatic reticulum) of rat liver.[83,84,125] The topographies of these carnitine acyltransferases are still only partially known, and it is unknown whether the endoplasmatic reticulum, like the mitochondria, contains a carnitine translocase. Still it is likely that these transferases, like the transferases of mitochondria and per-oxisomes, are active in transport of fatty acids. Cytosolic triacylglycerol in the liver is not secreted directly from the liver. A breakdown by lipolysis and re-esterification is assumed to take place as part of the transport into the lumen of the endoplasmatic reticulum before secretion as very low density lipoproteins (VLDL) by the Golgi apparatus.[126] The carnitine acyltransferases may take part in this process.[127] A function in the acylation of secreted pro-teins is also a possibility. The details of these processes remain to be eluci-dated.

Carnitine acyltransferases are also found in sarcoplasmatic reticu-lum,[85] in erythrocyte membranes,[86,87] and in neurons.[128] In neurons and in erythrocytes[129] the carnitine acyltransferases are assumed to have a function in the turnover of fatty acid in the membrane phospholipids.

### Nuclear Carnitine Acyltransferases?

A stress-regulated protein (54 kDa) with carnitine acyltranferase ac-tivity has been characterized. It is a member of the thioredoxin superfam-ily, has a nuclear localization signal and has been found in the nucleus.[88] (For discussion of possible regulatory functions of this carnitine acyltransferase, see chapter 2.)

## FATTY ACID OXIDATION IN LIVER

### Esterification or Oxidation?

Numerous studies have shown that a high rate of fatty acid oxidation and ketogenesis in the liver depends on a rapid rate of lipolysis in adipose tissues and a high level of free fatty acids in the blood which automatically give a high rate of fatty acid uptake in the liver. However, the distribution of the fatty acids taken up between esterification into phospholipids and triacylglycerol on one hand and carnitine-dependent oxidation in the mitochondria on the other depends on intrahepatic regulatory mechanisms. Extensive switches from esterification to oxidation and vice versa take place depending on fasting and feeding[130] as well as endocrine changes.[131] Evidently, the rate of esterification will influence the availability of fatty acids for oxidation. The endocrine regulation of lipolysis in adipose tissues and the regulation of re-esterification in the liver will not be further discussed here.

CPT-I AS GATE TO OXIDATION

A main control of fatty acid oxidation and ketogenesis takes place in the carnitine dependent transfer of activated fatty acids into the mitochondria. A high rate of fatty acid oxidation correlates with a high acylcarnitine/carnitine ratio, and with a high acetylcarnitine/carnitine ratio (Fig 1.2).[132] The great physiological importance of the control at this site will be clear from the following considerations: The complete oxidation of acylcarnitines to carbon dioxide and water can be seen as the result of two interacting cycles, the β-oxidation cycle and the citric acid cycle (Fig. 1.3). One turn of the β-oxidation cycle produces one acetyl-CoA, one turn of the citric acid cycle converts one acetyl-CoA to carbon dioxide. In muscle tissues the two cycles operate almost like two cogwheels because there is almost no use of acetyl-CoA outside the citric acid cycle. Therefore, if the citric acid cycle is blocked in muscle tissues, fatty acid oxidation is almost completely inhibited.[61] In liver the situation is different because the ketogenic enzymes have the capacity to convert acetyl-CoA to ketone bodies at a high rate, even in liver from carbohydrate-fed animals.

CHANNELING OF INTERMEDIATES

The carnitine translocase, CPT-II, and all the β-oxidation enzymes represent a highly integrated substrate channeling system for oxidation of acylcarnitines to acetyl-CoA. The acylcarnitines coming in over the carnitine translocase do not equilibrate with the whole carnitine pool of the mitochondrial matrix,[50] and even most of the tiny amounts of β-oxidation intermediates found in mitochondria oxidizing palmitoylcarnitine represent "leakage" from the "true" intermediates of the pathway to acetyl-CoA.[133] Ketogenesis permits this integrated β-oxidation cycle to turn over at a faster rate than the citric acid cycle (Fig. 1.3).

RESPIRATORY CONTROL

Why do we get ketogenesis only when liver oxidizes fatty acids, while we never see ketogenesis when it oxidizes carbohydrate (pyruvate)? One main reason is that β-oxidation of intramitochondrial acyl-CoA is under poor respiratory control. Usually mitochondrial oxidation of energy-yielding substrates, e.g. pyruvate and intermediates in the citric acid cycle, are under strict respiratory control. The rate of oxidation depends on the availability of ADP. A low work load results in a low level of ADP in the cell and a high mitochondrial NADH/NAD ratio, which inhibits pyruvate dehydrogenase[134] and the dehydrogenase reactions of the citric acid cycle.[135] However, a high NADH/NAD ratio gives only a weak inhibition of the β-oxidation of intramitochondrial acyl-CoA which is formed from extramitochondrial acylcarnitines.[136] In liver the excess acetyl-CoA gives a high acetyl-CoA/CoA ratio, a high equilibrium level of acetoacetyl-CoA in the thiolase reaction, and a substrate-stimulated activity of HMG-CoA synthase which is rate limiting in ketogenesis. The activity of this enzyme is also increased by its desuccinylation.[137]

REGULATION OF CPT-I AND ACYLTRANSFER

The regulation of the carnitine dependent transfer of fatty acids (Fig. 1.1) seems to depend mainly on the rate-limiting activity of CPT-I and its regulation by malonyl-CoA.[22] In addition, a regulated activity of the (acyl)carnitine translocase may also be important. Thus, the oxidation of preformed octanoylcarnitine in perfused livers is under similar regulation as the carnitine-dependent oxidation of oleate, while free octanoate is not regulated to any significant extent,[138] presumably because octanoate is activated inside the mitochondria and, therefore, bypasses the carnitine-dependent transport into these particles. It is also striking that the level of long-chain acylcarnitines in the liver can be increased several-fold by a carnitine load without increasing ketogenesis.[139] Thus the ratio of acylcarnitine/carnitine rather than the absolute level of acylcarnitines in the cells seems to determine the rate of transfer via the translocase into the mitochondria. More direct evidence for a regulatory function of the translocase has also been published. Its activity is increased under ketogenic conditions.[140] However, almost all studies on the regulation of carnitine-dependent transfer of fatty acids focus on CPT-I, which is assumed to be the main regulatory site. This is dramatically demonstrated when the rate of reduction of flavoproteins (acyl-CoA dehydrogenases and electron transfer protein) in mitochondria is compared with acyl-CoA and carnitine or palmitoylcarnitine as reducing substrates. With palmitoylcarnitine this rate is several hundred times faster than with palmitoyl-CoA + carnitine.[141]

Studies on fatty acid oxidation and CPT-I activity in liver in different physiological conditions have shown that increased rates of acylcarnitine formation and fatty acid oxidation may be explained by a) a decreased concentration of malonyl-CoA, b) an increased activity of CTP-I, and c) a de-

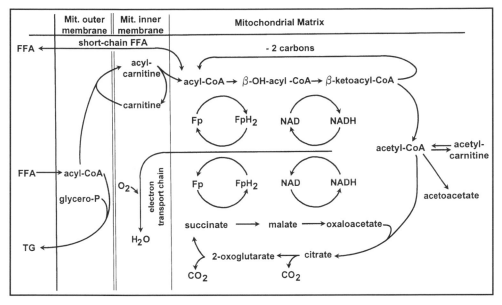

Fig 1.3. Interaction of the β-oxidation cycle with the citric acid cycle in the oxidation of fatty acids in mitochondria. FFA: free fatty acids; Glycero-P, glycerophosphate; β-OH-acyl-CoA, β-hydroxyacyl-CoA; Mit., mitochondrial.

creased sensitivity of CPT-I to malonyl-CoA. Table 1.2 describes how different treatments of live animals, isolated liver cells, or isolated liver mitochondria influence CPT-I activity, malonyl-CoA concentration, and the sensitivty of the enzyme to malonyl-CoA.

## What changes malonyl-CoA level?

The direction of malonyl-CoA changes in liver in a series of different physiological conditions is listed in Table 1.2. Malonyl-CoA is formed by acetyl-CoA carboxylase which is considered to be rate determining in fatty acid synthesis and in fatty acid elongation. The regulation of this enzyme has been extensively studied and treated in numerous reviews in the literature and does not need to be treated here. Suffice it to say that it is regulated at the gene level by hormones and transcription factors, by phosphorylation and dephosphorylation, and allosterically by metabolites. The enzyme is activated by citrate and inhibited by long-chain acyl-CoA esters. A main hormone in its regulation is insulin, which is involved in the activation of its gene, in its activation by dephosphorylation, and by lowering its inhibitor long-chain acyl-CoA by inhibiting lipolysis and stimulating esterification to triacylglycerol. Consequently, the activity of acetyl-CoA carboxylase and lipogenesis is high in carbohydrate-fed animals, low in fasting as well as diabetic animals. The level of malonyl-CoA varies accordingly, but the correlation of lipogenesis and malonyl-CoA level is qualitative rather than quantitative. Thus, the lipogenesis rate in obese Zucker rats was found to be 15-20-fold higher than in normal rats, but the level of malonyl-CoA was only about 1.5-fold higher.[166] It was already mentioned that rat heart[122] and sheep liver[115] with almost no lipogenesis have levels of malonyl-CoA not very different from that of rat liver with a high rate of lipogenesis. Evidently, the malonyl-CoA level is determined by the relative activities of the acetyl-CoA carboxylase and the malonyl-CoA utilizing fatty acid synthase and fatty acid elongases. As we shall see, there is also sometimes a poor correlation between malonyl-CoA level and rate of fatty acid oxidation and ketogenesis in the liver. This is explained by variations in the activity of CPT-I and its sensitivity to malonyl-CoA.

## What changes CPT-I activity?

Table 1.2 lists how different physiological conditions change the activity of CPT-I. Inspection of the table will show that the activity of liver CPT-I goes up in all conditions known to imply an increased rate of fatty acid oxidation and ketogenesis. The enzyme is "turned on" at birth when the pup becomes dependent on the high fat milk diet; it increases in fasting, diabetes and hyperthyroidism. In agreement with these observations thyroid hormone increases CPT-I activity, while it is decreased by insulin. Birth and these hormone effects imply alterations in the rate of enzyme synthesis.[167-169] (see chapter 2).

The activity of the CPT-I is not determined by the amount of enzyme only. Table 1.2 shows that a series of treatments of isolated liver cells or of isolated liver mitochondria, and even of extracted mitochondrial membranes,[160] changes the activity of CPT-I. It is evidently physiologically important that long-chain acyl-CoA inhibits acetyl-CoA carboxylase and, at the same time, displaces malonyl-CoA from CPT.[170] This physiology is illustrated by the effect of 3-thia fatty acids on fatty acid oxidation in hepatocytes (Fig. 1.4). 3-thia fatty acids cannot be β-oxidized because of the S-atom in the 3-position, but they are activated to their CoA esters. When fed to rats, the CoA ester accumulates in the liver and the level of malonyl-CoA is acutely lowered, presumably because acetyl-CoA carboxylase is inhibited.[148] In hepatocytes from fasted rats the 3-Thia fatty acids, as expected, inhibit fatty acid oxidation (Fig. 1.4). However, in hepatocytes from fasted carbohydrate refed rats the thia fatty acids stimulate fatty acid oxidation (Fig. 1.4). Evidently the nonmetabolizable thia fatty acid CoA ester lowers malonyl-CoA and displaces it from the inhibitory site on CPT-I, and this effect activates the enzyme sufficiently to more than compensate for the inhibition seen in cells from fasted rats where the CPT-I evidently already is fully "turned on."

The changes in CPT-I activity in liver have been called "activation and inactivation,"[160] "transition between states of low and high affinity for malonyl-CoA"[158] or "hysteretic behavior of carnitine palmitoyltransferase."[171] The last expression implies that the enzyme is allosteric with a slow transition from one state to another depending on the presence of malonyl-CoA, long-chain acyl-CoA, salts and other additions. With liver mitochondria from fed rats as little as 1 μM malonyl-CoA is sufficient to preserve the malonyl-CoA sensitivity of CPT-I when the mitochondria are incubated in a salt-containing medium.[160]

### What changes CPT-I's sensitivity to malonyl-CoA?

Cook et al[23] detected that malonyl-CoA is less inhibitory in liver mitochondria from fasted rats. This turned out to have a double explanation: fasting increases the activity of CPT-I and it decreases its sensitivity to malonyl-CoA.[24] It is striking that the "hysteresis," or change to a malonyl-CoA insensitive state is more rapid in mitochondria from fasted and/or hyperthyroid rats than in mitochondria from fed and/or hypothyroid rats (Fig. 1.5). Most dramatic is the effect of fasting on hypothyroid rats. The reason for this more rapid change to an insensitive state is uncertain. Since glucagon and cyclic AMP, activators of protein kinases, and okadaic acid, an inhibitor of protein phosphatases, all reduce the sensitivity of CTP-I, the postulated phosphorylation of CPT as a regulatory mechanism[172] seemed to be confirmed. But no phosphorylation of the CTP-I peptide has been detected.[173] If the enzyme peptide molecule remains unmodified, other components in the membrane must influence the sensitivity. Cholesterol uptake in macrophages decreases CPT-I sensitivity to malonyl-CoA.[157] Treatment of liver mitochondria with phospholipids increases the sensitivity of CPT-I to malonyl-COA.[164] Fasting and diabetes have been shown to increase the content of spingomyeline in the outer membrane 2-4-fold,[161] but any effect of sphingomyeline has not been demonstrated in vitro. It is still uncertain whether lipid changes and membrane fluidity changes in the outer membrane can explain the changes in CPT-I sensitivity to malonyl-CoA in vivo, or whether other (phospholylated?) membrane or cytosolic components are involved.

The importance of CPT-I sensitivity to malonyl-CoA is evident from the observation that sometimes changes of fatty acid oxidation occurs in the presence of high concentrations of malonyl-CoA. This is the case at weaning when a decrease in fatty acid oxidation in liver is brought about mainly by an increase in sensitivity of CPT-I.[143] In rats fed a single dose of a 3-thia fatty acid, the level of malonyl-CoA in the liver is initially decreased,

**Table 1.2. Factors changing CPT-I activity, CPT-I sensitivity to malonyl-CoA, and malonyl-CoA concentration in liver**

| | CPT activity | CPT sensitivity | Malonyl-CoA level |
|---|---|---|---|
| **IN VIVO** | | | |
| **Birth and diet** | | | |
| birth (milk diet) | ↑↑ | ↓↓ | ?[142] |
| weaning | | | |
| (carbohydrate diet) | ↑ | ↑ | ↑[143] |
| fasting | ↑ | ↓ | ↓[24] |
| carbohydrate diet | ↓ | ↑ | ↑?[144] |
| fish oil | ↑ | ↓ | ↓?[145-147] |
| 3-thia fatty acids | ↑ | ↓ | ↑[148] |
| ethanol | ↓ | ↑ | ?[149] |
| | | | |
| **Hormones** | | | |
| diabetes | ↑↑ | ↓↓ | ↓[150,151] |
| insulin | ↓ | ↑ | ↑[150,151] |
| thyroid hormones | ↑ | ↓? | ?[153] |
| estrogen | ↓ | ↑ | ?[153] |
| | | | |
| **IN VITRO** | | | |
| **Treatment of cells** | | | |
| glucagon | ↑ | ↓ | ?[154,155] |
| dibutyryl-cAMP | ↑ | ↓ | ?[154,155] |
| okadaic acid | ↑ | ? | ?[155] |
| swelling | ↓ | ? | ↑?[156] |
| cholesterol uptake | ↓ | ↓ | ?[157] |
| | | | |
| **Treatment of mitochondria** | | | |
| preincubation | | | |
| with malonyl-CoA ? | ? | ↑[158,159] | |
| with acyl-CoA | ↑ | ↓[160] | |
| with salts | ↑ | ↓[159-161] | |
| with sucrose | ? | ↑[92] | |
| with microsomes | ? | ↑[162] | |
| low pH | ↓ | ↑↑[163] | |
| phospholipids | ? | ↑[164] | |
| higher alcohols | ? | ↓[165] | |

↑ increase, ↓ decrease.

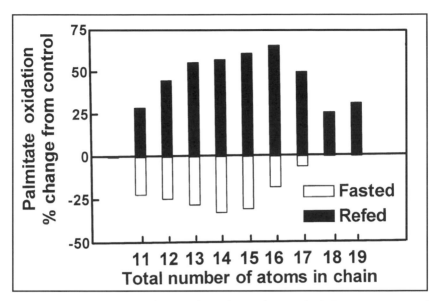

Fig 1.4. The effect of 3-thia fatty acids on the oxidation of 1-[14]C-palmitate to acid soluble products (mainly ketone bodies) in isolated liver mitochondria from rats fasted for 48 hours (white columns), or from rats fasted for 48 hours and then refed carbohydrate (white bread + 10% sucrose in the drinking water) for 24 hours (black columns). The isolated hepatocytes (3-4 mg protein/ml) were incubated with Krebs-carbonate buffer, bovine serum albumin (3.5%) and 1-[14]C-palmitate (0.5 mM) with and without thia fatty acids of different chain lengths (0.2 mM) for 30 min. The thia fatty acids used were octyl- to hexadecyl-thioacetic acid.

but after 24 hours the level is even higher than in control animals. In spite of this, isolated hepatocytes from these animals have an increased rate of fatty acid oxidation.[148] The CTP-I showed an increased activity and probably a decreased sensitivity to malonyl-CoA in these hepatocytes.

## FATTY ACID OXIDATION IN HEART

As in liver the mitochondrial β-oxidation of fatty acids in heart is under poor respiratory control. It is not inhibited to any significant extent by a high NADH/NAD ratio, while the citric acid cycle is easily inhibited. Since the acetyl-CoA formed in this tissue has to be disposed of in the citric acid cycle the β-oxidation cycle and the citric acid cycle are interlocked almost like two cogwheels.[174] If the citric acid cycle is inhibited in isolated heart mitochondria, e.g. by the formation of fluorocitrate or by lack of ADP (a high NADH/NAD ratio), fatty acid oxidation is also inhibited, not because of accumulated NADH, but because of lack of free CoA.[174] In the intact tissue the regulation is more complicated, and it is different from the regulation in the liver.

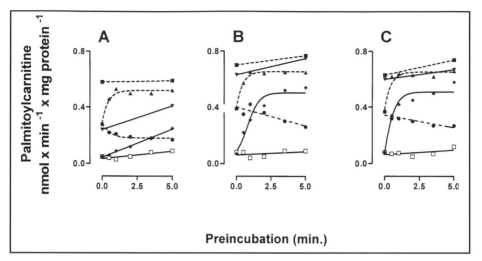

**Preincubation (min.)**

Fig. 1.5. The effects of thyroid state and of fasting on the loss of malonyl-CoA inhibition of CPT-I in liver mitochondria. Liver mitochondria were isolated in a sucrose medium from fasted or fed, normal, hypo- or hyperthyroid rats.
The mitochondria were preincubated in a salt containing medium (KCl 37 mM, Hepes buffer (pH 7.0) 25 mM, sucrose 120 mM) without or with malonyl-CoA (10 μM).
After dilution to assay conditions CPT-I was assayed with $^3$H-CH3-carnitine (0.5mM), palmitoyl-CoA (50 μM), albumin (1%), Hepes, 20 mM, KCl, 80 mM, sucrose 48 mM, and without or with malonyl-CoA (4 μM). Assay time, 2 min. Temperature, 30°C.
A, Hypothyroid rats; B, normal rats; C, hyperthyroid rats. Continuous curves, fed rats; dotted curves, fasted rats.
▼,■, no malonyl in preincubation or assay.
◆,▲, no malonyl-CoA in preincubation, 4 μM in assay.
●, ❑, 10 μM malonyl-CoA in preincubation, 4 μM in assay medium.
The curves represent the means of 4 different mitochondria preparations. The rate with which the inhibition by malonyl-CoA was lost in mitochondria from fed rats preincubated in the absence of malonyl-CoA (◆) was significantly slower ($P < 0.05$) in hypothyroid mitochondria (A) than in normal and hyperthyroid mitochondria (B and C).
Reproduced from ref. 159 with permission from Biochim Biophys Acta.

The very active reversible carnitine acetyltransferase of heart mitochondria will tranfer the increased acetyl-CoA/CoA ratio to a corresponding increased acetylcarnitine/carnitine ratio in the cytosol, possibly also to
an extramitochondrial high acetyl-CoA/CoA ratio. Less free CoA and free
carnitine remain for long chain acyl-CoA and acylcarnitine formation. This
explains the paradoxical observation of Neely et al[175] who found that a decreased work load in perfused hearts resulted in a decreased level of long-
chain acylcarnitine and an increased level of acetylcarnitine in the heart.
Since the oxidation of long-chain acyl-CoA to acetyl-CoA has to be slowed
down with a decreased work load, an accumulation of long-chain
acylcarnitines and a drop in acetyl-CoA and acetylcarnitine could be ex-

pected. These results show that the citric acid cycle is inhibited before β-oxidation.

Recently it has become clear that there is additional regulation of fatty acid entry into the mitochondria by malonyl-CoA.[176] The heart CPT-I activity or its sensitivity to malonyl-CoA is not altered by fasting,[105] but the activity is increased by endurance exercise.[177]

Surprisingly, heart contains malonyl-CoA at almost the same level as liver.[122] Since heart CPT-I apparently has a much lower $I_{50}$ than liver CTP-I,[114] a nearly complete inhibition of heart CPT-I might be expected almost under all conditions. However, a careful study of the kinetics of CPT-I in permeabilized heart myocytes showed that it retained 20-35% of its activity at malonyl-CoA concentrations at 50-100 times its estimated $K_i$ value.[178] This agrees with malonyl-CoA as an allosteric inhibitor which downregulates the enzyme without complete inhibition.

It is uncertain how muscle tissues produce cytosolic acetyl-CoA as substrate for the acetyl-CoA carboxylase. Mitochondria normally cannot acetylate cytosolic coenzyme A because the carnitine acetyltransferase is latent and cannot acetylate CoA in the cytosol.[57] However, a peroxisomal β-oxidation of fatty acids in the heart may be an alternative source of acetyl-CoA for the acetyl-CoA carboxylase.[179]

## CARNITINE IN INSULIN SECRETION

Long-chain fatty acids stimulate insulin secretion by a direct effect on the pancreas,[180] and they do so by potentiating the glucose-induced insulin secretion.[181] Pancreatic islets can oxidize fatty acids at a rate similar to that of liver[182] and as in liver the rate of oxidation evidently is regulated by a malonyl-CoA-sensitive CPT-I.[183] The effect of fatty acids on insulin secretion is reduced in islets from fasted rats, but restored by 2-bromopalmitate which inhibits CPT-I. Efficient stimulation of insulin secretion is obtained with nutrients which have the ability to elevate the level of malonyl-CoA in the cells.[184] Hydroxycitrate, which inhibits malonyl-CoA formation, stimulates fatty acid oxidation and inhibits insulin secretion. Again, bromostearate and etomoxir (a more specific inhibitor of CPT-I) stimulate insulin secretion. These studies indicate that insulin secretion is stimulated when elevated malonyl-CoA levels inhibit fatty acid oxidation and thus also elevate also the long-chain acyl-CoA level in the cytosol of the cells. How elevated levels of these CoA esters act on insulin secretion is not known.

## PERSPECTIVES

Fundamental carnitine research has come a long way since its role in fatty acid oxidation was detected more than 40 years ago.[5] The detection of malonyl-CoA as an inhibitor of CPT-I brought this enzyme into focus in studies on the regulation of fatty acid oxidation. Its regulation is still a challenge. What are the signal pathways and mechanisms which change its activity in liver? Its regulation by gene activation and suppression is being unravelled, but the variable malonyl-CoA sensitivity is still enigmatic. The enzyme itself seems not to undergo covalent modification, so its regulation must be sought in the effects of membrane lipids or other components.

The detection of specific carnitine acyltransferases in the endoplasmatic reticulum raises the question whether carnitine and its acyltranferases are also involved also in triacylglycerol secretion and VLDL production in liver. Is there also a microsomal carnitine translocase? Only a mitochondrial carnitine translocase has been isolated.

It is evident that the sodium-dependent transporters in uptake, and other transporters in release, are involved in carnitine homeostasis. Lack of knowledge of their regulation and specificities toward acylcarnitines makes it difficult to understand the development of carnitine deficiency in different metabolic conditions. And what are carnitine acyltransferase(s) doing in the cell nucleus?

REFERENCES

1. Fraenkel G, Friedman S. Carnitine. In: Harris RS, Marian GF, Thimann KV, eds. Vitamins and Hormones. Vol 15. New York: Academic Press, 1957:73-118.
2. Gulewitsch W, Krimberg R. Zur Kenntnis der Extraktivstoffe der Muskeln. Z Physiol Chem 1905; 45:326-330.
3. Tomita M, Sendju Y. Über die Oxyaminoverbindungen, welche die Biuretreaktion zeigen. III. Spaltung der m-amino-b-oxybuttersäure in die optisch-aktiven Komponenten. Hoppe-Zeyler's Z Physiol Chem 1927; 169:263-277.
4. Carter HE, Bhattacharrya PK, Weidman KR et al. Chemical studies on vitamin $B_T$ isolation and characterization as carnitine. Arch Biochem Biophys 1952; 38:405-416.
5. Fritz IB. The effects of muscle extracts on the oxidation on palmitic acid by liver slices and homogenates. Acta Physiol Scand 1955; 34:367-385.
6. Friedman S, Fraenkel G. Reversible enzymatic acetylation of carnitine. Arch Biochem Biophys 1955; 59:491-501.
7. Lindstedt G, Lindstedt S. On the biosynthesis and degradation of carnitine. Biochem Biophys Res Commun 1961; 6:319-323.
8. Bremer J. Carnitine precursors in the rat. Biochim Biophys Acta 1962; 57:327-335.
9. Bremer J. Carnitine in intermediary metabolism. Reversible acetylation of carnitine by mitochondria. J Biol Chem 1962; 237:2228-2231.

10. Bremer J. Carnitine in intermediary metabolism. The metabolism of fatty acid esters of carnitine by mitochondria. J Biol Chem 1962; 237:3628-3632.
11. Fritz IB, Yue KTN. Long-chain carnitine acyltransferase and the role of acylcarnitine derivatives in the catalytic increase of fatty acid oxidation induced by carnitine. J Lipid Res 1963; 4:279-288.
12. Marquis NR, Fritz IB. The distribution of carnitine, acetylcarnitine and carnitine acetyltransferase in rat tissues. J Biol Chem 1965; 240: 2193-2196.
13. Norum KR, Farstad M, Bremer J. The submitochondrial distribution of acid:CoA ligase (AMP) and palmityl-CoA: carnitine palmityltransferase in rat liver mitochondria. Biochem Biophys Res Commun 1966; 24:797-804.
14. Yates DW, Shepherd D, Garland PB. Organization of fatty-acid activation in rat liver mitochondria. Nature 1966; 209:1213-1215.
15. Solberg HE, Bremer J. Formation of branched chain acylcarnitines in mitochondria. Biochim Biophys Acta 1970; 222:372-380.
16. Horne DW, Tanphaichitr V, Broquist HP. Role of lysine in carnitine biosynthesis in Neurospora crassa. J Biol Chem 1971; 246:4373-4375.
17. Markwell MAK, McGroarty EJ, Bieber LL et al. The subcellular distribution of carnitine acetyltransferases in mammalian liver and kidney. A new peroxisomal enzyme. J Biol Chem 1973; 248:3426-3432.
18. DiMauro S, DiMauro PM. Muscle carnitine palmityltransferase deficiency and myoglobinuria. Science 1973; 182:929-931.
19. Engel AG, Angelini C. Carnitine deficiency of human muscle with associated lipid storage myopathy: a new syndrome. Science 1973; 179:899-902.
20. Ramsay RR, Tubbs PK. The mechanism of fatty acid uptake by heart mitochondria: an acylcarnitine-carnitine exchange. FEBS Lett 1975; 54:21-25.
21. Pande SV. A mitochondrial carnitine acylcarnitine translocase system. Proc Natl Acad Sci USA 1975; 72:883-887.
22. McGarry JD, Leatherman GF, Foster DW. Carnitine palmitoyltransferase I. The site of inhibition of hepatic fatty acid oxidation by malonyl-CoA. J Biol Chem 1978; 253:4128-4136.
23. Cook GA, Otto DA, Cornell NW. Differential inhibition of ketogenesis by malonyl-CoA in mitochondria from fed and starved rats. Biochem J 1980; 192:955-958.
24. Bremer J. The effect of fasting on the activity on liver carnitine pamitoyltransferase and its inhibition by malonyl-CoA. Biochim Biophys Acta 1981; 665:628-631.
25. Murthy MSR, Pande SV. Malonyl-CoA binding site and the overt carnitine palmitoyltransferase activity reside on the oppsite sides of the outer mitochondrial membrane. Proc Natl Acad Sci USA 1987; 84:378-382.

26. Jacobs BS, Wanders RJA. Fatty acid oxidation in peroxisomes and mitochondria: The first unequivocal evidence for the involvement of carnitine in shuttling propionyl-CoA from peroxisomes to mitochondria. Biochem Biophys Res Commun 1995; 213:1035-1041.

27. Cederblad G, Lindstedt S. Metabolism of labeled carnitine in the rat. Arch Biochem Biophys 1976; 175:173-180.

28. Bremer J. Carnitine, metabolism and functions. Physiol Rev 1984; 63:1420-1480.

29. Carter AL, Frenkel R. The role of the kidney in the biosynthesis of carnitine in the rat. J Biol Chem 1974; 254:10670-10674.

30. Erfle JD. Hydroxylation of -butyrobetaine by rat and ovine tissues. Biochem Biophys Res Commun 1975; 64:553-557.

31. Brooks DE, McIntosh JEA. Turnover of carnitine in rat tissues. Biochem J 1975; 148:439-445.

32. Cederblad G, Lindstedt S, Lundholm K. Concentration of carnitine in human muscle tissue. Clin Chim Acta 1974; 53:311-321.

33. Brooks DE. Carnitine in the male reproductive tract and its relation to the metabolism of the epididymis and spermatozoa. In: Frenkel RA, McGarry JD, Eds. Carnitine Biosynthesis, Metabolism, and Functions. New York: Academic Press 1980:219-2335.

34. Rebuche CJ, Lehman LJ, Olson AL. e-N-Trimethyllysine availability regulates the rate of carnitine biosynthesis in the growing rat. J Nutr 1986; 116:751-759.

35. Hokland BM, Bremer J. Metabolism and excretion of carnitine and acylcarnitines in the perfused rat kidney. Biochim Biophys Acta 1986; 886:223-230.

36. Hokland BM, Bremer J. Formation and excretion of branched-chain acylcarnitines and branched-chain hydroxy acids in the perfused rat kidney. Biochim Biophys Acta 1988; 961:30-37.

37. Engel AG, Rebouch CJ, Wilson DM et al. Primary systemic carnitine deficiency II. Renal handling of carnitine. Neurology 1981; 31: 819-825.

38. Vary TC, Neely JR. Sodium dependence of carnitine transport in isolated perfused adult rat hearts. Am J Physiol 1983; 244:H247-H252.

39. Shaw RD, Ulysses B, Hamilton JW et al. Carnitine transport in rat small intestine. Am J Physiol 1983; 245:G376-G381.

40. Rebouche CJ, Mack DL. Sodium gradient-stimulated transport of L-carnitine into renal brush border membrane vesicles: kinetics, specificity, and regulation by dietary carnitine. Arch Biochem Biophys 1984; 235:393-402.

41. Siliprandi N, Di Lisa F, Pivetta A et al. Transport and function of L-carnitine and L-propionylcarnitine: relevance to some cardiomyopathies and cardiac ischemia (Review). Z Cardiol 1987; 76 Suppl 5:34-40.

42. Rebouche CJ. Effect of dietary carnitine isomers and -butyrobetaine on L-carnitine biosynthesis and metabolism in the rat. J Nutr 1983; 113:1906-1913.

43. Lispal G, Melegh B, Sandor A. Effect of insulin and glucagon on the uptake of carnitine by perfused rat liver. Biochim Biophys Acta 1987; 929:226-228.

44. Snoswell AM, Koundajakin PP. Relationship between carnitine and coenzyme A esters in tissues of normal and alloxan-diabetic sheep. Biochem J 1972; 127:133-141.

45. Kispal G, Melegh B, Alkonyi I et al. Enhanced uptake of carnitine by perfused liver following starvation. Biochim Biophys Acta 1987; 896:96-102.

46. Hokland BM. Uptake, metabolism and release of carnitine and acylcarnitines in the perfused rat liver. Biochim Biophys Acta 1988; 961:234-241.

47. Marquis NR, Fritz IB. Effects of testosterone on the distribution of carnitine, acetylcarnitine, and carnitine acetyltransferase in tissues of the reproductive system of the male rat. J Biol Chem 1965; 240:2197-2200.

48. Indiveri C, Tonazzi A, Palmieri F. Identification and purification of the carnitine carrier from rat liver mitochondria. Biochim Biophys Acta 1990; 1020:81-86.

49. Noël H, Pande SV. An essential requirement of cardiolipin for mitochondrial carnitine acylcarnitine translocase activity. Lipid requirement of carnitine acylcarnitine translocase. Eur J Biochem 1986; 155:99-102.

50. Murthy MSR, Pande SV. Microcompartmentation of transported carnitine, acetylcarnitine and ADP occurs in the mitochondrial matrix. Implications for transport measurements and metabolism. Biochem J 1985; 230:657-663.

51. Mahadevan S, Sauer F. Carnitine ester hydrolase of rat liver. J Biol Chem 1979; 245:4448-4453.

52. Mentlein R, Reuter G, Heymann E. Specificity of two different purified acylcarnitine hydrolases from rat liver, their identity with other carboxylesterases, and their possible function. Arch Biochem Biophys 1985; 240:801-810.

53. Pande SV, Bhuiyan AKMJ, Murthy MSR. Carnitine palmitoyltransferases: How many and how to distinguish? In: Carter AL, ed. Current Concepts in Carnitine Research. Boca Raton: CRC Press 1992:165-178.

54. Farrel SO, Fiol CJ, Reddy CK et al. Properties of purified carnitine acyltransferases of mouse liver peroxisomes. J Biol Chem 1984; 259:13089-13095.

55. Markwell MAK, Tolbert NE, Bieber LL. Comparison of the carnitine acyltransferase activities from rat liver peroxisomes and microsomes. Arch Biochem Biophys 1976; 176:479-488.

56. DiDonato CO, Finocchiaro G. Divergent sequences in the 5' region of cDNA suggest alternative splicing as a mechanism for the generation of carnitine acetyltransferases with different cellular localizations. Biochem J 1994; 303:37-41.

57. Edwards YH, Chase JFA, Edwards MR et al. Carnitine acetyltransferase: the question of multiple forms. Eur J Biochem 1974; 46:209-215.

58. Chase JFA, Pearson DJ, Tubbs PK. The preparation of crystalline carnitine acetyltransferase. Biochim Biophys Acta 1965; 96:162-165.

59. Chase JFA. The substrate specificity of carnitine acetyltransferase. Biochem J 1967; 104:510-518.

60. Clarke PRH, Bieber LL. Isolation and purification of mitochondrial carnitine octanoyltransferase activities from beef heart. J Biol Chem 1981; 256:9861-9868.

61. Bremer J, Davis EJ. Flouroacetylcarnitine: metabolism and metabolic effects in mitochondria. Biochim Biophys Acta 1978; 326:262-271.

62. Chase JFA, Tubbs PK. Conditions for the self-catalyzed inactivation of carnitine acetyltransferase. A novel form of enzyme inhibition. Biochem J 1969; 111:225-235.

63. Chase JFA, Tubbs PK. Specific alkylation of a histidine residue in carnitine acetyltransferase by bromoacetyl-L-carnitine. Biochem J 1970; 116:713-720.

64. Brown NF, Anderson RC, Caplan SL et al. Catalytically important domains of rat carnitine palmitoyltransferase II as determined by site-directed mutagenesis and chemical modification. Evidence for a critical histidine residue. J Biol Chem 1994; 269:19157-19162.

65. Diep QN, Bøhmer T. Increased pivaloylcarnitine in the liver of the sodium pivalate treated rat exposed to clofibrate. Biochim Biophys Acta 1995; 1256:245-247.

66. Ueda M, Tanaka A, Fukui S. Peroxisomal and mitochondrial carnitine acetyltransferases in alkane-grown yeast Candida tropicalis. Eur J Biochem 1981; 124:205-210.

67. Kahonen MT. Effect of clofibrate treatment on carnitine acyltransferases in different subcellular fractions of rat liver. Biochim Biophys Acta 1976; 428:690-701.

68. Hovik R, Osmundsen H, Berge R et al. Effects of thia-substituted fatty acids on mitochondrial and peroxisomal β-oxidation. Studies in vivo and in vitro. Biochem J 1990; 270:167-173.

69. Leighton F, Bergseth S, Rørtveit T et al. Free acetate produced by rat hepatocytes during peroxisomal fatty acid and dicarboxylic acid oxidation. J Biol Chem 1989; 264:10347-10350.

70. Skorin C, Nechochea C, Johow V et al. Peroxisomal fatty acid oxidation and inhibitors on the mitochondrial carnitine palmitoyltransferase I in rat isolated hepatocytes. Biochem J 1992; 281:561-567.

71. Bøhmer T, Bremer J. Propionylcarnitine. Physiological variations in vivo. Biochim Biophys Acta 1968; 152:559-567.

72. Sandor A, Cseko J, Kispal G et al. Surplus acylcarnitines in the plasma of starved rats derive from the liver. J Biol Chem 1990; 265: 22313-22316.

73. Friolet R, Hoppeler H, Krähenbühl S. Relationship between the co-enzyme A and the carnitine pools in human skeletal muscle at rest and after exhaustive exercise under normic and acutely hypoxic conditions. J Clin Invest 1994; 94:1490-1495.

74. Brass EP, Fennesey PV, Miller LV. Inhibition of oxidative metabolism by propionic acid and its reversal by carnitine in isolated rat hepatocytes. Biochem J 1986; 236:131-136.

75. Lysiak W, Toth PP, Suelter CH et al. Quantitation of the efflux of acylcarnitines from rat heart, brain, and liver mitochondria. J Biol Chem 1986; 261:13698-13703.

76. Holme E, Jacobson C-E, Nordin I et al. Carnitine deficiency induced by pivampicillin and pivmecillinam therapy. Lancet 1989; ii:469-472.

77. Milkowski AL, Babcock DF, Lardy HA. Activation of bovine epidydimal sperm respiration by caffeine. Its transient nature and relationship to the utilization of acetyl carnitine. Arch Biochem Biophys 1976; 176:250-256.

78. Kurth L, Fraker P, Bieber L. Utilization of intracellular acylcarnitine pools by mononuclear phagocytes. Biochim Biophys Acta 1994; 1201:321-327.

79. Childress CC, Sacktor B, Traynor DR. Function of carnitine in the fatty acid oxidase-deficient insect flight muscle. J Biol Chem 1966; 242:754-760.

80. Barker PJ, Fincham NJ, Hardwick DC. The availability of carnitine acetyltransferase in mitochondria from guinea-pig liver and other tissues. Biochem J 1968; 110:739-746.

81. Ramsay RR, Derrick JP, Friend AS et al. Purification and properties of the soluble carnitine palmitoyltransferase from bovine liver mitochondria. Biochem J 1987; 244:271-278.

82. Derrick JP, Ramsay RR. L-Carnitine acyltransferase in intact peroxisomes is inhibited by malonyl-CoA. Biochem J 1989; 262:801-806.

83. Lilly K, Bugaisky GE, Umeda PK et al. The medium chain carnitine acyltransferase activity associated with rat liver microsomes is malonyl-CoA sensitive. Arch Biochem Biophys 1990; 280:167-174.

84. Broadway NM, Saggerson ED. Solubilization and separation of two distinct carnitine acyltransferases from hepatic microsomes: characterization of the malonyl-CoA-sensitive enzyme. Biochem J 1995; 310:985-995.

85. McMillin JB, Hudson EK, Van Winkle WB. Evidence for malonyl-CoA-sensitive carnitine acyl-CoA transferase in sarcoplasmic reticulum of canine heart. J Mol Cell Cardiol 1992; 24:259-268.

86. Wittels B, Hochstein P. The identification of carnitine palmityltransferase in erythrocyte membranes. J Biol Chem 1967; 242: 126-130.

87. Ramsay RR, Mancinelli G, Arduini A. Carnitine palmitoyltransferase in human erythrocyte membrane. Properties and malonyl-CoA sensitivity. Biochem J 1991; 275:685-688.
88. Murthy MSR, Pande SV. A stress regulated protein, GRP58, a member of thioredoxin superfamily, is a carnitine palmitoyltransferase isoenzyme. Biochem J 1994; 304:31-34.
89. Lund H. Carnitine palmitoyltransferase: Characterization of a labile detergent-extracted malonyl-CoA-sensitive enzyme from rat liver mitochondria. Biochim Biophys Acta 1987; 918:67-75.
90. Murthy MSR, Pande SV. Some differences in the properties of carnitine palmitoyltransferase activities of the mitochondrial outer and inner membranes. Biochem J 1987; 248:727-733.
91. Woeltje KF, Kuwajima, M, Foster DW et al. Characterization of the mitochondrial palmitoyltransferase enzyme system. II. Use of detergents and antibodies. J Biol Chem 1987; 262:9822-9827.
92. Bergseth S, Lund H, Bremer J. Is carnitine palmitoyltransferase inhibited by a malonyl-CoA-binding unit in the mitochondria? Biochem Soc Transactions 1986; 14:671-672.
93. Ghadiminejad I, Saggerson ED. Carnitine palmitoyltransferase (CPT$_2$) from liver mitochondrial inner membrane becomes inhibitable by malonyl-CoA if reconstituted with outer membrane malonyl-CoA binding protein. FEBS Lett 1990; 269:406-408.
94. Chung CH, Woldegiorgis G, Dai, G et al. Conferral of malonyl Coenzyme A sensitivity to purified rat heart mitochondrial carnitine palmitoyltransferase. Biochemistry 1992; 31:9777-9783.
95. Kerner J, Zaluzec E, Gage D et al. Characterization of the malonyl-CoA-sensitive carnitine palmitoyltransferase (CPT$_o$) of a rat heart mitochondrial particle. Evidence that the catalytic unit is CPT$_i$. J Biol Chem 1994; 269:8209-8219.
96. Brown NF, Esser V, Foster DW et al. Expression of a cDNA for rat liver carnitine palmitoyltransferase I in yeast establishes that catalytic activity and malonyl-CoA sensitivity reside in a single polypeptide. J Biol Chem 1994; 269:26438-26442.
97. Declercq PE, Falck JR, Kuwajima M et al. Characterization of the mitochondrial carnitine palmitoyltransferase enzyme system I. Use of inhibitors. J Biol Chem 1987; 262:9812-9821.
98. Murthy MSR, Pande SV. Characterization of a solubilized malonyl-CoA-sensitive carnitine palmitoyltransferase from the mitochondrial outer membrane as a protein distinct from the malonyl-CoA-insensitive carnitine palmitoyltransferase of the inner membrane. Biochem J 1990; 268:599-604.
99. Esser V, Britton CH, Weiss BC et al. Cloning, sequencing, and expression of a cDNA encoding rat liver carnitine palmitoyltransferase I. Direct evidence that a single polypeptide is involved in inhibitor interaction and catalytic function. J Biol Chem 1993; 268:5817-5822.

100. Kashfi K, Cook GA. Malonyl-CoA inhibits proteolysis of carnitine palmitoyltransferase. Biochem Biophys Res Commun 1991; 178: 600-605.
101. Esser V, Kuwajima M, Britton CH et al. Inhibitors of mitochondrial carnitine palmitoyltransferase I limit the action of proteases on the enzyme. Isolation and partial amino acid analysis of a truncated form of rat liver isozyme. J Biol Chem 1993; 268:5810-5816.
102. Kashfi K, Mynatt RL, Cook GA. Hepatic carnitine palmitoyl-transferase-I has two independent inhibitory binding sites for regulation of fatty acid oxidation. Biochim Biophys Acta 1994; 1212: 245-252.
103. Zierz S, Engel AG. Different sites of inhibition of carnitine palmitoyltransferase by malonyl-CoA, and by acetyl-CoA and CoA, in human skeletal muscle. Biochem J 1987; 245:205-209.
104. Solberg HE. Acyl group specificity of mitochondrial pools of carnitine acyltransferases. Biochim Biophys Acta 1974; 360:101-112.
105. Mynatt RL, Lappi MD, Cook GA. Myocardial carnitine palmitoyl-transferase of the mitochondrial outer membrane is not altered by fasting. Biochim BIophys Acta 1992; 1128:105-111.
106. Christiansen EN, Davis EJ. The effects of coenzyme A and carnitine on steady-state ATP/ADP ratios and the rate of long-chain free fatty acid oxidation in liver mitochondria. Biochim Biophys Acta 1978; 502:17-28.
107. Singh H, Beckman K, Poulos A. Peroxisomal beta-oxidation of branched chain fatty acids in rat liver. Evidence that carnitine palmitoyltransferase I prevents transport of branched chain fatty acids into mitochondria. J Biol Chem 1994; 269:9514-9520.
108. Pourfarzam M, Bartlett K. Skeletal muscle mitochondrial β-oxidation of dicarboxylates. Biochim Biophys Acta 1993; 1141:81-89.
109. Skrede S, Wu P, Osmundsen H. Effects of tetradecylthiopropionic acid and tetradecylthioacrylic acid on rat liver lipid metabolism. Biochem J 1995; 305:591-597.
110. Clarke RH, Bieber LL. Effect of micelles on the kinetics of purified beef heart mitochondrial carnitine palmitoyltransferase. J Biol Chem 1981; 256:9861-9868.
111. Bremer J, Norum KR. Palmitoyl-CoA: carnitine O-palmitoyl-transferase in the mitochondrial oxidation of palmitoyl-CoA. Eur J Biochem 1967; 1:427-433.
112. Bird MI, Saggerson ED. Interacting effects of L-carnitine and malonyl-CoA on rat liver carnitine palmitoyltransferase. Biochem J 1985; 230:161-167.
113. Bremer J, Norum KR. The mechanism of substrate inhibition of palmitoyl coenzyme A: carnitine acyltransferase in rat liver cells. J Biol Chem 1967; 242:1744-1748.
114. Mills SE, Foster DW, McGarry JD. Interaction of malonyl-CoA and related compounds with mitochondria from different rat tissues.

Relationship between ligand binding and inhibition of carnitine palmitoyltransferase I. Biochem J 1983; 214:83-91.

115. Brindle NPJ, Zammit VA, Pogson CI. Regulation of carnitine palmitoyltransferase activity by malonyl-CoA in mitochondria from sheep liver, a tissue with a low capacity for fatty acid synthesis. Biochem J 1985; 232:177-182.

116. Stephens TW, Cook GA, Harris RA. Two mechanisms produce tissue-specific inhibition of fatty acid oxidation by oxfenicine. Biochem J 1985; 227:651-660.

117. Kiorpes TC, Hoerr D, Ho W et al. Identification of 2-tetradecylglycidyl coenzyme A as the active form of methyl 2-tetradecylglycidate (methyl palmoxirate) and its characterization as an irreversible, active site-directed inhibitor of carnitine pamitoyltransferase A in isolated rat liver mitochondria. J Biol Chem 1984; 259:9750-9755.

118. Brown NF, Weis BC, Husti JE et al. Mitochondrial carnitine palmitoyltransferase I isoform switching in the developing rat heart. J Biol Chem 1995; 270:8952-9857.

119. Christiansen RZ, Christiansen EN, Bremer J. The stimulation of erucate metabolism in isolated rat hepatocytes by rape seed oil and hydrogenated marine oil-containing diets. Biochim Biophys Acta 1979, 573:417-429.

120. Saggerson ED, Carpenter CA. Carnitine palmitoyltransferase and carnitine octanoyltransferase activities in liver, kidney cortex, adipocyte, lactating mamary gland, skeletal muscle and heart. Relative activities, latency and effect of malonyl-CoA. FEBS Lett 1981; 129:229-232.

121. McGarry JD, Mills SE, Long CS et al. Observations on the affinity for carnitine, and malonyl-CoA sensitivity, of carnitine palmitoyltransferase I in animal and human tissues. Demonstration of the presence of malonyl-CoA in non-hepatic tissues of the rat. Biochem J 1983; 214:21-28.

122. Singh B, Stakkestad JA, Bremer J et al. Determination of malonyl-Coenzyme A in rat heart, kidney and liver: A comparison between acetyl-coenzyme A and butyryl-coenzyme A as fatty acid synthase primers in the assay procedure. Analytical Biochem 1984; 138: 107-111.

123. McGarry JD, Stark MJ, Foster DW. Hepatic malonyl-CoA levels of fed, fasted and diabetic rats as measured using simple radioisotopic assay. J Biol Chem 1978; 253:8291-8293.

124. Buechler KF, Loewenstein JM. The involvement of carnitine intermediates in peroxisomal fatty acid oxidation: A study with 2-bromofatty acids. Arch Biochem Biophys 1990; 281:233-238.

125. Murthy MS, Pande SV. Malonyl-CoA-sensitive and -insensitive carnitine palmitoyltransferase activities of microsomes are due to different proteins. J Biol Chem 1994; 269:18283-18286.

126. Wiggins D, Gibbons GF. The lipolysis/esterification cycle of hepatic triacylglycerol. Its role in the secretion of very-low-density lipoprotein and its response to hormones and sufphonylureas. Biochem J 1992; 284:457-462.
127. Broadway NM, Saggerson ED. Microsomal carnitine acyltransferases. Biochem Soc Transactions 1995; 23:490-494.
128. Arduini A, Denisova N, Virmani A et al. Evidence for the involvement of carnitine-dependent long-chain acyltransferases in neuronal triglyceride and phospholipid fatty acid turnover. J Neurochem 1994; 62:1530-1538.
129. Arduini A, Mancinelli G, Radatti GL et al. Role of carnitine and carnitine palmitoyltransferase as integral components of the pathway for membrane phopholipid fatty acid turnover in intact human erythrocytes. J Biol Chem 1992; 267:12673-12681.
130. Zammit VA, Moir AMB. Monitoring the partitioning of hepatic fatty acids in vivo: keeping track of control. Trends Biochem Sci 1994; 19:313-317.
131. Moir AMB, Zammit VA. Effects of insulin treatment of diabetic rats on hepatic partitioning of fatty acids between oxidation and esterification, phospholipid and acylglycerol synthesis, and on the fractional rate of secreting of triacylglycerol in vivo. Biochem J 1994; 304:177-182.
132. Bøhmer T. Tissue levels of activated fatty acids (acylcarnitines) and the regulation of fatty acid metabolism. Biochim Biophys Acta 1967; 144:259-270
133. Stanley KK, Tubbs PK. The role of intermediates in mitochondrial fatty acid oxidation. Biochem J 1975; 150:77-88.
134. Bremer J. Pyruvate dehydrogenase, substrate specificity and product inhibition. Eur J Biochem 1969; 8:535-540.
135. Bremer J. Comparison of acylcarnitines and pyruvate as substrates for rat-liver mitochondria. Biochim Biophys Acta 1966; 116:1-11.
136. Bremer J, Wojtczak AB. Factors controlling the rate of fatty acid β-oxidation in rat liver mitochondria. Biochim Biophys Acta 1972; 280:515-530.
137. Quant PA. Activity and expression of hepatic mitochondrial 3-hydroxy-3-methylglutaryl-CoA synthase during the starved-to-refed transition. Biochem Soc Trans. 1990; 18:994-995.
138. McGarry JD, Foster DW. The metabolism of (-)octanoylcarnitine in perfused livers from fed and fasted rats. Evidence for a possible regulatory role of carnitine acyltransferase in the control of ketogenesis. J Biol Chem 1974; 249:7984-7990.
139. Brass EP, Hoppel CL. Disassociation between acid insoluble acylcarnitines and ketogenesis following carnitine administration in vivo. J Biol Chem 1978; 253:5274-5276.
140. Parvin R, Pande SV. Enhancement of mitochondrial carnitine and carnitine acylcarnitine translocase-mediated transport of fatty acids

into liver mitochondria under ketogenic conditions. J Biol Chem 1979; 254:5423-5429.

141. Normann PT, Ingebretsen OC, Flatmark T. On the rate limiting step in the transfer of long-chain acyl groups across the inner membrane of brow adipose tissue mitochondria. Biochim Biophys Acta 1978; 501:286-295.

142. Saggerson ED, Carpenter CA. Regulation of hepatic carnitine palmitoyltransferase activity during foetal-neonatal transition. FEBS Lett 1982; 150:177-180.

143. Decaux J-F, Ferre P, Robin D et al. Decreased hepatic fatty acid oxidation at weaning in the rat is not linked to a variation of malonyl-CoA concentration. J Biol Chem 1988; 263:3284-3289.

144. Borrebaek B. Acylation of carnitine and glycerophosphate in suspensions of rat liver mitochondria at varying levels of palmitate and coenzyme A. Acta Physiol Scand 1975; 95:448-456.

145. Wong SH, Nestel PJ, Trimble RP et al. The adaptive effects of dietary fish and safflower oil on lipid and lipoprotein metabolism in perfused rat liver. Biochim Biophys Acta 1984; 792:103-109.

146. Berge RK, Nilsson A, Husøy A-M. Rapid stimulation of liver palmitoyl-CoA synthetase, carnitine palmitoyltransferase and glycerophosphate acyltransferase compared to peroxisomal β-oxidation and palmitoyl-CoA hydrolase in rats fed high-fat diets. Biochim Biophys Acta 1988; 960:417-426.

147. Clouet P, Niot I, Gresti J et al. Polyunsaturated n-3 and n-6 fatty acids at a low level in the diet alter mitochondrial outer membrane parameters in Wistar rat liver. Nutritional Biochem 1995; 6:626-634.

148. Skrede S, Bremer J. Acylcarnitine formation and fatty acid oxidation in hepatocytes from rats treated with tetradecylthioacetic acid (a 3-thia fatty acid). Biochim Biophys Acta 1993; 1167:189-196.

149. Guzman M, Geelen MJH. Effects of ethanol feeding on the activity and regulation of hepatic carnitine palmitoyltransferase I. Arch Biochem Biophys 1988; 267:580-588.

150. Cook GA, Gamble MS. Rergulation of carnitine palmitoyltransferase by insulin results in decreased activity and decreased apparent $K_i$ values for malonyl-CoA. J Biol Chem 1987; 262:2050-2055.

151. Penicaud L, Robin D, Robin P et al. Effect of insulin on the properties of liver carnitine palmitoyltransferase in the starved rat: Assessment by the euglycemic hyperinsulinemic clamp. Metabolism 1991; 40:873-876.

152. Stakkestad JA, Bremer J. The outer carnitine palmitoyltransferase and regulation of fatty acid metabolism in rat liver in different thyroid states. Biochim Biophys Acta 1983; 750:244-252.

153. Weinstein I, Cook GA, Heimberg M. Regulation by oestrogen of carnitine palmitoyltranferase in hepatic mitochondria. Biochem J 1986; 237:593-596.

154. Pegorier J-P, Garcia-Garcia M-V, Prip-Buus C et al. Induction of ketogenesis and fatty acid oxidation by glucagon and cyclic AMP in cultured hepatocytes from rabbit fetuses. Evidence for a decreased sensitivity of carnitine palmitoyltransferase I to malonyl-CoA inhibition after glucagon or cyclic AMP treatment. Biochem J 1989; 264:93-100.

155. Guzman M, Castro J. Okadaic acid stimulates carnitine palmitoylttransferase I and palmitate oxidation in isolated rat hepatocytes. FEBS Lett 1991; 291:105-108.

156. Guzman M, Velasco G, Castro J et al. Inhibition of carnitine palmitoyltransferase I by hepatocyte swelling. FEBS Lett 1994; 344:239-241.

157. Kashfi K, Dory L, Cook GA. Effects of cholesterol loading of mouse macrophages on carnitine palmitoyltransferase activity and sensitivity to inhibition by malonyl-CoA. Biochem Biophys Res Commun. 1991; 177:1121-1126.

158. Zammit VA. Increased sensitivity of carnitine palmitoyltransferase I activity to malonyl-CoA inhibition after preincubation of intact rat liver mitochondria with micromolar concentrations of malonyl-CoA in vitro. Biochem J 1983; 210:953-956.

159. Bergseth S, Lund H, Poisson J-P et al. Carnitine palmitoyltransferase: Avtivation and inactivation in liver mitochondria from fed, fasted, hypo- and hyperthyroid rats. Biochem Biophys Acta 1986; 876: 551-558.

160. Bremer J, Woldegiorgis G, Schalinske K et al. Carnitine palmitoyltransferase. Activation by palmitoyl-CoA and inactivation by malonyl-CoA. Biochim Biophys Acta 1985; 833:9-16.

161. Ghadiminejad I, Saggerson D. Physiological state and the sensitivity of liver mitochondrial outer membrane carnitine palmitoyltransferase to malonyl-CoA. Correlations with assay temperature, salt concentration and membrane lipid composition. Int J Biochem 1992; 24:1117-1124.

162. Niot I, Pacot F, Bouchard P et al. Involvement of microsomal vesicles in part of the sensitivity of carnitine palmitoyltransferase I to malonyl-CoA inhibition in mitochondrial fractions of rat liver. Biochem J 1994; 304:577-584.

163. Stephens TW, Cook GA, Harris RA. Effect of pH on malonyl-CoA inhibition of carnitine palmitoyltransferase I. Biochem J 1983; 212:521-524.

164. Mynatt RL, Greenhaw JJ, Cook GA. Cholate extracts of mitochondrial outer membranes increase inhibition by malonyl-CoA of carnitine palmitoyltransferase-I by a mechanism involving phospholipids. Biochem J 1994; 299:761-767.

165. Kolodziej MP, Zammit VA. Sensitivity of inhibition of rat liver mitochondrial outer membrane carnitine palmitoyltransferase by

malonyl-CoA to chemical- and temperature-induced changes in membrane fluidity. Biochem J 1990; 272:421-425.

166. Malewiak M-I, Griglio S, Le Liepvre X. Relationship between lipogenesis, ketogenesis, and malonyl-CoA content in isolated hepatocytes from the obese Zucker rat adapted to a high-fat diet. Metabolism 1985; 34:604-611.

167. Mynatt RL, Park EA, Thorngate FE et al. Changes in carnitine palmitoyltransferase-I mRNA abundance produced by hyperthyroidism and hypothyroidism. Parallel changes in activity. Biochim Biophys Res Commun 1994; 201:932-937.

168. Thumelin S, Esser V, Charvy D et al. Expression of liver carnitine palmitoyltransferase I and II genes during development in the rat. Biochem J 1994; 300:583-587.

169. Park EA, Mynatt RL, Cook GA et al. Insulin regulates enzyme activity, malonyl-CoA sensitivity and mRNA abundance of hepatic carnitine palmitoyltranferase I. Biochem J 310:853-858.

170. Kolodziej MP, Zammit VA. Re-evaluation of the interaction of malonyl-CoA with rat liver mitochondrial carnitine palmitoyltransferase system by using purified outer membranes. Biochem J 1990; 267:85-90.

171. Cook GA, Cox KA. Hysteretic behaviour of carnitine palmitoyltransferase. The effect of preincubation with malonyl-CoA. Biochem J 1986; 236:917-919.

172. Harano Y, Kashiwagi A, Kojima H et al. Phosphorylation of carnitine palmitoyltransferase and activation by glucagon in isolated rat hepatocytes. FEBS Lett 1985; 188:267-272.

173. Guzman M, Kolodziej MP, Caldwell A et al. Evidence against direct involvement of phosphorylation in the activation of carnitine palmitoyltransferase by okadaic acid in rat hepatocytes. Biochem J 1994; 300:693-699.

174. Bremer J. The carnitine-dependent pathways in heart muscle. In: De Jong JW, Ferrari R, eds. The carnitine system. A new therapeutical approach to cardiovascular diseases. Kluwer Academic Publishers, Dordrecht 1995; 7-20.

175. Oram JF, Bennetch SL, Neely JR. Regulation of fatty acid utilization in isolated perfused rat hearts. J Biol Chem 1973; 248:5299-5309.

176. Saddik M, Gamble J, Witters LA et al. Acetyl-CoA carboxylase regulation of fatty acid oxidation in the heart. J Biol Chem 1993; 268:25836-25845.

177. Guzman M, Castro J. Effect of endurance excercise on palmitoyltransferase I from rat heart, skeletal muscle and liver mitochondria. Biochim Biophys Acta 1988; 963:562-565.

178. McMillin JB, Wang D, Witters LA et al. Kinetic properties of carnitine palmitoyltransferase I in cultured neonatal rat cardiac myocytes. Arch Biochem Biophys 1994; 312:375-384.

179. Kvannes J, Eikhom TS, Flatmark T. The peroxisomal β-oxidation enzyme system of rat heart. Basal level and effect of the peroxisome proliferator clofibrate. Bichim Biophys Acta 1994; 12o1:203-216.
180. Crespin SR, Greenough WG, Steinberg D. Stimulation of insulin secretion by long-chain free fatty acids. A direct pancreatic effect. J Clin Invest 1973; 52:1979-1984.
181. Prentki M, Vischer S, Glennon MC et al. Malonyl-CoA and long chain acyl-CoA esters as metabolic coupling factors in nutrient-induced insulin secretion. J Biol Chem 1992; 267:5802-5810.
182. Malaisse WJ, Best L, Kawazu S et al. Fuel metabolism in islets. Arch Biochem Biophys 1983; 224:102-110.
183. Shrago E, MacDonald MJ, Woldegiorgis G et al. The role of carnitine palmitoyltransferase and carnitine in the metabolism of pancreatic islets. In: Borum PR, Ed. Clinical aspects of human carnitine deficiency. New York: Pergamon Press 1986:28-37.
184. Chen S, Ogawa A, Ohneda M et al. More direct evidence for a malonyl-CoA-carnitine palmitoyltransferase I interaction as a key event in pancreatic β-cell signaling. Diabetes 1994; 43:878-883.

# CHAPTER 2

# Molecular Biology of Carnitine Palmitoyltransferases and Role of Carnitine in Gene Transcription

Madiraju S. R. Murthy and Shri V. Pande

## INTRODUCTION

Much available information indicates that carnitine influences a variety of processes in the body; this is attested to by the nature of diverse carnitine related topics covered in the other chapters of this volume. In terms of mechanisms, the best understood function of carnitine is its participation as an essential component in the process of mitochondrial fatty acid oxidation. In this process, as shown in Figure 2.1, carnitine, with the cooperation of two carnitine palmitoyltransferases (CPT) and a transporter for carnitine and acylcarnitines, acts as a carrier of acyl groups across the inner mitochondrial membrane. The ability of carnitine together with carnitine acyltransferases to modulate the cellular acyl-CoA to free CoA ratio is believed to be involved somehow in most if not all the other functions of carnitine. The recognition that distinct CPT isozymes occur in various subcellular locations (Table 2.1) heightens the hope that clarification of 'the other functions of carnitine' may now be around the corner. Applications of the tools of molecular biology to the characterization of the various CPTs and of the mutations involved in related genetic diseases are greatly aiding our understanding of the structure-function relationships. The information available on these aspects forms the subject of the present chapter, together with indications of possible role(s) of carnitine in the nucleus. Several other aspects of carnitine acyltransferases are covered in chapter 1. For the sake of unambiguity and brevity, here we are referring to the various CPTs as described in the first column of Table 2.1.

---

*Carnitine Today,* edited by Claudio De Simone and Giuseppe Famularo.
© 1997 Landes Bioscience.

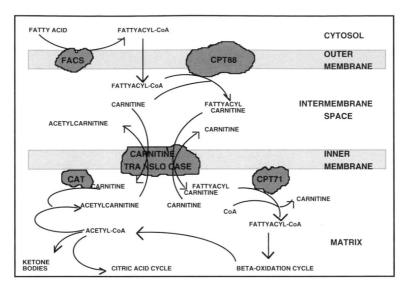

Fig. 2.1. Organization of the mitochondrial carnitine shuttle system. The reactions catalyzed by CPT71, CPT88, CAT and the carnitine acylcarnitine translocase are reversible and the translocase enables the entry and exit of free and acyl (short, medium and long chain) carnitines across the inner membrane. CPT, carnitine palmitoyl transferase; CAT, carnitine acetyltransferase; FACS, fatty acyl-CoA synthetase.

## MITOCHONDRIAL CPTS

Mitochondrial outer CPT has been found to be highly sensitive to inhibition by malonyl-CoA, the first intermediate of fatty acid biosynthesis, as part of a feedback regulatory mechanism.[1] Although initially it was thought that the malonyl-CoA-sensitivity is an exclusive property of the mitochondrial outer CPT, different malonyl-CoA- sensitive CPTs from other organelles have been described.[2] More recently, we have provided evidence that in both peroxisomes and microsomes of rat liver the malonyl-CoA-sensitive CPTs are novel CPT isoenzymes.[2,3] A malonyl-CoA-sensitive CPT has also been described in the erythrocyte membranes.[4]

The existence of an outer CPT and an inner CPT localized in different locations in mitochondria was proposed some 25 years ago.[5,6] These two activities were thought to reside, respectively, on the outer and inner aspects of the inner mitochondrial membrane, and the outer activity was thought to be the one loosely associated with the membrane.[7] Subsequently, we showed that the outer CPT is a firmly attached protein of the outer mitochondrial membrane[8,9] and data of others indicated that the loosely associated CPT with mitochondrial preparations that was at times mistaken for

*Table 2.1. Nomenclature of the subcellular location specific CPTs*

| Used presently | Other names used in literature | Malonyl-CoA inhibition | Localization | Molecular wt., kDa[*] |
|---|---|---|---|---|
| CPT71[*] | CPT-II, $CPT_i$, mitochondrial inner CPT, CPT-B | No | Inner membrane of mitochondria | 71.5 |
| L-CPT88 | CPT-I, $CPT_o$, CPT-A, and 90 kDa mitochondrial outer CPT of liver | Yes | Outer membrane of liver mitochondria | 88.1 |
| H-CPT88 | CPT-I, $CPT_o$, CPT-A, and 84 kDa mitochondrial outer CPT of heart | Yes | Outer membrane of heart mitochondria | 88.2 |
| CPT54 | Microsomal soluble CPT, GRP58, ERp61 | No | Microsomal lumen | 54.2 |
| CPT70 | Carnitine octanoyltransferase, soluble 66 kDa CPT of peroxisomes | No | Peroxisomal matrix | 70.3 |
| CPT~88P?[†] (Putative) | Membrane-bound CPT of liver peroxisomes | Yes | Peroxisomal membrane | |
| CPT~47?[†] (Putative) | Membrane-bound CPT of liver microsomes | Yes | Microsomal membrane | |

[*] The numeral without ~ refers to the molecular weight deduced from the cDNA-derived amino acid sequence for the mature protein.

[†] The '?' mark indicates that the designation is putative; a '~' indicates the assessed approximate subunit molecular size from SDS-PAGE.

the mitochondrial outer CPT was of peroxisomal origin.[10,11] The two differentially located CPT catalytic activities were initially assumed to reside in the same protein, as classical purification procedures from liver and heart mitochondria yielded only one protein having CPT activity (current designation CPT71) of apparent subunit molecular weight, on SDS-PAGE of ~68 kDa.[12,13] Indications that these two CPTs were dissimilar at least in details appeared from the discoveries that malonyl-CoA potently inhibits the outer CPT selectively and that the two mitochondrial CPT activities reside in separate mitochondrial membranes.[1,8] The ability to physically separate the outer malonyl-CoA sensitive CPT in preparations of the outer membrane vesicles from the malonyl-CoA insensitive CPT of the inner membrane vesicles allowed clear demonstration[9] that the outer CPT is detergent labile, whereas detergents enhance the activity of the inner membrane associated CPT; the former was independently deduced by Declercq et al[14] and Lund[15] also. These findings appeared to rationalize the finding that in purification protocols using detergents only one protein with CPT activity was obtained from mitochondria.

The observations of Kiorpes et al[16] that 2-tetradecyl glycidyl-CoA, a potent, specific and irreversible inhibitor of outer CPT in liver mitochondria covalently tagged a ~90 kDa protein implied that this protein could be the outer CPT itself or that it constituted a component of the outer CPT system. The following findings strengthened this idea further: a marked difference in the properties of the outer and inner CPT of mitochondria as monitored in outer and inner membrane vesicles; the ability eventually to separate under appropriate conditions the two activities in purification protocols, with the demonstration that the malonyl-CoA inhibitable activity associated with a protein fraction containing the etomoxir-CoA labeled ~90 kDa protein but not with the CPT71 protein containing fraction;[9,17] the apparent size difference of the malonyl-CoA sensitive and insensitive CPTs in irradiation inactivation experiments;[18] an antibody raised against a 90 kDa protein band from the liver mitochondrial outer membrane specifically precipitated the octylglucoside-solubilized malonyl-CoA sensitive CPT activity from liver mitochondrial outer membrane, but not the malonyl-CoA insensitive CPT from the inner membrane;[19] and the recognition of clearly identifiable different deficiency diseases associated with the loss of malonyl-CoA-insensitive and malonyl-CoA-sensitive CPT activities.[20] Conclusive evidence that the two mitochondrial CPTs are different proteins has emerged from the characterization of their distinct cDNAs, largely from the laboratory of Denis McGarry, and these are described below.

CPT71: THE MALONYL-CoA-INSENSITIVE CPT OF MITOCHONDRIA

Woeltje et al,[21] employing oligonucleotide probes, designed on the basis of peptide amino acid sequences obtained from the purified rat liver

CPT71, isolated the cDNA of rat liver CPT71. The full length clone contained an open reading frame of 1,974 bases coding for a protein of 658 amino acids with a calculated molecular weight of 74.119 kDa. The first 25 amino acid stretch from the predicted sequence of this protein was found to possess the characteristics of a mitochondrial targeting leader peptide; subsequently, it was shown that this leader peptide is cleaved off during the import of CPT71 in mitochondria.[22] Transfection of COS cells with the CPT71 cDNA led to an ~6-fold increase in the malonyl-CoA-insensitive mitochondrial CPT activity and this increased CPT activity was immunoprecipitated by the anti-CPT71 antibody. Later, Finocchiaro et al[23] isolated the human liver CPT71 cDNA and showed that the predicted amino acid sequences of rat liver and human liver CPT71 shared ~82% homology.

Gelb[24] in 1993 reported a cardiac promoter for the CPT71 in mouse and showed that the same promoter is active also in hepatoma cells, and on the basis of highly conserved 5'-UTR sequences (untranslated regions) of mouse heart and rat liver CPT71 cDNAs, it was suggested that the same promoter is responsible for the expression of the CPT71 in murine liver. Recently, Montermini et al[25] reported that the 5'- regulatory sequences of human CPT71 gene show ~52% homology with the corresponding sequence of the mouse CPT71 gene.

Brady et al[26] have described that the N-terminal of CPT71 includes the sequence "pyro Glu-Lys-Gly-Val-Gln-Thr-Gly-Gln." Employing DNA probes/primers coding for this putative sequence, they have described many hormonal and dietary effects on the mRNA levels of liver CPT71[26-29] and have also reported[13] the isolation of a promoter sequence for the rat liver CPT71. However in the closely matching cDNA derived CPT71 amino acid sequences of the rat liver[21] and of human liver,[23] the above N-terminal sequence, as described by Brady et al,[26] was not found. Moreover, the sequence of the CPT71 gene promoter as reported by Brady et al[13] is also entirely different from that described by Gelb[24] and Montermini et al.[25] To clarify this situation, Weis et al[30] performed a PCR analysis of the poly(A)+ RNA of rat liver, using either a 19mer from the 5'-UTR of Woeltje et al[21] or a 24mer from the 5'-UTR sequence reported by Brady et al[13] as the 5'-primers and a 25mer from base 516 to 540 of CPT71 coding sequence as the 3'-primer. Southern analyses of the PCR products using a DNA probe corresponding to the first 25 bases of the CPT71 coding region showed that the PCR product obtained using the 5'-primer of Woeltje et al[21] strongly hybridized with the CPT71 probe, while there was little hybridization with the small amount of PCR product formed using the 5'-primer of Brady et al.[13] These results established the authenticity of the CPT71 cDNA reported by Woeltje et al[21] and Finocchiaro et al[23] and have put to question the validity of the various results obtained by Brady et al.[26-29] The possibility that the promoter sequences described by Brady et al[13] could be a cloning artifact has been suggested.[25]

In all tissues, to the extent examined, CPT71 appears to be the same protein on the basis of molecular size, immuno-crossreactivity, Northern hybridization and in some cases cDNA sequence information.[21,23,24,31] Analysis of the mouse CPT71 gene showed its size to be ~19.5 kb, with 5 exons and 4 introns ranging from 1.6 to 8.6 kb.[24] The transcription start site for the CPT71 gene in mouse heart was found to be at 73 nucleotides upstream of the initiating codon;[24] for human CPT71 gene it was 516 nucleotides upstream.[25] No evidence for alternate splicing of the CPT71 mRNA or of multiple transcription initiation sites was found. The 386 nt region upstream of the transcription start site in mouse heart CPT71 gene when cloned into the promoter-less pCAT vector increased the chloramphenicol acetyltransferase expression 22-fold in Hepa 1-6 cells,[24] indicating that this region acts as a promoter. Similarly, Montermini et al[25] showed that the 100 nt region upstream of the transcription start site for the human CPT71 gene, when cloned in the pCAT enhancer vector, increased the chloramphenicol acetyltransferase expression 15-fold in COS cells. The mechanism of transcriptional regulation of CPT71, the promoter region boundaries and the transcription factors involved remain to be identified. Initially the CPT71 gene was localized to chromosome 1q12-pter[23] but further work has led to refinement of this position to the 1p32 region of chromosome 1.

### Structural requirements for CPT71 catalytic activity

Involvement of a histidine residue in the active site of carnitine acetyltransferase was indicated in the experiments of Chase and Tubbs.[32] For CPT71 a histidine at position 372 likewise appears important. Brown et al[33] have shown that the treatment of recombinant CPT71 with diethyl pyrocarbonate, a specific histidine-binding agent, led to the loss of activity that was reversed on subsequent exposure to hydroxylamine. A 'catalytic triad' involving histidine appears functional in lipases, esterases, proteases and acyltransferases, and the realization that the amino acid sequence around His-372 is conserved among the nine carnitine/choline acyltransferases indicates that this may be true also for the CPT71. In line with this it was observed that the site-directed mutagenesis of CPT71 causing the mutations His372Ala, His372Lys, and Asp376Ala led to a complete loss of CPT71 activity. It was accordingly suggested that in CPT71's catalysis, histidine-372-induced deprotonation of the hydroxyl group of carnitine facilitates a nucleophilic attack on the carbonyl carbon of the acyl moiety of acyl-CoA, leading to the transfer of the acyl group to the oxygen of the carnitine's hydroxyl and the release of free CoASH.[33] The "adenine binding loop" of citrate synthase is involved in acetyl-CoA binding and this region includes the amino acid sequence motif of G, F/Y, G; a similar sequence is present also in the carnitine and choline acyltransferase family. Site-directed mutagenesis of the corresponding amino acids in CPT71, namely of Val605Ala, Gly609Ala and Gly611Ala, indicated, surprisingly, that they are not involved in the palmitoyl-CoA binding but are involved in carnitine binding, inasmuch as these mutations increased the $K_m$ for carnitine 4-5-fold.

## Expression of CPT71 cDNA

For obtaining a catalytically active protein in *E. coli*, the human CPT71 required expression as a fusion protein with glutathione-S-transferase, unlike that for the rat CPT71 expression.[34] Both the precursor and mature forms of the rat CPT71 were found to show catalytic activity, whereas the N-terminally truncated (the first 18 amino acids deleted from the mature CPT71) form did not.[34] This study also revealed that despite similar molecular weights the rat CPT71 migrates faster on SDS-PAGE than the human counterpart. Expression of larger quantities using the baculovirus expression system in Sf9 insect cells enabled demonstration that the properties of the recombinant protein closely matched those of the CPT71 purified from liver.[35]

Several disease-causing mutations to CPT71 deficiency have been recognized[36-39] (Table 2.2). In the infantile form of the inner CPT deficiency disease which accompanies severe loss of CPT71 activity, the Arg631Cys change appears commonly involved; this activity loss is found more marked when accompanied with the polymorphic mutations Val368Ile and Met647Val, which on their own do not affect the CPT activity. CPT71 with the three mutations, when expressed in COS cells, did not show significant differences in affinity for substrates but the approximate half-life of the mutant enzyme was lowered (from ≈14 h to ≤5 h); thus the enhanced proteolytic degradation of the improperly folded mutant enzyme is likely involved here.[36] In the less severe adult form of the CPT71 deficiency disease, the Ser113Leu is the commonly identified mutation,[37] but in this case the loss of activity is not further aggravated by the other common polymorphic mutations. Here also the mutation appears to lead to unstable protein (Table 2.2).

## CPT88: The Malonyl-CoA Sensitive CPT of Mitochondria

The molecular cloning of the liver mitochondrial malonyl-CoA-sensitive CPT was described by Esser et al.[40,41] These workers observed that dinitrophenyl-etomoxir labeled an ~90 kDa protein in liver mitochondria that on controlled proteolysis with a mixture of trypsin and chymotrypsin became converted into an ~82 kDa protein; amino acid sequences for 4 peptides derived from this truncated protein were used to construct degenerate oligonucleotide probes for screening a rat liver cDNA library.[41] A clone

**Table 2.2. Mutations in CPT71 identified as deficiency disease in humans**

| Mutations in CPT71 | Mutant activity (% of normal) | Affinities for substrates | Stability of the mutant CPT71 | Reference |
|---|---|---|---|---|
| Adult form deficiency: | 5- 26% | Not affected | Decreased | |
| Ser113Leu; | | | | Taroni et al[37] |
| Pro50His; | | | | Verderio et al[39] |
| Asp553Asn | | | | Verderio et al[39] |
| | | | | |
| Infantile form deficiency: | 4- 10% | Not affected, | Decreased | |
| Arg631Cys; | | except for | | Taroni et al[36] |
| Tyr628Ser; | | Pro227Leu | | Bonnefont et al[38] |
| Pro227Leu | | | | Bonnefont et al[38] |

with an open reading frame of 2319 bases coding for a 773 amino acid protein (Mr = 88150) was isolated and the derived amino acid sequence from this clone was found to house all of the 4 peptide sequences obtained from the truncated ~82 kDa protein.[41] Northern analysis of the liver mRNA with a 0.9 kb DNA fragment of the above cDNA revealed a single mRNA species of ~4.7 kb. (Similar Northern analysis with a probe for the CPT71 revealed a ~2.5 kb mRNA). The authenticity of the isolated cDNA was established when transient expression in COS cells was found to lead to 10-fold increase in malonyl-CoA sensitive CPT activity (Table 2.3) without any significant change in the malonyl-CoA insensitive CPT activity.[41] Comparison of amino acid sequence of L-CPT88 with CPT70 and CPT71 showed an ~30% overall identity and a similarity of ~50% with allowance for conservative amino acid changes. Hydropathy plot revealed at least two probable membrane-spanning regions, at amino acids 48-75 and 103-122. Conversely, CPT71 does not possess any defined membrane spanning regions, consistent with the known easily solubilizable nature of CPT71.[41]

Kolodziej and Zammit[42] reported that when the L-CPT88 band (obtained by Con-A sepharose chromatography and then SDS-PAGE) was subjected to limited proteolysis using V8-protease, one of the resultant peptides had the N-terminal sequence corresponding to position 4-18 of the cDNA predicted sequence of L-CPT88. This indicated that there is no proteolytic processing of L-CPT88 on its import in common with that known for the majority of the other outer membrane proteins. The N-terminus of the mature L-CPT88 appears to be blocked (V. Zammit, personal communication). These authors also suggested that amino acid residues 48-73, flanked on both sides by highly charged amino acids, most likely serve as

**Table 2.3. Expression of rat L-CPT88 and H-CPT88 cDNAs in COS and human 293 cells**

| Transfection with plasmids | Relative CPT Activity | | $K_m$ for carnitine | $IC_{50}$ for malonyl-CoA | Reference |
|---|---|---|---|---|---|
| | Total | Malonyl-CoA sensitive | | | |
| In COS cells | | | | | |
| Control | 1 | 0.84 | — | — | Esser et al[41] |
| pCMV6-L-CPT88 | 6.9 | 4.8 | ~0.25 mM | 8 µM | |
| pCMV6-H-CPT88 | 5.1 | 5.0 | 0.4-0.6 mM | 0.15 µM | Esser et al[55] |
| In human 293 cells | | | | | |
| Control | 1 | 0.92 | — | — | Murthy and |
| pcDNAI(neo)-L- | 6.7 | 6.2 | — | — | Pande |
| CPT88 | | | | | (Unpublished) |

Transfection and expression plasmids are as indicated below. The plasmid pcDNAI(neo)-L-CPT88 was constructed by ligating the L-CPT88 cDNA from pCMV6-L-CPT88 plasmid[41] into the BamH I site of the pcDNAI(neo). On the third day after transfection, the cells were homogenized, a mitochondrial fraction was obtained and CPT activity without and with malonyl-CoA was assayed using palmitoyl-CoA as a substrate. CPT relative activity is expressed with the control cell activity being assigned as 1.

the transmembrane domain, with the N-terminal region protruding in the cytosol.[42] Consistent with our initial suggestion[8] Cook et al[43] provided evidence that L-CPT88 has two inhibitor binding sites; one is located on the cytoplasmic side of the outer membrane and binds malonyl-CoA, while the other one is at the active site; kinetic analyses confirmed that the binding of malonyl-CoA and the substrate acyl-CoA are 'mutually exclusive' and account for the apparent competitive kinetics. These investigators suggested that the first 102 amino acid portion of the L-CPT88 likely protrudes into the cytosol and houses the malonyl-CoA binding site.

In spite of the formidable evidence that the inner and outer CPTs of mitochondria are different proteins, there have been lingering arguments favoring the concept that the catalytic subunit of outer CPT is identical to that of the inner CPT and that the etomoxir-binding protein of 88 kDa is a regulatory subunit that confers malonyl-CoA sensitivity to the catalytic subunit.[44-47] This possibility was unequivocally eliminated by the demonstration that the expression of the cDNA for the 88 kDa protein in *Saccharomyces cerevisiae*, which does not have any endogenous CPT activity, led to the emergence of both malonyl-CoA and etomoxir-CoA inhibitable CPT activity.[48] L-CPT88 has two hydrophobic domains at amino acid residues 48-75 (H1) and 103-122 (H2). When L-CPT88 constructs lacking either H1 (resultant protein has amino acids 83-773) or both H1 and H2 (this construct

Fig. 2.2. Malonyl-CoA inhibition of the wild-type L-CPT88 and ΔH1-L-CPT88 expressed in yeast (modified from Brown et al[48]).
Full length form of L-CPT88 (met1-L-CPT88) and 1-83 amino acids truncated L-CPT88 (ΔH1-L-CPT88) were expressed separately in *Saccharomyces cerevisiae*. Mitochondrial fraction was isolated and CPT activity was assayed using palmitoyl-CoA. Malonyl-CoA was present as indicated.

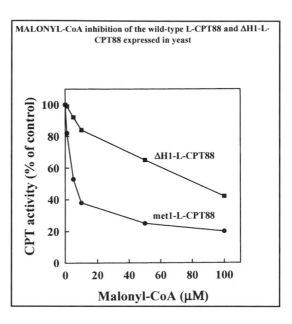

MALONYL-CoA inhibition of the wild-type L-CPT88 and ΔH1-L-CPT88 expressed in yeast

has amino acids 1-30 followed by 149-773) were expressed in yeast, the ΔH1-L-CPT88 product showed CPT activity. However, the ΔH1 H2-L-CPT88 was not made in any significant amount. Whereas the normal L-CPT88 expressed in yeast showed an $IC_{50}$ for malonyl-CoA of ~5 μM, this was ~ 80 μM for the ΔH1-L-CPT88 (Fig. 2.2). At 100 μM malonyl-CoA, the observed maximal inhibition of the normal L-CPT88 was ~80% whereas the ΔH1 construct could be inhibited by only ~50%. These results indicated that the amino acid residues 1-83 of L-CPT88, though not needed for catalytic activity, play a role in determining the malonyl-CoA inhibitability.[48] This observation further demonstrated that the 88 kDa protein coded by the cDNA clone[41] expresses both the CPT activity and malonyl-CoA inhibitability. This information, when taken together with the observations that controlled exposure of outer membrane vesicles or mitochondria to proteases leads to loss of malonyl-CoA sensitivity of L-CPT88 and of malonyl-CoA binding[8,49,50] indicates that the amino acid residues 1-83 of L-CPT88 may form part of the malonyl-CoA binding site on the cytosolic side of the outer membrane. The second hydrophobic domain (amino acids 103-122) of L-CPT88 may form the membrane spanning region with the rest of the protein housing the catalytic site, facing the intermembrane space. This fits the model we proposed earlier.[8] More recently, the cDNA for human liver L-CPT88 has also been cloned and its derived primary structure is 88% identical to that of the rat liver CPT88.[51] Using a panel of somatic cell hybrids, Britton et al[51] found that the human L-CPT88 gene is located on the q-region of chromosome 11. Thus the two genes coding outer and inner CPTs of mitochondria are located on separate chromosomes.

The mitochondrial outer CPT in heart and skeletal muscle tissues is a protein that is different from its liver counterpart. Two important kinetic differences were the first to indicate that the liver and muscle enzymes are probably distinct.[52] The liver outer CPT shows a higher affinity for carnitine ($K_m \approx 30 \ \mu M$) than the heart and the muscle enzymes ($K_m \approx 200$ and $500 \ \mu M$, respectively). And the sensitivity to malonyl-CoA inhibition is lower for the liver enzyme ($IC_{50} \approx 3 \ \mu M$) as compared to the enzyme from heart and skeletal muscle ($IC_{50} \approx 0.1$ and $0.03 \ \mu M$, respectively). Later, it was found that [$^3$H]-tetradecyl glycidyl-CoA, an irreversible inhibitor of outer CPT, covalently labeled a ~90 kDa protein in liver mitochondria whereas in heart mitochondria the labeled protein shows a lower (~82 to 84 kDa) apparent molecular size,[14,17] again suggesting that the liver and heart mitochondrial outer CPTs are different.[52] Studies employing Northern hybridization using the L-CPT88 cDNA probe, anti-L-CPT88 antibody and [$^3$H]-deschloroetomoxir labeling revealed that rat heart, but not skeletal muscle, expresses small amounts of liver type CPT88 also.[31] The L-CPT88 makes a minor contribution (initially assessed as ~10% but later revised[33] to 2-3%) to the total outer CPT activity in adult rat heart with the major activity being due to the muscle type outer CPT. These findings suggest an explanation for the finding that in heart the overall outer CPT shows kinetic parameters intermediate to those for liver and skeletal muscle isoenzymes.[31]

Experiments in developing rats showed that in the neonatal stage, ~25% of the total outer CPT activity of heart is due to L-CPT88; this value then steadily declines during growth to reach the adult level of 2-3% by weaning.[33] The decline in the level of L-CPT88 expression in the developing rat heart was found inversely correlated with the simultaneous increase in the carnitine content of this organ.[33] This is of interest, as Uenaka et al[53] have reported that in the genetically carnitine deficient JVS mice, which suffer from cardiac hypertrophy, the L-CPT88 mRNA levels in the heart are ~6-fold higher than in the controls and that this is promptly normalized on carnitine administration. Thus, carnitine appears to play a role in the expression of L-CPT88 in heart during development.

While looking for the proteins specifically expressed in the brown but not the white adipose tissue by subtractive cloning strategy, Yamazaki et al[54] isolated a rat cDNA clone with an open reading frame of 2316 bases coding for a protein with 772 amino acids. This protein of calculated Mr of 88200 was found to show ~62.6% homology with the rat L-CPT88 and ~27.6% homology with CPT71 and was accordingly described as the putative muscle type outer CPT. The mRNA corresponding to this cDNA was predominantly expressed in the brown adipose tissue and in heart muscle. However,

Yamazaki et al[54] did not express this protein to ascertain whether it would show any CPT activity. Esser et al[55] later isolated this cDNA clone from a rat heart cDNA library and showed that its expression in COS cells led to ~5-fold increase in the malonyl-CoA sensitive CPT activity (Table 2.3). The expressed protein was found to resemble the muscle mitochondrial outer CPT in its $K_m$ for carnitine and $IC_{50}$ for malonyl-CoA. Since the protein made in vitro by transcription and translation from the heart cDNA migrated relatively faster (at the position of 82 kDa) in SDS-PAGE, similarly to the [³H]-etomoxir labeled protein from muscle mitochondria as well as from COS cells expressing the above rat heart cDNA clone, it became evident that the rat heart outer CPT migrates anomalously in SDS-PAGE gels at ~82 kDa position, despite having a calculated molecular weight of 88.2 kDa (H-CPT88).

REGULATION OF THE EXPRESSION OF MITOCHONDRIAL CPTs

It has been known for a while that feeding and fasting profoundly affect mitochondrial β-oxidation of fatty acids in liver, and that fasting increases the L-CPT88 activity while lowering its sensitivity to malonyl-CoA inhibition.[56] The fasting mediated increase in the activity of L-CPT88 accompanies elevated levels of the L-CPT88 protein itself.[19,57] Fasting mediated changes in L-CPT88 levels were once related to alterations in insulin/ glucagon levels but no clear supporting evidence to this effect has emerged.[58] During development in rats, from 21 day fetus to a day after birth, L-CPT88 activity increases 4-6-fold.[59,60] Asins et al[61] recently showed that the liver L-CPT88 mRNA reaches adult values by 3 days postnatally; similar increase in L-CPT88 expression in the small intestine from birth to weaning was also observed.

Dibutyryl-cAMP and long-chain fatty acids were found to enhance L-CPT88 gene transcription through independent pathways in cultured hepatocytes from 20-day-old rat fetus; these effects were blocked by insulin.[62] The transcription of CPT71 was not affected. Perturbations leading to the accumulation of long-chain acyl-CoA esters, viz., use of 2-bromo-palmitate or linoleate + tetradecylglycidate (inhibitor of L-CPT88) led to the induction of L-CPT88 mRNA like that known for certain peroxisomal proteins,[52] but they had no effect on the CPT71 mRNA levels. However, clofibrate, a known peroxisome proliferator, increased the mRNAs of both L-CPT88 and CPT71. These results suggest that L-CPT88 induction by long chain fatty acids involves a pathway distinct from that of the classical peroxisome proliferator activated receptor pathway. It appears that the high fat content of the mother's milk plays a role in the developmental increase in the liver L-CPT88 expression during suckling, as the L-CPT88 mRNA levels remain low when the pups are weaned on a high carbohydrate diet.[62]

L-CPT88, which comprises ~25% of the outer CPT activity in the neonatal rat hearts, declines steadily during growth, reaching the adult level of 2-3% by weaning; this decline inversely correlates with the simultaneous increase in the carnitine content of heart, indicating that carnitine may negatively modulate L-CPT88 expression in developing heart.[33] This possibility is further strengthened by the observation of Uenaka et al[53] in the genetically carnitine deficient JVS mice heart ventricles, as mentioned earlier. Thus, it is possible that the L-CPT88 gene expression is upregulated through long chain acyl-CoA (or a related metabolite) while carnitine downregulates it.

Recently, Xia et al[64] reported that when the neonatal rat heart myocytes are subjected to electrical contractile stimulation in the absence of added growth factors, there is a marked proliferation of mitochondria and this accompanies ~50% decrease in the mRNA level of L-CPT88 and about 2.5-fold increase in the mRNA level of H-CPT88. These mRNA changes were reflected in the activity levels of L- and H-CPT88 isoenzymes. Thus, Xia et al[64] argued that the "isoform switch" from the L-CPT-88 to H-CPT88 in the heart myocyte during development is likely due to the increased contractile activity of the myocardium at this period. The exact mechanism of the electrical stimulation mediated transcriptional repression of L-CPT88 and transcriptional activation of H-CPT88 genes remains to be investigated.

Thyroid status is known to affect the activity of L-CPT88;[65] in rats L-CPT88 activity is lowered on administration of propyl thiouracil, an inhibitor of thyroid hormone production, and is elevated by triiodothyronine ($T_3$).[66] These changes in the L-CPT88 activity correlate with the corresponding mRNA levels in livers that are ~40-fold lower in hypothyroid versus hyperthyroid state. This strongly indicates that thyroid hormone status plays a role in the transcriptional control of L-CPT88. Although both fasting and thyroid hormone can elevate the liver L-CPT88 gene transcription, unlike fasting, the $T_3$-induction does not lead to diminished sensitivity to malonyl-CoA.[66] The possibility that liver CPT may be controlled by its phosphorylation/dephosphorylation was indicated by Harano et al[67] and Guzman and Geelen.[68] However, the latter work has undergone reinterpretation, and convincing data to support the phosphorylation hypothesis have not emerged.[69]

Most peroxisomal proliferators are known to induce carnitine acyltransferase activities not only in peroxisomes of liver, particularly of rodents, but also in mitochondria. Thus, clofibrate markedly induces carnitine acetyltransferase of mitochondria and peroxisomes, CPT70 of peroxisomes and CPT71 of mitochondria. This indicates that the genes coding for these enzymes could be under the control of peroxisomal proliferator activated receptors. In adult rats the induction of L-CPT88 by clofibrate is not as marked as that of CPT71,[70] although in cultured fetal hepatocytes the L-CPT88 mRNA level is elevated ~4-fold.[62] In the promoter region of many peroxisomal proteins the response elements for the peroxisomal proliferator activated receptors, known as Direct Repeat-1, (i.e. a repeat of AGGTCA or its variants separated by one base), have been identified as being involved in the peroxisomal proliferator mediated induction.[71] It is of interest that the promoter region of CPT71 from human liver appears to contain an imperfect Direct Repeat-1 between nucleotides -125 and -85 upstream of the TATA box.[25] The promoter regions of the L-CPT88 and H-CPT88 genes are yet to be characterized.

Genetic deficiency disease due to the loss of L-CPT88 has also been identified.[72,73] Assays in skin fibroblasts helped identify this disorder, and it has now been shown that indeed in fibroblasts the outer mitochondrial CPT expressed is the L-CPT88 form.[51] In most deficiency cases described, the outer CPT activity and the rates of fatty acid oxidation were found to have declined to ~10-15 % of the normal values while the serum free and total carnitine levels were found elevated; the latter contrast with the reverse situation is found in CPT71 deficiency disorder.[72,74]

## PEROXISOMAL CPTS

### CPT70: THE MALONYL-CoA INSENSITIVE CPT OF PEROXISOMES

The existence of a β-oxidation system in peroxisomes distinct from the one in mitochondria is well established. Markwell et al[75] reported that peroxisomes contain carnitine acyltransferase activities; subsequently purification of a soluble carnitine acyltransferase from rat and mouse liver peroxisomes, of ~66 kDa on SDS-PAGE, was achieved.[76,77] This soluble peroxisomal enzyme was referred to as carnitine octanoyltransferase; it shows high activity with both medium and long-chain acyl-CoA esters, and accordingly we are referring to it as a CPT,[2] more precisely as CPT70 (Table 2.1).

Employing a polyclonal antibody raised against the purified mouse liver peroxisomal (readily solubilizable) CPT, Chatterjee et al[78] isolated a cDNA clone from rat liver λgt11 cDNA expression library. Sequence analysis showed that it codes for a 523 amino acid protein with a calculated molecular weight of 60.269 kDa. Unlike many soluble peroxisomal proteins which generally have a peroxisomal targeting sequence (PTS-I), Ser-Lys-Leu or its variants ([Ser/Ala/Cys]-[Lys/Arg/His]-[Leu/Val/Ile/Phe]) at their carboxy terminus,[79] the cDNA derived amino acid sequence of this CPT ended with Ser-Lys-Arg-Cys. Chatterjee et al[78] mentioned that the cDNA clone they had isolated may code for most or all of the peroxisomal soluble CPT despite the fact that the cDNA derived molecular weight appeared to be smaller than that assessed as ~66 kDa by SDS-PAGE for the purified enzyme. Whether the protein expressed by their cDNA clone showed CPT activity was not verified.[78]

More recently, Chatterjee's group[80] reported that their cDNA sequence published earlier[78] was incomplete and that, indeed, it had some sequencing errors both at the 5' and the 3' end of the open reading frame. The updated now full-length cDNA sequence for the peroxisomal CPT is 2681 bp long, and is expected to code for a protein with 613 amino acids having a calculated molecular weight of 70.301 kDa (CPT70) with the C-terminal peroxisomal targeting signal, Ala-His-Leu.[80] That the expression product of this cDNA indeed shows CPT activity has been ascertained (Adler E and Ramsay RR, personal communication).

In rat liver, the CPT70 gene appears to be at least 40 kb long with 16 small exons (sizes range from 30 bp to 124 bp) and one large exon (912 bp). Analysis of the upstream, up to 1140 bp, promoter region of the CPT70 gene indicated the presence of a peroxisomal proliferator activated receptors consensus binding site, TGACCT, at the -737 position.[80] It is well established that peroxisomal CPT70 is induced several-fold by a variety of peroxisomal proliferators. This promoter region, when cloned in a promoterless pGL2-basic vector, was able to increase the luciferase expression by about 100-fold. However, the responsiveness of this promoter to peroxisome proliferators was not examined.[80]

### CPT~88P? THE MALONYL-CoA SENSITIVE CPT OF PEROXISOMES

The purified peroxisomal CPT was reported as not inhibited by malonyl-CoA.[76] However, Derrick and Ramsay[81] showed that in intact peroxisomes 10 μM malonyl-CoA inhibited the CPT activity by up to 90% and that this sensitivity to malonyl-CoA inhibition was lost on CPT purification. It was speculated that part of the CPT70 associates with the peroxisomal membrane and then shows inhibition by malonyl-CoA.[81] Subsequently, evidence that the peroxisomal membrane associated CPT is distinct from the CPT70 emerged in our experiments when the results showed[2] that the peroxisomal membranes containing the malonyl-CoA inhibitable CPT activity did not show presence of any CPT70 protein monitored by sensitive Western blotting using antibody to the CPT70. Our more recent evidence indicates that the malonyl-CoA sensitive CPT of the peroxisomal membrane is an ~88 kDa protein (CPT ~88P) and that it resembles the L-CPT88 in: (a) inhibition by malonyl-CoA, etomoxir-CoA and 2-tetradecyl glycidyl-CoA; (b) partial inactivation upon octylglucoside solubilization; (c) covalent labeling by [³H]-etomoxir-CoA; and (d) positive immunoreactivity with an anti- L-CPT88 antibody against the whole L-CPT88 protein.[70] However, the following indicate that the malonyl-CoA sensitive ~88 kDa CPT of peroxisomal membrane is distinct from the L-CPT88: (a) the CPT ~88P (both activity and protein content) is induced several-fold by clofibrate feeding while the L-CPT88 is induced only modestly; (b) in Western blots two antibodies raised against peptides of L-CPT88 (one against a 115 amino acid recombinant L-CPT88 peptide raised by us and the other against a 13- amino acid L-CPT88 peptide raised by Dr. V. Zammit), recognized only the L-CPT88 and not the CPT ~88P of peroxisomes.[70] A further molecular characterization of the CPT ~88P and its cDNA cloning are presently underway in our laboratory.

## MICROSOMAL CPTS

### CPT54: THE MALONYL-CoA INSENSITIVE CPT OF MICROSOMES

Markwell et al[75] showed the presence of CPT activity in microsomal fractions and Lilly et al[82] showed that the CPT activity associated with freshly made liver microsomes is strongly inhibited by malonyl-CoA and etomoxir-CoA. While working in the laboratory of Dr. Loran Bieber one of us (Madiraju Murthy) purified and characterized a microsomal CPT as a monomeric protein of ~54 kDa.[83] The purified CPT was not inhibited by malonyl-CoA and showed no cross reactivity in Western blots with either anti-CPT70 or anti-CPT71 antibodies. N-terminal amino acid sequence analysis of this microsomal CPT revealed the sequence as (S)DVLELTDEN and a database search showed that this same protein had previously been described as a phosphoinositide specific phospholipase-C, a protein disulfide isomerase, a protease[84] and that originally[85] this protein had been described as GRP58 (Glucose Regulated Protein, with a molecular weight of ~58 kDa). The corresponding cDNA was cloned by Bennet et al[86] from rat basophilic leukemia cell cDNA library and later by Mazzarella et al[87] from mouse fibroblasts. To ascertain the activity associated with this protein, we expressed the mouse cDNA in human 293 cells both transiently and stably and found that this led to a marked increase in the CPT specific activity (Fig. 2.3) of the cell extracts.[88] No increase in the protein disulfide isomerase activity was found, in agreement with Mazzarella et al.[87] Moreover, synthesis of this protein by the in vitro transcription and translation system also showed an increase in CPT activity (Fig. 2.4) demonstrating that this 54 kDa microsomal protein is a CPT isoenzyme (CPT54). A sequence comparison between the GRP58/CPT54 and CPT71, L-CPT88 and CPT70 shows 39-45% similarity with ~20% identity; this indicates that the CPT54 differs markedly from the other previously characterized CPT isozymes.

More recently, Bourdi et al[89] have cloned the cDNA for the human GRP58 and have reported that the purified recombinant GRP58 expressed in the baculovirus system did not show any CPT activity when assayed with 17 μM acetyl-CoA and carnitine; however, these investigators did not real-

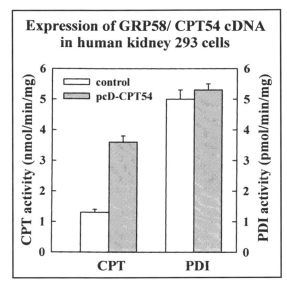

**Expression of GRP58/ CPT54 cDNA in human kidney 293 cells**

Fig. 2.3. Expression of GRP58/ CPT54 cDNA in human kidney 293 cells. Mouse GRP58/ CPT54 cDNA was cloned into pCD plasmid and expressed transiently. For control transfections, plasmid without the cDNA was used. Three days after transfection, cells were homogenized and a 110,000xg membrane fraction was obtained and assayed for CPT and protein disulfide isomerase. CPT was assayed using [1-[14]C] decanoyl-CoA plus carnitine and protein disulfide isomerase was assayed using [125]I-insulin. (modified from Murthy and Pande[88]).

ize that acetyl-CoA is not a suitable substrate[83,90] for monitoring carnitine palmitoyltransferase activity. More recently, we have expressed the rat GRP58 in *E. coli* as a hexa-histidine tagged protein. After purification and removal of the hexa histidine tag (by cleavage with enterokinase), this recombinant protein showed CPT activity when assayed with [1-[14]C]decanoyl-CoA plus carnitine (Murthy and Pande, manuscript in preparation). Using this assay, we have also found CPT activity in the recombinant human GRP58 of Bourdi et al[89] (obtained as a gift). However, these recombinant GRP58/CPT54 proteins showed lower specific activities compared to the freshly obtained batches of the CPT54 purified from rat liver microsomes. We are presently examining whether this results from the known marked instability of the CPT activity in the purified CPT54 preparations that we observe despite the presence of carnitine as a stabilizer[83,84] or whether the folding of the recombinant GRP58 may not be optimal for CPT activity to begin with. The possibility that the recombinant GRP58 protein does show protein disulfide isomerase activity as described by others[89,91] is also being re-examined.

CPT54/GRP58 is known to be a stress-regulated protein; it is induced by low glucose availability, exposure to calcium ionophore A23187, thiol binding agents and heat stress.[85,87] Mobb et al[92] studied this protein as a hormone induced protein-70 and reported that in the hippocampus region of brain this protein is induced several-fold by estrogens. Initially this protein is synthesized as a 57 kDa precursor that, following targeting to the endoplasmic reticulum, undergoes loss of the N-terminal signal peptide of the first 24 amino acids to yield the 54 kDa mature protein.[87,88] The mature

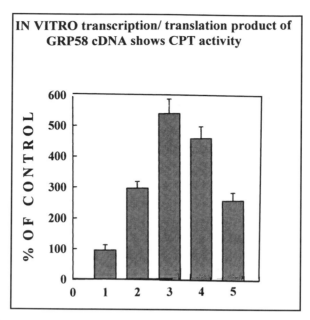

Fig. 2.4. In vitro transcription/translation product of GRP58 cDNA shows CPT activity. GRP58/CPT54 cDNA was cloned next to the $T_7$-promoter in the pcDNAI(neo) plasmid and was used for in vitro transcription and translation (TNT of Promega). Formation of the protein product was verified using [35]S-methionine (not shown). For measuring CPT activity nonradioactive amino acids were employed and where indicated (see below) rat liver microsomes (22 μg) were present for the import and processing of the GRP58/CPT54 precursor. The TNT reaction mix was centrifuged at 110,000xg for 30 min and the pellet was monitored for CPT activity using [14C]-decanoyl-CoA plus carnitine. 1, Control (with pcDNAI(neo) without CPT54 cDNA); 2, 1 μg pcDNAI(neo)-CPT54; 3, 2 μg pcDNAI(neo)-CPT54; 4, 1 μg pcDNAI(neo)-CPT54 plus microsomes; 5, control plus microsomes (modified from Murthy and Pande[88]).

CPT54 has a Gln-Glu-Asp-Leu sequence at its C-terminus which acts as a (weak) luminal retention sequence[93] to help keep it in the lumen of endoplasmic reticulum;[87] Hirano et al[91] in experiments with NIH3T3 cells stably transfected with the bovine GRP58 expression vector and Kozaki et al,[94] working with hybridoma cells secreting monoclonal antibodies have reported that this protein is secreted in the culture medium. The genetic elements responsible for the control of the CPT54 expression and the mechanism of its secretion have not been identified. CPT54 also has a potential nuclear localization signal near its C-terminus and the presence of this protein in the nuclei from different sources has been demonstrated.[95,96]

## CPT~47? The Malonyl-CoA Sensitive CPT of Microsomes

Although microsomes contain a malonyl-CoA sensitive CPT, as mentioned above, the purified microsomal CPT54 does not show any inhibition by malonyl-CoA.[83] Evidence for the presence of a distinct malonyl-CoA sensitive CPT in rat liver microsomes emerged when subfractionation of microsomes revealed that the malonyl-CoA-sensitive CPT activity associated with their membrane preparation where no CPT54 protein could be detected.[3] Western blot results with microsomal membrane preparations using antibodies to CPT54 and L-CPT88 did not identify any positive band, indicating that the malonyl-CoA sensitive microsomal CPT is an immunologically distinct CPT isozyme. Moreover, 2-tetradecyl glycidyl-CoA was found to preferentially inhibit the membrane-associated CPT activity. Incubation with [³H]-etomoxir with ATP + CoA specifically labeled a ~47 kDa protein putatively identifying it as the malonyl-CoA inhibitable CPT of microsomes.[3] Recently, Broadway and Saggerson[97] have also reached the conclusion that microsomes have malonyl-CoA sensitive and insensitive forms of CPTs and that the former is membrane associated; they observed that following solubilization with deoxycholate and fractionation, a fraction was obtained that had CPT activity but did not show malonyl-CoA inhibition; the latter was restored on reconstitution in liposomes, matching the situation we had described[17] earlier for the L-CPT88.

The evidence thus obtained shows that the CPT system in microsomes and peroxisomes is similar to that in mitochondria; in all these organelles, there is at least one CPT activity that is weakly membrane-associated or is soluble and is interior localized, and there is another CPT that is exterior localized, is membrane bound and is sensitive to inhibition by malonyl-CoA and oxirane acyl-CoAs. The malonyl-CoA sensitive and insensitive CPTs of these organelles are different proteins. Based on analogy to the mitochondrial system, it is possible that in microsomes and peroxisomes a carnitine/acylcarnitine translocase is also present to facilitate the transport of carnitine and acylcarnitines across their membrane; we do know that transporters exist in the microsomal membrane for the movement of small charged molecules like glucose-6-phosphate, ATP and glutathione.[98-100] Wander's group[101,102] has presented evidence for the possible presence of a carnitine transport system in the peroxisomal membrane in yeast and in human fibroblasts. While the functional significance of the mitochondrial carnitine system, composed of the inner and outer CPTs and a translocase, is now fairly well understood, the physiological significance of the related system in microsomes and peroxisomes is presently a matter of conjecture. An inhibition of microsomal CPTs by the sulfonyl urea drug, tolbutamide, has been described and it has been suggested that the microsomal CPTs may play a part in the assembly of very low density lipoprotein triacylglycerol.[58,103]

## NUCLEAR CPTS

The reported presence of GRP58/CPT54 in the nuclei of chick livers[95] and in epididymal spermatozoa[96] prompted us to examine whether nuclei show any CPT activity. We isolated highly purified nuclei from livers and kidneys of rat and from different cell lines (293, HepG2, HeLa, COS7 and human skin fibroblasts). The mitochondrial, microsomal and peroxisomal contamination of these nuclei was monitored and proved to be less than 2-3% on the basis of various marker enzymes analyzed both in terms of catalytic activity and immunoblots using appropriate specific antibodies.[104] Both soluble extracts and membrane preparations of these nuclei were found to show significant CPT activity that could not be attributed to contamination by other subcellular organelles. The CPT activity associated with the nuclear membrane was found sensitive to inhibition by malonyl-CoA and 2-tetradecyl glycidyl-CoA while the nuclear matrix CPT was not comparably inhibited.[104] Moreover, although ~80% of the liver nuclear matrix CPT activity could be immunoprecipitated by anti-CPT71 antibody, in Western blots, instead of a reactive band corresponding to CPT71, a new reactive ~55 kDa band was found. Immunologically, the nuclear membrane CPT does not appear to be similar to L-CPT88. In rat liver and kidney nuclei, two proteins seem to contribute to the matrix CPT activity: one is reactive to anti-CPT71 antibody but appears to be smaller in size (~55 kDa) than the purified CPT71; the other reacts positively in Western blots with the anti-CPT54 antibody (manuscript in preparation). Hemipalmitoyl-carnitinium, known to inhibit the CPTs from mitochondria, microsomes and peroxisomes with an $IC_{50}$ of 3-5 $\mu M$[105] was found to inhibit the nuclear matrix CPT, but with an $IC_{50}$ of ~0.4 $\mu M$.

## A ROLE FOR CARNITINE IN TRANSCRIPTIONAL REGULATION

Our preliminary findings indicate that there are nuclear specific forms of CPTs as described above. Based on the information described above and what follows, we suggest that the nuclear CPTs may have a role in the regulation of acyl-CoA levels intranuclearly and thereby affect the transcriptional regulation of relevant genes. Evidence that fatty acyl-CoA esters affect the transcriptional regulation of certain genes appears firm.[106,107] For example, in *E. coli*, fatty acid degradation/biosynthetic genes are regulated reciprocally by a repressor protein, FadR. Fatty acyl-CoAs bind FadR with high affinity, causing its dissociation from DNA and this, in turn, leads to the activation of the fatty acid oxidation genes and repression of the fatty acid biosynthesis genes.[108,109] Whether any FadR counterparts exist in mammalian cells is not known. In mammalian cells, peroxisomal proliferator activated receptors are transactivated by fatty acids and their analogues, such as tetradecylthioacetic acid and 2-bromo-palmitic acid. Fatty acids are now known to regulate not only the enzymes and certain other proteins involved in their metabolism but also a wide variety of genes related to the control of adipogenesis, glycolysis and gluconeogenesis.[110,111] It is possible that some of these effects of fatty acids on gene transcription are exercised through fatty acyl-CoA ester formation. In rat primary hepatocytes, the presence of oleic acid and tetradecyl glycidic acid (an inhibitor of L-CPT88) together causes an induction of the various peroxisomal proteins, cytosolic fatty acid binding protein and microsomal P-450-4A1; the observations that oleic acid alone had no such effect indicates that an accumulation of oleyl-CoA may be necessary for the above inductions.[63] Likewise, a combination of linoleate plus tetradecylglycidate was found to enhance the transcription of the L-CPT88 gene in fetal hepatocytes.[62] Recently, prostaglandin derivatives have been identified as the ligands for peroxisomal proliferator activated receptors[112,113] but whether diverse peroxisomal proliferators and various fatty acids and their analogues exert their pleotropic effects exclusively through these ligands alone is not known.

More recently, in *Saccharomyces cerevisiae*, unsaturated fatty acids have been shown to repress the Δ-9-desaturase but this effect was found dependent upon the activation of the fatty acids.[114] The $T_3$-nuclear receptor binds long-chain acyl-CoA esters with high affinity competitively with respect to $T_3$ binding.[115] Whether long-chain acyl-CoAs influence the $T_3$-receptor's function in vivo is not known. Thus there is a growing number of genes whose transcription seems influenced directly or indirectly by fatty acyl-CoAs. Inasmuch as dietary fat alters the expression of various enzyme activities, fatty acids or fatty acyl-CoAs may also be involved in the repression/derepression of mammalian genes. Nuclear CPTs and carnitine could conceivably contribute to the transcriptional regulation of such genes by modulating the availability of fatty acyl-CoA.[116] Carnitine's possible involvement in the control of transcription of certain nuclear genes is suggested by the work of Roncero and Goodridge;[117] in experiments with chick embryo hepatocytes these investigators found that carnitine modulated the abundance of malic enzyme and fatty acid synthase through the enhanced responsiveness of these genes to $T_3$.

That carnitine offers protection against hyperammonemia is well recognized now. Hyperammonemia, described as a 'silent killer', is a hallmark[118] of the metabolic disorders that result in/or accompany free carnitine deficiency.[119] Examples include a wide range of primary disorders, viz., primary carnitine deficiency,[120] carnitine-acylcarnitine translocase deficiency,[121-123] mitochondrial inner carnitine palmitoyltransferase deficiency,[20] various organic acidurias,[118] the medium chain acyl-CoA dehydrogenase deficiency[121-123] and secondary disorders like valproate therapy,[124] pivampicillin therapy[125] and sulfadiazine/pyrimethamine therapy.[126] Recent findings strongly indicate that carnitine has a role in the transcriptional control of urea cycle enzymes. Thus in genetically carnitine deficient and hyperammonemic JVS mice, the liver mRNA levels of urea cycle enzymes are abnormally low[127] while the mRNAs levels of c-jun and c-fos are elevated.[128] Administration of small doses of carnitine to these mice was found to restore to normal the mRNA levels of the urea cycle enzymes and to enhance their survival.[127] It would be of interest to know whether the levels of the mRNAs of the urea cycle enzymes in the primary carnitine-deficient patients are low and if so whether carnitine therapy normalizes their levels. Tomomura et al[128] have suggested that the increased amounts of jun and fos may interfere with the action of glucocorticoid hormone receptors which are known to regulate the urea cycle enzymes. Horiuchi et al[127] discussed the possibility of an inhibitory effect of fatty acyl-CoA esters on the expression of urea cycle enzymes but speculated that the beneficiary role of carnitine in normalizing the urea cycle enzymes is perhaps not related to the sequestration of the acyl-CoAs. However, since there is hepatic lipid accumulation in both hyperammonemia and carnitine deficiencies, it would be of interest to ascertain whether the effect of carnitine on urea cycle enzyme expression may be mediated through its ability to sequester fatty acyl-CoAs in the nuclear matrix.

As mentioned above, in JVS mice which suffer from cardiac hypertrophy, the L-CPT88 expression in the heart is nearly 6-fold higher than in controls and these are normalized upon carnitine administration.[53] It is possible that the lowered β-oxidation causes a rise in the steady state levels of fatty acids and their CoA esters, causing in turn the induction of L-CPT88 in the myocardium; that fatty acids appear to induce the L-CPT88 in hepatocytes from neonatal rats is known.[62] Also in the livers of rats made carnitine deficient by feeding D-carnitine and mildronate, an inhibitor of -butyrobetaine hydroxylase, peroxisomal fatty acid oxidation and L-CPT88 activity were found enhanced.[129] Whether the carnitine-mediated antagonization of the L-CPT88 expression is related to the sequestration of fatty acyl-CoA to fatty acylcarnitine has not been examined.

## PERSPECTIVES

As summarized above, significant advances have been made recently in the understanding of the structure/function relationships and regulation of mitochondrial carnitine acyltransferases. The recognition that several distinct CPT genes have been retained in cells, and that malonyl-CoA sensitive CPT resides not only in the mitochondrial outer membrane but also in membranes of other subcellular organelles as distinct isozymes, points to more general pivotal role(s) for this metabolic/regulatory step in cell metabolism. Whether the overall carnitine systems in endoplasmic reticulum and the peroxisomal network would turn out to be similar to that in mitochondria, and what their organelle specific functions would be, remain to be established. Much evidence also indicates that the metabolic roles of carnitine and CPT likely extend to the nucleus; the potential of the carnitine system to modulate the intranuclear fatty acyl-CoA levels is one possible way by which this system may influence the fatty acid mediated control of gene transcription. More direct effects of carnitine and acylcarnitines on transcriptional control, however, also remain possible and deserve to be explored.

REFERENCES

1. McGarry JD, Leatherman GF, Foster DW. Carnitine palmitoyl transferase I. The site of inhibition of hepatic fatty acid oxidation by malonyl-CoA. J Biol Chem 1978; 253:4128-4136.
2. Pande SV, Bhuiyan AKJM, Murthy MSR. Carnitine Palmitoyltransferases: How many and how to discriminate? In: Carter L, ed. Current Concepts in Carnitine Research, Atlanta, GA:CRC Press, 1992:165-178.
3. Murthy MSR, Pande SV. Malonyl-CoA sensitive and -insensitive carnitine palmitoyl transferase activities are due to different proteins. J Biol Chem 1994; 269:18283-18286.
4. Ramsay RR, Mancinelli G, Arduini A. Carnitine palmitoyl transferase in human erythrocyte membrane. Properties and malonyl-CoA sensitivity. Biochem J 1991; 275:685-688.
5. Fritz IB, Yue KTN. Long-chain carnitine acyltransferase and the role of acylcarnitine derivatives in the catalytic increase of fatty acid oxidation induced by carnitine. J Lipid Res 1963; 4:279-288.
6. Bremer J. Carnitine in intermediary metabolism. The biosynthesis of palmitoylcarnitine by cell fractions. J Biol Chem 1963; 238:2774-2779.
7. Hoppel CL, Brady LJ. Carnitine palmitoyl transferase and transport of fatty acids. In: Martonosi AN. ed. The enzymes of biological membranes, vol. 2. New York: Plenum Press, 1985:139.
8. Murthy MSR, Pande SV. Malonyl-CoA binding site and overt carnitine palmitoyl transferase activity reside on the opposite sides of the outer mitochondrial membrane. Proc Nat Acad Sci USA 1987; 84:378-382.
9. Murthy MSR, Pande SV. Some differences in the properties of carnitine palmitoyl transferase activities of the outer and the inner mitochondrial membranes. Biochem J 1987; 248:727-733.
10. Ramsay RR. The soluble carnitine palmitoyl transferase from bovine liver. Biochem J 1988; 249:239-245.
11. Healy MJ, Kerner J, Biber LL. Enzymes of carnitine acylation. Biochem J 1988; 249:231-238.

12. Bieber LL. Carnitine. Ann Rev Biochem 1988; 57:261-283.
13. Brady PS, Park EA, Liu JS et al. Isolation and characterization of the promoter for the gene coding for the 68 kDa carnitine palmitoyl transferase from the rat. Biochem J 1992; 286:779-783.
14. Declercq PE, Falck JR, Kuwajima M et al. Characterization of the mitochondrial carnitine palmitoyl transferase enzyme system. I. Use of inhibitors. J Biol Chem 1987; 262:9812-9821.
15. Lund H. Carnitine palmitoyl transferase: characterization of a labile detergent extracted malonyl-CoA sensitive enzyme from rat liver mitochondria. Biochim Biophys Acta 1987; 918:67-73.
16. Kiorpes TC, Hoerr D, Weaner L et al. Identification of 2-tetradecylglycidate (methyl palmitate) and its characterization as an irreversible active site directed inhibitor of carnitine palmitoyl transferase A in isolated rat liver mitochondria. J Biol Chem 1984; 259:9750-9762.
17. Murthy MSR, Pande SV. Characterization of a solubilized malonyl-CoA sensitive carnitine palmitoyl transferase from the mitochondrial outer membrane as a protein distinct from the malonyl-CoA insensitive enzyme of the inner membrane. Biochem J 1990; 268:599-604.
18. Zammit VA, Corstorphine CG, Kolodziej MP. Target size analysis by radiation inactivation of carnitine palmitoyl transferase activity and malonyl-CoA binding in outer membranes from rat liver mitochondria. Biochem J 1989; 263:89-95.
19. Kolodziej MP, Crilly PJ, Corstorphine CG et al. Development and characterization of a polyclonal antibody against rat liver mitochondrial overt carnitine palmitoyl transferase (CPT I). Biochem J 1992; 282:415-421.
20. Demaugre F, Bonnefont J-P, Cepanec C et al. Immunoquantitative analysis of human carnitine palmitoyl transferase I and II defects. Pediatr Res 1990; 27:497-500.
21. Woeltje KF, Esser V, Weis BC et al. Cloning, sequencing, and expression of a cDNA encoding rat liver mitochondrial carnitine palmitoyl transferase II. J Biol Chem 1990; 265:10720-10725.
22. Brown NF, Esser V, Gonzalez AD et al. Mitochondrial import and processing of rat liver carnitine palmitoyl transferase II defines the amino terminus of the mature protein. J Biol Chem 1991; 266:15446-15449.
23. Finocchiaro G, Taroni F, Rocchi M et al. cDNA cloning, sequence analysis, and chromosomal localization of the gene for human carnitine palmitoyl transferase. Proc Natl Acad Sci USA 1991; 88:661-665.
24. Gelb B. Genomic structure of and a cardiac promoter for the mouse carnitine palmitoyl transferase II gene. Genomics 1993; 18:651-655.
25. Montermini L, Wang H, Verderio E et al. Identification of 5' regulatory regions of the human carnitine palmitoyl transferase II gene. Biochim Biophys Acta 1994; 1219:237-240.

26. Brady PS, Feng Y-X, Brady LJ. Transcriptional regulation of carnitine palmitoyl transferase synthesis in riboflavin deficiency in rats. J Nutr 1988; 118:1128-1136.
27. Brady PS, Brady LJ. Regulation of carnitine palmitoyl transferase *in vivo* by glucagon and insulin. Biochem J 1989; 258:677-682.
28. Brady PS, Marine KA, Brady LJ et al. Co-ordinate induction of hepatic mitochondrial and peroxisomal carnitine acyltransferase synthesis by diet and drugs. Biochem J 1989; 260:93-100.
29. Brady LJ, Ramsay RR, Brady PS. Regulation of carnitine acyltransferase synthesis in lean and obese Zucker rats by dehydroepiandrosterone and clofibrate. J Nutr 1991; 121:525-531.
30. Weis BC, Foster DW, McGarry JD. Clarification of the nucleotide sequence at the 5'-end of the cDNA for rat liver carnitine palmitoyl transferase II. Biochem J 1993; 296:271-272.
31. Weis BC, Esser V, Foster DW et al. Rat heart expresses two forms of mitochondrial carnitine palmitoyl transferase I. J Biol Chem 1994; 269:18712-18715.
32. Chase JF, Tubbs PK. Specific alkylation of a histidine residue in carnitine acetyltransferase by bromoacetyl-L-carnitine. Biochem J 1970; 116:713-720.
33. Brown NF, Weis BC, Husti JE et al. Mitochondrial carnitine palmitoyl transferase I isoform switching in the developing rat heart. J Biol Chem 1995; 270:8952-8957.
34. Brown NF, Sen A, Soltis DA et al. Expression of precursor and mature carnitine palmitoyl transferase II in *Escherichia coli* and *in vitro*: differential behaviour of rat and human isoforms. Biochem J 1993; 294:79-86.
35. Johnson TM, Mann WR, Dragland CJ et al. Over-expression and characterization of active recombinant rat liver carnitine palmitoyl transferase II using baculovirus. Biochem J 1995; 309:689-693.
36. Taroni F, Verderio E, Fiorucci F et al. Molecular characterization of inherited carnitine palmitoyl transferase II deficiency. Proc Nat Acad Sci USA 1992; 89:8429-8433.
37. Taroni F, Verderio E, Dworzak F et al. Identification of a common mutation in the carnitine palmitoyl transferase II gene in familial recurrent myoglobinuria patients. Nature Genetics 1993; 4:314-319.
38. Bonnefont J-P, Taroni F, Cavadini P et al. Molecular analysis of carnitine palmitoyl transferase II deficiency with hepatocardiomuscular expression. Am J Hum Genet 1996; 58:971-978.
39. Verderio E, Cavadini P, Monermini L et al. Carnitine palmitoyl transferase II deficiency: structure of the gene and characterization of two novel disease-causing mutations. Hum Mol Genet 1995; 4:19-29.
40. Esser V, Kuwajima M, Britton CH et al. Inhibitors of mitochondrial carnitine palmitoyl transferase I limit the action of proteases on the enzyme. J Biol Chem 1993; 268:5810-5816.

68. Guzman M, Geelen MJH. Activity of carnitine palmitoyl transferase in mitochondrial outer membranes and peroxisomes in digitonin-permeabilized hepatocytes. Biochem J 1992; 287:487-492.

69. Guzman M, Kolodziej MP, Caldwell A et al. Evidence against direct involvement of phosphorylation in the activation of carnitine palmitoyl transferase by okadaic acid in rat hepatocytes. Biochem J 1994; 300:693-699

70. Murthy MSR, Esser V, McGarry JD et al. The malonyl-CoA sensitive carnitine palmitoyl transferase (CPT) of peroxisomes resembles the mitochondrial outer CPT but is a distinct protein. FASEB J 1996; 10:Abst.# 2916.

71. Green S, Wahli W. Peroxisome proliferator-activated receptors: finding the orphan home. Mol Cell Endocrinol 1994; 100:149-153.

72. Haworth JC, Demaugre F, Booth FA et al. Atypical features of the hepatic form of carnitine palmitoyl transferase deficiency in a Hutterite family. J Pediatr 1992; 121:553-557.

73. Bergman AJIW, Donckerwolcke RAMG, Duran M et al. Rate-dependent distal renal tubular acidosis and carnitine palmitoyl transferase I deficiency. Pediatr Res 1994; 36:582-588.

74. Stanley CA, Sunaryo F, Hale DE et al. Elevated plasma carnitine in the hepatic form of carnitine palmitoyl transferase-1 deficiency. J Inher Metab Dis 1992; 15:785-789.

75. Markwell MA, McGroaty EJ, Bieber LL et al. The subcellular distribution of carnitine acyltransferases in mammalian liver and kidney. A new peroxisomal enzyme. J Biol Chem 1973; 248:3426-3432.

76. Miyazawa S, Ozasa H, Osumi T et al. Purification and properties of carnitine octanoyl transferase and carnitine palmitoyl transferase from rat liver. J Biochem (Tokyo) 1983; 94:529-542.

77. Farrell SO, Fiol CJ, Reddy JK et al. Properties of purified carnitine acyltransferases of mouse liver peroxisomes. J Biol Chem 1984; 259:13089-13095.

78. Chatterjee B, Song CS, Kim JM et al. Cloning, sequencing and regulation of rat liver carnitine octanoyltransferase: transcriptional stimulation of the enzyme during peroxisome proliferation. Biochemistry 1988; 27:9000-9006.

79. Subramani S. Protein import in to peroxisomes and biogenesis of the organelle. Ann Rev Cell Biol 1993; 9:445-478.

80. Choi SJ, Oh DH, Song CS et al. Molecular cloning and sequence analysis of the rat liver carnitine octanoyltransferase cDNA, its natural gene and the gene promoter. Biochim Biophys Acta 1995; 1264:215-222.

81. Derrick JP, Ramsay RR. L-Carnitine acyl transferase in intact peroxisomes is inhibited by malonyl-CoA. Biochem J 1989; 262:801-806.

82. Lilly K, Bugaisky JE, Umeda PK et al. The medium-chain carnitine acyltransferase activity associated with the rat liver microsomes is malonyl-CoA sensitive. Arch Biochem Biophys 1990; 280:167-174.

83. Murthy MSR, Bieber LL. Purification of the medium chain/long chain carnitine acyltransferase (COT/CPT) from rat liver microsomes. Protein Expr and Purif 1992; 3:75-79.

84. Murthy MSR, Pande SV. Carnitine medium/long chain acyltransferase of microsomes seems to be the previously cloned ~54 kDa protein of unknown function? Mol Cell Biochem 1993; 122:133-138.

85. Lee AS. The accumulation of three specific proteins related to glucose-regulated proteins in a temperature-sensitive hamster mutant cell line K12. J Cell Physiol 1981; 106:119-125.

86. Bennet CF, Balcarek JM, Varrichio A et al. Molecular cloning and complete amino acid sequence of form-I phosphoinositide-specific phospholipase C. Nature 1988; 334:268-270.

87. Mazzarella RA, Marcus N, Haugejorden SM et al. ERp61 is GRP58, a stress-inducible luminal endoplasmic reticulum protein, but is devoid of phosphoinositide-specific phospholipase C activity. Arch Biochem Biophys 1994; 308:454-460.

88. Murthy MSR, Pande SV. A stress regulated protein, GRP58, a member of thioredoxin superfamily, is a carnitine palmitoyltransferase isoenzyme. Biochem J 1994; 304:31-34.

89. Bourdi M, Demady D, Martin JL et al. cDNA cloning and baculovirus expression of the human liver endoplasmic reticulum P58: Characterization as a protein disulfide isomerase isoform, but not as a protease or a carnitine acyltransfcrase. Arch Biochem Biophys 1995; 323:397-403.

90. Chung CD, Bieber LL. Properties of the medium chain/long chain carnitine acyltransferase purified from rat liver microsomes. J Biol Chem 1993; 268:4519-4524.

91. Hirano N, Shibasaki F, Sakai R et al. Molecular cloning of the human glucose-regulated protein Erp57/GRP58, a thiol-dependent reductase. Eur J Biochem 1995; 234:336-342.

92. Mobb CV, Fink G, Pfaff DW. HIP-70: a protein induced by estrogen in the brain and LH-RH in the pituitary. Science 1990; 247:1477-1479.

93. Pelham HR. The retention signal for the soluble proteins of the endoplasmic reticulum. Trends Biochem Sci 1990; 15:483-486.

94. Kozaki K, Miyaishi O, Asai N et al. Tissue distribution of ERp61 and association of its increased expression with IgG production in hybridoma cells. Expression Cell Res 1994; 213:348-358.

95. Altieri F, Maras B, Eufemi M et al. Purification of a 57 kDa nuclear matrix protein associated with thiol: protein disulfide oxidoreductase and phospholipase C activities. Biochem Biophys Res Commun 1993; 194:992-1000.

96. Ohtani H, Wakui H, Ishino T et al. An isoform of protein disulfide isomerase is expressed in the developing acrosome of spermatids during rat spermiogenesis and is transported into the nucleus of

mature spermatids and epididymal spermatozoa. Histochemistry 1993; 100:423-429.

97. Broadway NM, Saggerson ED. Solubilization and separation of two distinct carnitine acyltransferases from hepatic microsomes: characterization of the malonyl-CoA-sensitive enzyme. Biochem J 1995; 310:989-995.

98. Ballas LM, Arion WJ. Measurement of glucose-6-phosphate penetration into liver microsomes. Confirmation of substrate transport in the glucose-6-phosphatase system. J Biol Chem 1977; 252:8512-8518.

99. Clairmont CA, De Maio A, Hirschberg CB. Translocation of ATP into the lumen of rough endoplasmic reticulum-derived vesicles and its binding to luminal proteins including BiP (GRP78) and GRP94. J Biol Chem 1992; 267:3983-3990.

100. Hwang C, Sinskey AJ, Lodish HF. Oxidized redox state of glutathione in the endoplasmic reticulum. Sciene 1992; 257:1496-1502.

101. van Roermund CWT, Elgersma Y, Singh N et al. The membrane of peroxisomes in *Saccharomyces cerevisiae* is impermeable to NAD(H) and acetyl-CoA under *in vivo* conditions. EMBO J 1995; 14:3480-3486.

102. Jakobs BS, Wanders RJA. Fattyacid b-oxidation in peroxisomes and mitochondria: The first unequivocal evidence for the involvement of carnitine in shuttling propionyl-CoA from peroxisomes to mitochondria. Biochem Biophys Res Commun 1995; 213:1035-1041.

103. Broadway NM, Saggerson ED. Inhibition of liver microsomal carnitine acyltransferases by sulfonylurea drugs. FEBS Lett 1995; 371:137-139.

104. Pande SV, Murthy MSR. New carnitine acyltransferase isoenzymes in nuclei. FASEB J 1995; 9:Abst.# 92.

105. Nic a'Bhaird N, Kumaravel G, Gandour RD et al. Comparison of the active sites of the purified carnitine acyltransferases from peroxisomes and mitochondria by using a reaction-intermediate analogue. Biochem J 1993; 294:645-651.

106. Tomaszewski KE, Melnick RL. In vitro evidence for the involvement of CoA esters in the peroxisome proliferation and hypolipidemia. Biochim Biophys Acta 1994; 1220:118-124.

107. Nishimaki-Mogami T, Takahashi A, Hayashi Y. Activation of a peroxisome-proliferating catabolite of cholic acid to its CoA ester. Biochem J 1993; 296:265-270.

108. DiRusso CC, Heimert TL, Metzger AK. Characterization of FadR, a global transcriptional factor of fatty acid metabolism in Escherichia coli. J Biol Chem 1992; 267:8685-8691.

109. Henry MF, Cronan Jr JE. A new mechanism of transcriptional regulation:release of an activator triggered by small molecule binding. Cell 1992; 70:671-679.

110. Jump DB, Clarke SD, Thelen A et al. Coordinate regulation of glycolytic and lipogenic gene expression by polyunsaturated fatty acids. J Lipid Res 1994; 35:1076-1084.

111. Tontonoz P, Hu E, Devine J et al. PPARγ2, regulates adipose expression of the phosphoenolpyruvate carboxykinase gene. Mol Cell Biol 1995; 15:351-357.

112. Forman BM, Tontonoz P, Chen J et al. 15-Deoxy-$\Delta^{12, 14}$-prostaglandin $J_2$ is a ligand for the adipocyte determination factor PPARγ. Cell 1995; 83:803-812.

113. Hertz R, Berman I, Keppler D et al. Activation of gene transcription by prostacyclin analogues is mediated by the peroxisome-proliferators-activated receptor (PPAR). Eur J Biochem 1996; 235:242-247.

114. Choi J-Y, Stukey J, Hwang S-Y, Martin CE. Regulatory elements that control transcription activation and unsaturated fatty acid-mediated repression of the Saccharomyces cerevisiae OLE1 gene. J Biol Chem 1996; 271:3581-3589.

115. Li Q, Yamamoto N, Morisawa S et al. Fatty acyl-CoA binding activity of the nuclear thyroid hormone receptor. J Cell Biochem 1993; 51:458-464.

116. Murthy MSR, Pande SV. A role for acyl-CoA and carnitine in gene transcription. FASEB J 1995; 9:Abst.# 91.

117. Roncero C, Goodridge AG. Hexanoate and octanoate inhibit transcription of the malic enzyme and fatty acid synthetase genes in chick embryo hepatocytes in culture. J Biol Chem 1992; 267:14918-14927.

118. Miga DE, Roth KS. Hyperammonemia: The silent killer. South Med J 1993; 86:742-747.

119. Quereshi IA. Animal models of heriditary hyperammonemia In:Boulton AA, Backer GB, Butterworth R. eds. Neuromethods: Animal models of neurological disease II: Metabolic encephalopathies and the epilepsies. vol. 22. Totawa, NJ: Humana Press, 1991:329-356.

120. Stanley CA. New genetic defects in mitochondrial fatty acid oxidation and carnitine deficiency. Adv Pediatr 1987; 34:59-88.

121. Stanley CA, Hale DE, Berry GT et al. Brief report: A deficiency of carnitine-acylcarnitine translocase in the inner mitochondrial membrane. N Engl J Med 1992; 327:19-23.

122. Pande SV, Brivet M, Slama A et al. Carnitine-acylcarnitine translocase deficiency with severe hypoglycemia and auriculoventricular block. Translocase assay in permeabilized fibroblasts. J Clin Invest 1993; 91:1247-1252.

123. Pande SV, Murthy MSR. Carnitine acylcarnitine translocase deficiency: Implications in human pathology. Biochim Biophys Acta 1994; 1226:269-276.

124. Coulter DL. Carnitine deficiency in epilepsy: Risk factors and treatment. J Child Neurol 1995; 10-Suppl 2:S32-S39.

125. Holme E, Greter J et al. Carnitine deficiency induced by pivampicillin and pivmecillinam therapy. Lancet 1989; 2:469-473.
126. Sekas G, Paul HS. Hyperammonemia and carnitine deficiency in a patient receiving sulfadiazine and pyrimethamine. Am J Med 1993; 95:112-113.
127. Horiuchi M, Kobayashi K, Kuwajima M et al. Carnitine administration to juvenile visceral steatosis mice corrects the suppressed expression of the urea cycle enzymes by normalizing their transcription. J Biol Chem 1992; 267:5032-5035.
128. Tomomura M, Imamura Y, Tomomura A et al. Abnormal gene expression and regulation in the liver of *jvs* mice with systemic carnitine deficiency. Biochim Biophys Acta 1994; 1226:307-314.
129. Tsoko M, Beuseigneur F, Gresti J et al. Enhancement of activities relative to fatty acid oxidation in the liver of rats depleted of L-carnitine by D-carnitine and a γ-butyrobetaine hydroxylase inhibitor. Bichem Pharmacol 1995; 49:1403-1410.

# CHAPTER 3

# Carnitine and Myocardial Glucose Metabolism

Gary D. Lopaschuk

## INTRODUCTION

L-carnitine has an important role in the integrated regulation of energy metabolism in muscle. While the role of L-carnitine as a cofactor in the oxidation of long-chain fatty acids has been well established, it is only recently that L-carnitine has been recognized to have an additional important role in the regulation of carbohydrate metabolism. Studies primarily performed in heart tissue have shown that increasing myocardial carnitine concentration can dramatically increase both glucose and lactate oxidation. This effect of carbohydrate metabolism appears to be partly responsible for the observed beneficial effects of L-carnitine in treating a number of pathological conditions. For instance, in hypertrophied hearts and in diabetic hearts increasing tissue levels of carnitine can improve both mechanical function and glucose oxidation. In addition, during reperfusion of hearts following ischemia, L-carnitine also improves heart function and increases glucose oxidation. In many of these pathologies the benefits of L-carnitine occur even though fatty acid oxidation is not impaired, and the effects of L-carnitine are accompanied by an increase in glucose oxidation. Whether the effects of L-carnitine on myocardial metabolism are related to an increase in fatty acid oxidation or to an increase in glucose oxidation probably depends to a large extent on whether a severe tissue carnitine deficiency exists, in which case the primary effect of L-carnitine treatment is probably via an increase in fatty acid oxidation rates. If L-carnitine treatment increases tissue carnitine levels, above relatively normal levels we believe that the primary metabolic effects of L-carnitine are on glucose oxidation. In this chapter, the mechanisms by which L-carnitine alters

*Carnitine Today,* edited by Claudio De Simone and Giuseppe Famularo.
© 1997 Landes Bioscience.

carbohydrate metabolism will be discussed, as well as the resultant effects on contractile function.

## REVIEW OF THE LITERATURE

### ENERGY SUBSTRATE PREFERENCE OF THE HEART

The mammalian heart primarily meets its requirements for energy through the oxidation of fatty acids.[1] The oxidation of glucose and lactate provide most of the remaining energy needs, with glycolysis providing an additional small amount of ATP production.[2,3] An overview of the pathway for fatty acid oxidation in the heart is shown in Figure 3.1. The main source of fatty acids for the heart is supplied by free fatty acids bound to albumin, fatty esters present in chylomicrons and very low density lipoproteins. Once the fatty acids cross the sarcolemmal membrane they bind to fatty acid binding proteins in the cytoplasm, followed by subsequent activation to long-chain acyl-CoA by acyl-CoA synthetase. The acyl moieties are then transferred into the mitochondria by a complex of enzymes involving carnitine palmitoyltransferase 1 (CPT 1), carnitine:acylcarnitine translocase, and carnitine palmitoyltransferase 2 (CPT 2). As will be discussed, L-carnitine has a critical role in the mitochondrial uptake of fatty acids. Once in the mitochondrial matrix long-chain acyl-CoA passes through the β-oxidation enzyme system (or spiral) to produce acetyl-CoA. Each successive cycle of the β-oxidation spiral results in a 2 carbon shortening of the fatty acid and formation of 1 NADH and 1 $FADH_2$.

The other major source of mitochondrial acetyl-CoA production is from the oxidation of carbohydrates (glucose and lactate). Extracellular glucose uptake is the primary source of glucose for glycolysis, and is regulated both by the transmembrane glucose gradient and the activity of sarcolemmal glucose transporters. This glucose is rapidly phosphorylated to glucose-6-P, where it subsequently passes through glycolysis to form 2 pyruvate, 2 NADH, and 2 ATP. The pyruvate is then taken up by the mitochondria for subsequent oxidation, or is converted to lactate by lactate dehydrogenase and released from the heart. It should be recognized that lactate can also be taken up by heart cells and converted to pyruvate also via lactate dehydrogenase. The pyruvate derived from both glycolysis or lactate dehydrogenase then enters the mitochondria, where it is acted upon by the pyruvate dehydrogenase complex to form acetyl-CoA, NADH and $CO_2$. The pyruvate dehydrogenase complex is a multi-enzyme complex which is the key irreversible rate-limiting step in carbohydrate oxidation.[4,5] The activity of pyruvate dehydrogenase (PDH) is highly regulated by a phosphorylation-dephosphorylation cycle involving PDH kinase and PDH phosphatase. The phosphorylated state of PDH and the rate of pyruvate oxidation is very dependent on a number of factors (see refs. 4 and 5 for reviews), with the

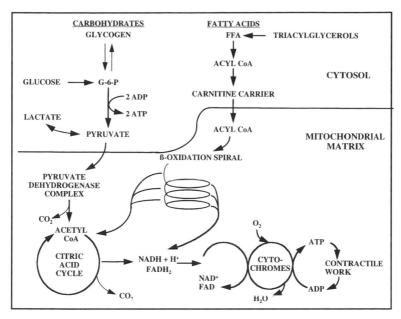

Fig. 3.1. Overview of pathways involved in fatty acid and carbohydrate metabolism in the heart.

concentrations of substrates (pyruvate, CoA, NAD$^+$) and products (acetyl CoA, NADH) being particularly important. With respect to the effects of L-carnitine on this enzyme (see below), increases in the intramitochondrial ratio of acetyl CoA to CoA will result in an activation of PDH kinase, resulting in an increased phosphorylation and inhibition of PDH. This will then result in a decrease in glucose oxidation rates. An important determinant of the ratio of acetyl CoA/CoA is both the rate of removal of intramitochondrial acetyl-CoA by the TCA cycle, and the rate of fatty acid β-oxidation, which is an alternate source of acetyl-CoA (i.e. the Randle cycle).[6,7]

The acetyl-CoA derived from either PDH or fatty acid β-oxidation enters the tricarboxylic acid (TCA) cycle, resulting in the liberation of 2 $CO_2$, 3 NADH and 1 FADH$_2$. The NADH derived from glycolysis, the pyruvate dehydrogenase complex (PDC), the TCA cycle, and β-oxidation, as well as FADH$_2$ from the TCA cycle and β-oxidation, then enter the electron transport chain. The hydrogen on NADH and FADH$_2$ is transferred to $H_2O$ in the presence of $O_2$, and ADP is converted to ATP.

ROLE OF CARNITINE IN REGULATING FATTY ACID OXIDATION

Once activated in the aqueous cytoplasm, long-chain acyl-CoAs are transferred into the mitochondrial matrix by the concerted efforts of three carnitine-dependent enzymes. The first of these enzymes, CPT 1, catalyzes the formation of long-chain acylcarnitine to form long-chain acyl-CoA. This enzyme is located on the inner surface of the outer mitochondrial membrane.[8] The second enzyme, carnitine:acylcarnitine translocase transports long-chain acylcarnitine across the inner mitochondrial membrane. The third enzyme, CPT 2, is associated with the inner mitochondrial membrane and catalyzes the reverse reaction ultimately regenerating long-chain acyl-CoA within the mitochondrial matrix. A scheme showing this pathway is provided in Figure 3.2.

CPT 1 represents a key regulatory point in the oxidation of fatty acids, and is the rate-limiting step involved in the transfer of fatty acyl groups into the mitochondria.[9,10] L-carnitine is an important cofactor of CPT 1, acting as an acceptor of fatty acyl groups from acyl-CoA to form long chain acylcarnitine. Recent evidence has shown that the heart contains two isoforms of CPT 1, designated L-CPT 1 and M-CPT 1, indicative of the tissue in which these isoforms were first characterized (i.e. liver and muscle).[11-13] These two isoforms of CPT 1 have different kinetic charateristics for L-carnitine, with a $K_m$ for L-carnitine of 30 and 500 µM for L-CPT 1 and M-CPT 1, respectively. Since the M-CPT 1 isoform predominates in heart,[11,12] L-carnitine deficiencies have a greater potential to limit mitochondrial fatty acid uptake than in tissues where L-CPT 1 predominates. As a result, decreases in myocardial carnitine levels can result in a significant impairment of fatty acid oxidation, which is associated with the development of cardiomyopathies.[14-17]

ROLE OF CARNITINE IN REGULATING GLUCOSE METABOLISM

In addition to its critical role in mitochondrial fatty acid uptake, L-carnitine can also transport acetyl groups from within the mitochondrial matrix to the cytoplasm.[18-20] Carnitine acetyltransferase catalyzes the transfer of acetyl groups from acetyl-CoA to carnitine, forming acetylcarnitine (Fig. 3.2). The acetylcarnitine can then be transported into the cytoplasm, where the acetyl groups are transferred back onto CoA. A number of studies have proposed a role for carnitine as a modulator of the intramitochondrial acetyl-CoA/CoA ratio.[18-23] In isolated heart mitochondria, carnitine has been shown to increase CoA levels and reduce acetyl-CoA levels, resulting in a 10- to 20-fold decrease in the ratio of acetyl-CoA/CoA.[18,19] In human skeletal muscle mitochondria, this decrease in acetyl-CoA/CoA stimulates pyruvate oxidation, secondary to an increase in PDC activity.[23] Changes in the ratio of acetyl-CoA/CoA in the presence of L-carnitine are also associated with an increased efflux of acetylcarnitine from the mitochondria,[18] which is consistent with the suggestion that carnitine increases the activity of the carnitine acetyltransferase present on mitochondrial membranes.

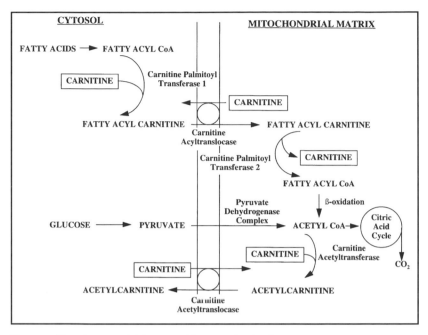

Fig. 3.2. Key sites at which L-carnitine acts in the heart.

A role for L-carnitine in regulating the intramitochondrial acetyl CoA/ CoA ratio is supported by direct measurements of carbohydrate oxidation in the intact heart. We have shown that carnitine supplementation of isolated working rat hearts will substantially increase glucose oxidation rates.[21] This increase in glucose oxidation probably occurs secondary to an increase in PDC activity, which results from the lowering of the intramitochondrial acetyl-CoA/CoA ratio (Fig. 3.2). Of interest is the observation that this L-carnitine-induced increase in glucose oxidation is accompanied by a concomitant decrease in fatty acid oxidation rates, such that overall ATP production rates remain similar.[21] While this effect of L-carnitine on fatty acid oxidation would appear paradoxical, it does not if one considers that the primary role of L-carnitine is to ensure an adequate supply of acetyl CoA for the tricarboxylic acid (TCA) cycle. As shown in Figure 3.2, L-carnitine has a critical role in regulating the supply of acetyl-CoA from both PDC and from β-oxidation of fatty acids. Since the primary supply of acetyl-CoA is normally derived from fatty acid oxidation, an increase in TCA cycle activity (i.e. such as by increasing myocardial workload) will increase the supply of acetyl-CoA derived from fatty acid oxidation.[1] Provided that intramitochondrial acetyl CoA supply from fatty acid oxidation is not limited, we propose that the primary effect of L-carnitine supplementation is to regulate the supply of TCA cycle acetyl CoA that is derived from PDC. By shuttling intramitochondrial acetyl-CoA out of the mitochondria and into the cytosol, via the carnitine acetyltransferase and carnitine acetyltranslocase pathway, intramitochondrial levels of acetyl-CoA will decrease (Figure 3.2). The decrease in the acetyl CoA/CoA ratio will result in a stimulation of PDC activity.[4,5] This in turn will result in increased rates of glucose oxidation.[21]

An example of the effects of L-carnitine supplementation on glucose oxidation rates in intact hearts is shown in Figure 3.3. Isolated working rat hearts were perfused with 10 mM L-carnitine for a 60 minute period, resulting in a 2.3-fold increase in tissue carnitine levels. This resulted in a significant increase in glucose oxidation rates. It is of interest is that fatty acid oxidation rates were significantly decreased in the L-carnitine treated hearts.[21] This can be explained by the observation that if the need for ATP at a given workload is constant, an increase in acetyl CoA derived from PDC would be expected to result in a decrease in the requirements of acetyl-CoA derived from β-oxidation. This would explain the observed decrease in myocardial fatty acid oxidation that accompanies the increase in glucose oxidation following L-carnitine supplementation to isolated perfused hearts. As a result, combined with the increase in glucose oxidation, the primary effect of L-carnitine treatment in these hearts is to increase the proportion of acetyl-CoA derived from glucose oxidation (i.e. increase the ratio of glucose oxidation to fatty acid oxidation) (Fig. 3.3).

CARNITINE DEFICIENCY VERSUS CARNITINE SUPPLEMENTATION

It is clear that the role of L-carnitine is complex in its regulation of fatty acid and carbohydrate metabolism. We believe that in severe tissue carnitine deficiencies the effects of L-carnitine supplementation on overall myocardial metabolism differ from the effects of L-carnitine supplementation to tissue where a carnitine deficiency does not exist. Whether the primary effect of L-carnitine is to stimulate fatty acid oxidation or to stimulate glucose oxidation is primarily dependent on the intramitochondrial acetyl CoA/CoA ratio.

Alterations in the metabolism of fatty acids and carbohydrates can occur when perturbations such as tissue carnitine depletion occur.[14-17,24-27] These perturbations can lead to an impairment of myocardial function (see refs. 14 and 24 for reviews). Most known situations associated with myocardial carnitine deficiencies are also associated with a depression in myocardial function.[14-17,24-27] Whether fatty acid oxidation rates are depressed in carnitine-deficient hearts probably depends to a large extent on the severity of the carnitine deficiency, as well as the presence of circulating carbon substrates.

In primary and secondary carnitine deficiencies the depressed myocardial function is presumed to occur secondary to a depression of fatty acid oxidation. Experimentally induced carnitine deficiencies, such as those following sodium pivalate treatment of rats, also result in a depression of fatty acid oxidation.[28] Long-term treatment with sodium pivalate can result in a 50-60% reduction in myocardial carnitine content. This severe carnitine deficiency results in a depression of cardiac function when the treatment is extended for periods of 24-26 weeks. These results suggest that in severe carnitine deficiencies CPT 1 activity is inhibited, resulting in a decrease in fatty acid oxidation.

Accompanying the decreased rates of fatty acid oxidation in sodium pivalate treated hearts is an increase in glucose oxidation rates.[28,29] An increase in glucose oxidation in carnitine deficient hearts would appear to contradict the observations that L-carnitine supplementation to normal

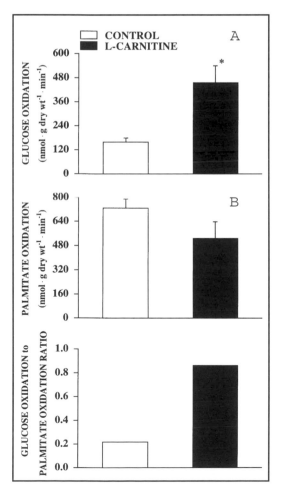

Fig. 3.3. Effects of L-carnitine supplementation on glucose and palmitate oxidation in the heart. Isolated working rat hearts were perfused at a 11.5 mm Hg left atrial preload and 80 mm Hg aortic afterload, with either; A) 11 mM $^{14}$C-glucose, 1.2 mM palmitate, and 3% albumin, or B) 11 mM glucose, 1.2 mM $^{14}$C-palmitate, and 3% albumin. Hearts were initially subjected to a 60 min perfusion in the absence or presence of 10 mM L-carnitine prior to measurement of glucose or palmitate oxidation. Glucose and palmitate oxidation were measured by quantitatively measuring $^{14}$CO$_2$ production from either $^{14}$C-glucose or $^{14}$C-palmitate, respectively. Values are the mean ± S.E. of 6 to 10 hearts in each group. The Figure is derived from data originally presented in ref. 21.
* significantly different from appropriate Control group.

hearts also increases glucose oxidation rates.[21,30] However, these apparent contradictions can again be readily explained by the importance of intramitochondrial acetyl-CoA/CoA in regulating glucose oxidation. In severe carnitine deficiencies where fatty acid oxidation is inhibited, acetyl CoA supply from β-oxidation will decrease. This will decrease the ratio of intramitochondrial acetyl-CoA/CoA, relieving the inhibition of PDC. The end result is that the activity of PDC will increase and rates of glucose oxidation will also increase. In normal hearts where fatty acid oxidation rates are not depressed, the effects of L-carnitine on the intramitochondrial acetyl CoA/CoA ratio would be expected to parallel what is seen in a severe carnitine deficiency, resulting a similar increase in glucose oxidation (Fig. 3.2). As a result, the effects of a carnitine deficiency on glucose oxidation probably depends on whether the deficiency is severe enough to inhibit fatty acid oxidation.

Decreased myocardial carnitine content can also be seen in hearts obtained from diabetic animals.[31] However, despite this decrease in tissue carnitine, almost all of the ATP requirements of the heart are met by the oxidation of fatty acids.[32-34] This is primarily due to the high circulating levels of fatty acids seen in uncontrolled diabetics. As a result, we believe that the mild carnitine deficiency seen in hearts from diabetic animals, when

**Table 3.1. Effects of carnitine deficiencies on energy metabolism**

| Reason for Carnitine Deficiency | Effect on Energy Metabolism | Reference |
|---|---|---|
| Primary and secondary carnitine deficiencies | Depression of fatty acid oxidation | see 14,16, 17 & 24 for review |
| Experimental Depletion: Na⁺ pivalate | Depressed fatty acid oxidation Enhanced glucose oxidation rates | 28, 29 |
| Myocardial Hypertrophy | Fatty acid oxidation depressed Glycolysis enhanced Glucose oxidation depressed | 26,27,36 |
| Diabetes | Primary source of ATP from fatty acid oxidation Depressed carbohydrate metabolism | 32-34 |
| Reperfusion following ischemia | Fatty acid oxidation increased Glucose oxidation depressed | 63-70 |

coupled to elevations in circulating fatty acids, is insufficient to cause a depression of fatty acid oxidation. Despite this observation, many studies have demonstrated that L-carnitine treatment can improve heart function in hearts from diabetic rats. We believe that the primary benefit of L-carnitine in these hearts is related to an increase in glucose oxidation. In isolated working hearts obtained from diabetic rats L-carnitine treatment will dramatically increase glucose oxidation rates (Table 3.2).

Decreased myocardial carnitine levels are also seen in hypertrophic hearts.[35] In severely hypertrophic hearts, carnitine depletion results in decreased rates of fatty acid oxidation.[26,27] In situations of mild hypertrophy, fatty acid oxidation can be depressed, but this is dependent on the perfusion conditions. In isolated working hypertrophied rat hearts performing low work, fatty acid oxidation is depressed with a concomitant increase in glycolysis.[26] If these hearts are perfused with high levels of fatty acids, no decrease in fatty acid oxidation is observed.[36] However, if tissue carnitine levels are increased 1.75-fold by PLC treatment a significant increase in glucose oxidation occurs (Table 3.3). This is also accompanied by an increase in contractile function in the hypertrophied hearts.[26,36] This suggests that the benefits of increasing carnitine in hypertrophied hearts can be explained by an increase in glucose oxidation. As a result, the carnitine deficiency seen in mild hypertrophy may only limit fatty acid oxidation if other sources of energy, such as carbohydrate metabolism, can be used as an alternate supply of ATP. In contrast, el Alaoui-Talibi et al[27] have found that the carnitine deficiency occurring in hypertrophic hearts does result in a decrease in fatty acid oxidation at both low and high work loads. Differences between our results and those of el Alaoui-Talibi et al[27] probably relate to differences in the severity of hypertrophy between the two experimental models used. Our model of pressure-overload hypertrophy resulted in a 38% increase in heart size,[26,36] whereas the latter model of volume-overload hypertrophy resulted in nearly a 100% increase in heart size.[27]

POTENTIAL LINK BETWEEN THE REGULATION OF FATTY ACID OXIDATION
AND CARBOHYDRATE OXIDATION

As discussed, L-carnitine supplementation to intact hearts increases glucose oxidation and decreases fatty acid oxidation, such that overall ATP production is maintained.[21] As shown in Figure 3.2, the effects of L-carnitine on glucose oxidation can be explained by a decrease in the intramitochondrial acetyl-CoA/CoA ratio. However, the effects of L-carnitine supplementation on fatty acid oxidation are less obvious, since a decrease in the acetyl CoA/CoA ratio should also act as a stimulus to increase $\beta$-oxidation of fatty acids. However, increasing both glucose and fatty acid oxidation at a given myocardial workload would decrease myocardial efficiency, since ATP production (and $O_2$ consumption) would increase in the absence of additional demands for ATP. To explain this apparent contradiction, we hypothesize that L-carnitine can inhibit fatty acid oxidation by increasing cytosolic acetyl CoA supply to acetyl CoA carboxylase, which by producing malonyl CoA will inhibit CPT 1 activity (Figure 3.4).

As discussed, CPT 1 is a key regulatory point in the oxidation of fatty acids, and is the rate-limiting step of long-chain acyl-CoA translocation into mitochondria.[9,10,37] The fact that CPT 1 in the heart is extremely sensitive to inhibition by malonyl-CoA (Ki = 50 nM),[10,38] and that malonyl-CoA is present in measurable quantities (10-15 nmol/g dry wt) in the heart,[10,39] suggests that malonyl-CoA may be an important effector for the entry of long-chain acyl-CoAs into the mitochondria and therefore a potentially important regulator of myocardial fatty acid oxidation. In support of this, we have now shown that malonyl CoA is an important regulator of fatty acid oxidation in the intact heart.[40-43]

The important role of malonyl-CoA in regulating energy metabolism suggests that changes in the absolute levels of cytoplasmic malonyl-CoA may be responsible for the changes in myocardial fatty acid oxidation that occur following L-carnitine supplementation. We hypothesize that increasing the concentration of carnitine in the heart will facilitate the export of intramitochondrial acetyl CoA into the cytoplasm (Fig. 3.4). The increased cytosolic levels of acetyl-CoA will then increase the activity of acetyl-CoA

*Table 3.2. Effect of L-carnitine treatment on glucose oxidation in control and diabetic rat hearts*

|  | Glucose Oxidation (nmol · g dry wt$^{-1}$ · min$^{-1}$) |
|---|---|
| **Control:** |  |
| No Treatment | 142 ± 29 |
| L-Carnitine Treated | 532 ± 121 * |
| **Diabetic:** |  |
| No Treatment | 33 ± 7 |
| L-Carnitine Treated | 272 ± 83 * |

Hearts were obtained from control rats or rats which were injected with 100 mg/kg streptozotocin i.v. 48 hour prior to experimentation (see reference 60 for details). Isolated working rat hearts perfused at a 11.5 mm Hg left atrial preload and 80 mm Hg aortic afterload were perfused with 11 mM $^{14}$C-glucose, 1.2 mM palmitate, and 3% albumin. Hearts were initially subjected to a 60 min perfusion in the absence or presence of 10 mM L-carnitine prior to measurement of glucose oxidation. Glucose oxidation was measured by quantitatively measuring $^{14}$CO$_2$ production from $^{14}$C-glucose. Values are the mean ± S.E. of 7 to 8 hearts in each group. The table is derived from data originally presented in Reference 60.
* significantly different than appropriate No Treatment group

carboxylase (ACC). ACC catalyzes the transfer of $CO_2$ from bicarbonate to acetyl-CoA to form malonyl-CoA,[44,45] and is widely distributed in a number of different mammalian tissues, including those where fatty acid oxidation is prominent, e.g. heart, brown adipose tissue, and skeletal muscle.[40,46-48] While ACC in liver and white adipose tissue primarily acts as the rate-limiting step in fatty acid biosynthesis, in heart it appears that ACC primarily acts to regulate fatty acid oxidation.[40] Myocardial ACC has a low affinity for acetyl-CoA[40] and cytoplasmic acetyl-CoA levels are very low in the heart.[49] This suggests that cytoplasmic acetyl-CoA levels may be an important determinant of ACC activity in the heart. We hypothesize that stimulation of carnitine acetyltransferase by L-carnitine increases cytoplasmic acetyl CoA levels, increasing ACC production of malonyl-CoA (Fig. 3.4). This would then inhibit CPT I activity, thereby decreasing fatty acid oxidation.

A role of L-carnitine and carnitine acetyltransferase as a link between glucose and fatty acid oxidation is a particularly attractive hypothesis to explain how the heart ensures an adequate supply of acetyl-CoA for the TCA cycle. When intramitochondrial acetyl CoA demand is high, both fatty acid and carbohydrate oxidation would increase to meet this demand. However, as supply exceeds demand and the acetyl-CoA/CoA ratio increases, acetyl CoA would be shuttled out of the mitochondria via carnitine

*Table 3.3. Effect of propionyl L-carnitine treatment on glucose oxidation in hypertrophied hearts*

|  | Glucose Oxidation (nmol · g dry wt$^{-1}$ · min$^{-1}$) |
| --- | --- |
| **Control:** | |
| No Treatment | $217 \pm 26$ |
| PLC Treated | $858 \pm 192$ * |
| **Hypertrophy:** | |
| No Treatment | $137 \pm 25$ [t] |
| PLC Treated | $627 \pm 110$ * |

Hearts were obtained from sham operated rats (control) or rats in which a 0.4 mm minimally occlusive clip was placed around the descending aorta (see ref 36 for details). Animals were used 8 weeks following surgery. Isolated working rat hearts perfused at a 11.5 mm Hg left atrial preload and 80 mm Hg aortic afterload were perfused with 11 mM 14C-glucose, 1.2 mM palmitate, and 3% albumin. Hearts were initially subjected to a 60 min perfusion in the absence or presence of 1 mM propionyl L-carnitine. Glucose oxidation was measured by quantitatively measuring $^{14}CO_2$ production from $^{14}C$-glucose. Values are the mean ± S.E. of 7 to 10 hearts in each group. The table is derived from data originally presented in Reference 36.
* significantly different than appropriate No Treatment group
[t] significantly different than Control No Treatment group

acetyltransferase and carnitine acetyltranslocase. This would increase malonyl-CoA production from ACC, resulting in a decrease in fatty acid oxidation. Carbohydrate oxidation would decrease by a direct inhibition of PDC as the levels of intramitochondrial acetyl-CoA/CoA increase.

This link between glucose and fatty acid oxidation is supported by our recent evidence demonstrating that when the supply of acetyl-CoA in the mitochondria is increased, a resultant decrease in fatty acid oxidation occurs.[40] Furthermore, we have observed a close relationship between myocardial acetyl-CoA levels and malonyl CoA levels, with a close inverse correlation between malonyl-CoA levels and fatty acid oxidation. Evidence for the involvement of carnitine acetyltransferase in this process comes from recent studies in which we increased myocardial carnitine content in hypertrophied rat hearts and found an increase of glucose oxidation to ATP production, with a concomitant decrease in fatty acid oxidation rates, and a marked increase in malonyl CoA. This is consistent with an increase in carnitine acetyltransferase activity (Fig. 3.4).

COMPARISON OF L-CARNITINE AND PROPIONYL L-CARNITINE ON GLUCOSE METABOLISM

In addition to L-carnitine, other derivatives of L-carnitine have been shown to have beneficial effects on heart function. One of these derivatives, propionyl L-carnitine (PLC), has shown efficacy in treating a number of cardiovascular disorders, which include ischemic heart disease, congestive heart failure, and hypertrophic heart disease (see refs. 50 and 51 for reviews). In a number of studies, PLC has shown superior efficacy compared to L-carnitine.[51] The actual mechanism(s) by which PLC exerts its effects on the heart have yet to be completely defined. Two possibilities are: increasing glucose oxidation by increasing tissue L-carnitine levels and providing propionyl groups as a source of carbon for the TCA cycle.

As discussed, increasing tissue carnitine levels will increase the rate of glucose oxidation in fatty acid perfused hearts.[21] Similar results have been obtained upon acute supplementation of isolated working hearts with PLC, which increases the contribution of carbohydrate oxidation to ATP production both in control and hypertrophied hearts.[36] As shown in Figure 3.5, acute treatment of isolated working rat hearts with 1 mM PLC for 60 min results in a significant increase in glucose oxidation rates. This probably occurs secondary to its effect of increasing carnitine levels (which increased by 1.7-fold), resulting in a stimulation of the PDC complex in these hearts. As with L-carnitine, PLC supplementation also increased the ratio of glucose oxidation to palmitate oxidation (Fig. 3.4). In hypertrophied hearts a similar increase in glucose oxidation is observed (Table 3.3).

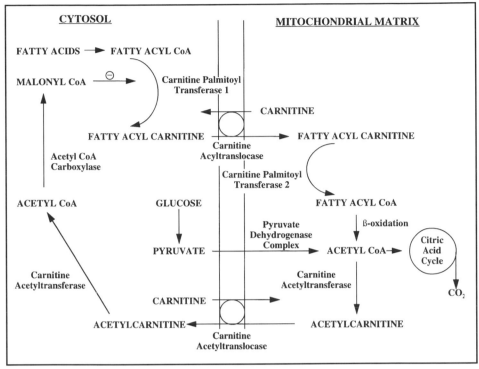

Fig. 3.4. Potential role of L-carnitine in supplying cytoplasmic acetyl CoA for acetyl CoA carboxylase. L-carnitine ensures an adequate supply of intramitochondrial acetyl CoA from fatty acid β-oxidation. In situations of adequate acetyl CoA supply for β-oxidation, carnitine can also act to lower the intramitochondrial acetyl CoA/CoA ratio at the level of carnitine acetyltransferase. This will increasing pyruvate dehydrogenase complex activity, and therefore glucose oxidation. Increasing the activity of carnitine acetyltransferase and acetylcarnitine will also increase cytoplasmic acetyl-CoA levels, resulting in an increase in acetyl CoA carboxylase activity. Increased malonyl-CoA production will then inhibit carnitine palmitoyltransferase 1 activity, resulting in a decrease in fatty acid oxidation.

Since PLC has been shown to be more effective than L-carnitine in treating a variety of pathologies, this suggests that, in addition to increasing tissue L-carnitine levels, other mechanisms of action must occur. The different results obtained with PLC compared to L-carnitine may be explained by an anaplerotic action. The propionyl moiety of PLC may be important in the maintenance of adequate levels of TCA cycle intermediates. The anaplerosis of PLC was initially documented in rat liver mitochondria.[52] Unlike propionate, PLC is converted into propionyl CoA without energy expenditure. The anaplerotic effect of PLC has also been demonstrated in rat heart mitochondria utilizing [2-$^{14}$C] pyruvate in the presence of either PLC or carnitine.[53,54] Pyruvate oxidation was increased more by PLC than by equimolar amounts of carnitine. As a result, the utilization of the propionyl moiety is a conceivable mechanism underlying the actions of PLC.

EFFECTS OF CARNITINE SUPPLEMENTATION ON MYOCARDIAL OXIDATIVE
METABOLISM AND CONTRACTILE FUNCTION

L-carnitine and PLC have previously been shown to improve heart function in pathological conditions such as diabetes and myocardial hypertrophy.[55-59] Because of the potential role of L-carnitine as a regulator of both carbohydrate and fatty acid oxidation we examined the effects of L-carnitine in isolated fatty acid perfused hearts obtained from normal and diabetic rats. In diabetic rat hearts, where fatty acid oxidation provides almost all of the ATP requirements,[6,32,33] L-carnitine is able to markedly increase glucose oxidation.[60] A similar phenomenon can be seen in hypertrophied hearts treated with PLC. PLC pretreatment is able to substantially increase carbohydrate oxidation in hypertrophied hearts.[36] As a result, stimulation of carbohydrate oxidation may partly explain the beneficial effects of L-carnitine and PLC in diabetes and hypertrophy.

If the heart is in a carnitine deficient state it would be expected that supplementation with carnitine or carnitine derivatives should result in a normalization of carnitine levels and, therefore, a normalization of fatty acid oxidation. However, we have found that in situations such as diabetes and mild myocardial hypertrophy, where decreases in tissue carnitine content are seen, the primary effect of increasing tissue carnitine content is to increase carbohydrate oxidation. Following acute PLC administration to hypertrophic hearts, the major metabolic response is an increased supply of ATP from the oxidation of glucose and lactate, suggesting that PDC activity is enhanced.[36] In severely hypertrophic hearts, where a decrease in fatty acid oxidation occurs even in the presence of high levels of fatty acids, it is possible that increasing carnitine levels in the heart will result in an increase in fatty acid oxidation. El Alaoui-Talibi and Moravec have shown that PLC treatment will increase fatty acid oxidation rates (Z. el Alaoui-Talibi, personal communication). Regardless of whether PLC acts to increase carbohydrate or fatty acid oxidation, in both studies PLC treatment improves mechanical function in the hypertrophic hearts.

The reason why stimulation of glucose oxidation by L-carnitine and PLC benefits the hypertrophied heart has still to be completely delineated. One possibility is that L-carnitine and PLC improve the coupling between glycolysis and glucose oxidation in the heart. It has recently been demonstrated that a significant increase in glycolysis occurs in the hypertrophied heart.[26,36] Despite this increase in glycolysis, rates of glucose oxidation are unchanged[26] or decreased[36] in the hypertrophied hearts compared to control hearts. As discussed, these metabolic alterations create a dramatic uncoupling of glycolysis from glucose oxidation, resulting in a greater amount of pyruvate derived from glycolysis being converted to lactate. Uncoupling of glycolysis from glucose oxidation is also a major source of $H^+$ production, which can contribute to a decreased efficiency of the heart.[61] As a result, stimulation of glucose oxidation with PLC has the potential not only to increase overall ATP production,[36] but also to improve cardiac efficiency.[62]

Increasing myocardial tissue content can also alter heart metabolism even if a carnitine deficiency is not present. This can be seen in isolated working rat hearts which are perfused under conditions where fatty acid oxidation is the major source of ATP production. Increasing tissue carnitine content by L-carnitine pre-treatment results in a marked increase in glucose oxidation, with a parallel decrease in fatty acid oxidation.[21] Addition of PLC to hearts perfused under similar conditions also results in an increase in carbohydrate oxidation (both glucose and lactate).[36] However, the effects of PLC on fatty acid oxidation rates are not as dramatic as they are with L-carnitine supplementation. This may be related to the observation that an increase in mechanical function occurs following administration of PLC. However, if rates of ATP production are normalized for differences in work,

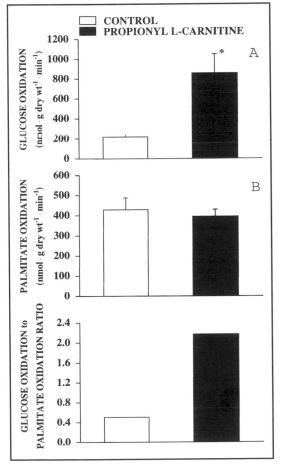

Fig. 3.5. Effects of propionyl L-carnitine on glucose and palmitate oxidation in the heart. Isolated working rat hearts were perfused at a 11.5 mm Hg left atrial preload and 80 mm Hg aortic afterload, with either; A) 11 mM $^{14}$C-glucose, 1.2 mM palmitate, 0,5 mM lactate and 3% albumin, or B) 11 mM glucose, 1.2 mM 9,10-$^3$H-palmitate, 0.5 mM lactate and 3% albumin. Hearts were initially subjected to a 60 min perfusion in the absence or presence of 1 mM propionyl L-carnitine prior to measurement of glucose or palmitate oxidation. Glucose oxidation was measured by quantitatively measuring $^{14}$CO$_2$ production from either $^{14}$C-glucose, while palmitate oxidation was measured by quantitatively collecting $^3$H$_2$O from $^3$H-palmitate. Values are the mean ± S.E. of 6 to 10 hearts in each group. The Figure is derived from data originally presented in ref.36. * significantly different from appropriate Control group.

PLC does cause a shift in the metabolic profile away from fatty acid oxidation and towards carbohydrate oxidation. However, even when differences in work are considered, the major effect of PLC is to increase the amount of ATP derived from the oxidation of glucose and lactate.

### BENEFICIAL EFFECT OF L-CARNITINE ON GLUCOSE OXIDATION IN THE REPERFUSED ISCHEMIC HEART

High levels of fatty acids have a detrimental effect on reperfusion recovery of hearts subjected to a severe episode of ischemia.[63-66] While the exact mechanism by which fatty acid oxidation contributes to ischemic injury is not clear, our studies suggest that this may be related to their ability to inhibit glucose oxidation.[63,67-69] High levels of fatty acid increase the intramitochondrial acetyl-CoA/CoA and $NADH/NAD^+$ ratios,[1,4,6] which in turn inhibit PDC through the activation of a pyruvate dehydrogenase kinase.[4,6,7] This inhibition of glucose oxidation during reperfusion can lead to a substantial imbalance between glycolysis and glucose oxidation during the actual reperfusion period.[69,70] This increases the production of $H^+$ formed by the hydrolysis of glycolytically derived ATP. It is this imbalance and exaggerated production of $H^+$ ions that we believe is mediating the detrimental effects of high levels of fatty acids on post-ischemic functional recovery. The production of $H^+$ during ischemia and early in reperfusion could lead to increased activity of the $Na^+/H^+$ and the $Na^+/Ca^{2+}$ exchangers and result in a potentially damaging $Ca^{2+}$ overload.[71]

Supplementation of the myocardium with carnitine or PLC results in an increased tissue carnitine content, which lessens the severity of ischemic injury and improves the recovery of heart function during reperfusion.[57,59,72-74] However, although myocardial carnitine content decreases during ischemia,[75,76] the actions of carnitine and PLC cannot be explained secondary to a stimulation of fatty acid oxidation. This is because fatty acid oxidation rates are not depressed during reperfusion of ischemic hearts. In fact, due to the high circulating levels of fatty acids normally seen during reperfusion,[77] fatty acid oxidation provides over 90% of ATP production during reperfusion.[63-66,78] In the presence of high levels of fatty acids, glucose oxidation provides only 5 to 10% of the ATP requirements. As previously mentioned, if glucose oxidation is stimulated during reperfusion it is possible to overcome the detrimental effect of high levels of fatty acids. Compounds which stimulate glucose oxidation directly by inhibiting the action of PDC kinase, such as dichloroacetate,[68-70] or indirectly such as CPT 1 inhibitors,[63,67] have the potential to improve post-ischemic functional recovery. Recently, we have demonstrated that the beneficial effects of L-carnitine on the functional recovery of post-ischemia are also associated with a marked increase in glucose oxidation.[30] The effects of L-carnitine on glucose oxidation during reperfusion of hearts subjected to severe ischemic

**Table 3.4. Effect of L-carnitine treatment on glucose oxidation in reperfused ischemic hearts**

|  | Glucose Oxidation (nmol · g dry wt$^{-1}$ · min$^{-1}$) |
| --- | --- |
| **Aerobic:** |  |
| No Treatment | 162 ± 32 |
| L-Carnitine Treated | 489 ± 84 * |
| **Reperfused Following Ischemia:** |  |
| No Treatment | 133 ± 12 |
| L-Carnitine Treated | 289 ± 49 * |

Isolated working rat hearts perfused at a 11.5 mm Hg left atrial preload and 80 mm Hg aortic afterload were perfused with 11 mM 14C-glucose, 1.2 mM palmitate, and 3% albumin. Hearts were initially subjected to a 60 min perfusion in the absence or presence of 10 mM L-carnitine. Hearts were then perfused for a further 30 min aerobic perfusion, followed by 30 min of global no flow ischemia and 60 min of aerobic reperfusion. Glucose oxidation was measured by quantitatively measuring $^{14}CO_2$ production from $^{14}$C-glucose. Values are the mean ± S.E. of 7 hearts in each group. The table is derived from data originally presented in ref. 30.
* significantly different than appropriate No Treatment group

injury are shown in Table 3.4. L-carnitine significantly increased glucose oxidation in the critical period of reperfusion. As a result, we hypothesize that the beneficial effects of L-carnitine and PLC in reperfused ischemic hearts occur secondary to a stimulation of glucose oxidation.

## CONCLUSIONS

Carnitine is an essential cofactor for the transportation of fatty acyl groups into the mitochondrial matrix where they undergo β-oxidation and result in the production of ATP. It is now evident that carnitine also has an important role in the regulation of glucose oxidation. Secondary to facilitating the intramitochondrial transfer of acetyl groups from acetyl CoA to acetylcarnitine, L-carnitine can relieve the inhibition of PDC, the rate-limiting enzyme for glucose oxidation. This role of L-carnitine may explain some of the beneficial effects associated with L-carnitine and PLC treatment in various pathological conditions. Furthermore, we believe that the well documented beneficial effects of L-carnitine and PLC in ischemic hearts are best correlated with its ability to overcome fatty acid inhibition of glucose oxidation during reperfusion.

REFERENCES
1. Neely JR, Morgan HE. Relationship between carbohydrate and lipid metabolism and the energy balance of heart muscle. Ann Rev Physiol 1974; 36:413-459.

2. Saddik M, Lopaschuk GD. Myocardial triglyceride turnover and contribution to energy substrate utilization in isolated working rat hearts. J Biol Chem 1991; 266:8162-8170.
3. Bing RJ, Siegel A, Vitale A. Metabolic studies on the human heart in vivo. Studies on carbohydrate metabolism of the human heart. 1953; 15:284-296.
4. Patel MS, Roche TE. Molecular biology and biochemistry of pyruvate dehydrogenase complex. FASEB J 1990; 4:3224-3233.
5. McCormack JG, Denton RM. Role of $Ca^{2+}$ ions in the regulation of intramitochondrial metabolism in rat heart. Biochem J 1984; 218:235-247.
6. Randle PJ. Fuel selection in animals. Biochem Soc Trans 1986; 14:799-806.
7. Kerbey AL, Vary TC, Randle PJ. Molecular mechanisms regulating myocardial glucose oxidation. Basic Res Cardiol 1985; 80(suppl 2):93-96.
8. Murthy MSR, Pande SV. Malonyl-CoA binding site and the overt carnitine palmitoyltransferase activity reside on the opposite sides of the outer mitochondrial membrane. Proc Natl Acad Sci USA 1988; 84:378-382.
9. McGarry JD, Woeltje KF, Kuwajima M, Foster DW. Regulation of ketogenesis and the renaissance of carnitine palmitoyltransferase. Diabetes/Metabolism Reviews 1989; 5:271-284.
10. McGarry JD, Mills SE, Long CS, Foster DW. Observations on the affinity for carnitine, and malonyl-CoA sensitivity, of carnitine palmitoyltransferase I in animal and human tissues. Biochem J 1983; 214:21-28.
11. Weis BC, Cowan AT, Brown N, Foster DW, McGarry JD. Use of a selective inhibitor of liver carnitine palmitoyltransferase I (CPT I. allows quantification of its contribution to total CPT I activity in rat heart. J Biol Chem 1994; 269:25443-26448.
12. Brown NF, Weis BC, Husti JE, Foster DW. Mitochondrial carnitine palmitoyltransferase I isoform switching in the developing rat heart. J Biol Chem 1995; 270:8952-8957.
13. Weis BC, Esser V, Foster DW, McGarry JD. Rat heart expresses two forms of mitochondrial carnitine palmitoyltransferase I. J Biol Chem 1994; 269:18712-18715.
14. Regitz-Zagrosek V, Fleck E. Myocardial carnitine deficiency in human cardiomyopathy. In: The Carnitine System. JW de Jong, R Ferrari Eds. Kluwer Academic Publishers: Dordrecht, The Netherlands, 1995; 145-166.
15. Regitz V, Shug AL, Fleck E. Defective myocardial carnitine metabolism in congestive heart failure secondary to dilated cardiomyopathy and to coronary, hypertensive and vascular heart diseases. Am J Cardiol 1990; 65:755-760.

16. Engel AG. Possible causes and effects of carnitine deficency in man. In: Frenkel RS, McGarry JD, eds. Carnitine Biosynthesis, Metabolism and Functions. NY: Academic Press, 1980; 271-286.
17. Boudin G, Mikol J, Guillard A, Engel AG. Fatal systemic carnitine deficiency with lipid storage in skeletal muscle, heart, liver and kidney. J Neurol Sci 1976; 30:56-60.
18. Lysiak W, Lilly K, Di Lisa F, Toth PP, Bieber LL. Quantification of the effect of L-carnitine on the levels of acid-soluble short-chain acyl CoA and CoA in rat heart and liver mitochondria. J Biol Chem 1988; 263:1511-1516.
19. Lysiak W, Toth PP, Suelter CH, Bieber LL. Quantitation of the efflux of acylcarnitines on the levels of acid-soluble short-chain acyl CoA and CoASH in rat heart and liver mitochondria. J Biol Chem 1986; 261:10698-13703.
20. Pearson DJ, Tubbs PK. Carnitine and derivatives in rat tissues. Biochem J 1967; 105:953-963.
21. Broderick TL, Quinney HA, Lopaschuk GD. Carnitine stimulation of glucose oxidation in the fatty acid perfused isolated working rat heart. J Biol Chem 1992; 267(6):3758-3763.
22. Fritz IB, Schultz SK, Srere PA. Properties of partially purified carnitine acetyl transferase. J Biol Chem 1963; 236:2509-2517.
23. Uziel G, Garaveaglia B, DiDonato S. Carnitine stimulation of pyruvate dehydrogenase complex (PDHC) in isolated human skeletal muscle mitochondria. Muscle and Nerve 1988; 11:720-724.
24. Di Lisa F, Barbato R, Manabo R, Siliprandi N. Carnitine and carnitine esters in mitochondrial metabolism and function. In: The Carnitine System. de Jong JW, Ferrari R, eds. Kluwer Academic Publishers: Dordrecht, The Netherlands, 1995; 21-38.
25. Pierpont MEM, Judd D, Goldenberg IF, Rings WS, Olivari MT, Pierpont GL. Myocardial carnitine in end-stage congestive heart failure. Am J Cardiol 1989; 64:56-60.
26. Allard MF, Schönekess BO, Henning SL, English DR, Lopaschuk GD. The contribution of oxidative metabolism and glycolysis to ATP production in the hypertrophied heart. Am J Physiol 1994; 267: H742-H750.
27. el Alaoui-Talibi Z, Landormy S, Loireau A, Moravec J. Fatty acid oxidation and mechanical performance of volume-overloaded rat hearts. Am J Physiol 1992; 262:H1068-H1074.
28. Broderick TL, DiDomenico D, Shug AL, Paulson DJ. Fatty acid oxidation and cardiac function in the sodium pivalate model of secondary carnitine deficiency. Metabolism 1995; 44:499-505.
29. Broderick TL, Panagakis G, DiDomenico D, Gamble J, Lopaschuk GD, Shug AL, Paulson DJ. L-carnitine improvement of cardiac function is associated with a stimulation in glucose but not fatty acid metabolism in carnitine-deficient hearts. Cardiov Res 1995; 30: 815-820.

30. Broderick TL, Quinney HA, Barker CC, Lopaschuk GD. Beneficial effect of carnitine on mechanical recovery of rat hearts reperfused after a transient period of global ischemia is accompanied by a stimulation of glucose oxidation. Circulation 1993; 87:972-981.

31. Vary TC, Neely JR. A mechanism for reduced myocardial carnitine content in diabetic animals. Am J Physiol 1982; 243:H154-H158.

32. Garland PB, Randle PJ. Regulation of glucose uptake by muscle. 10. Effects of alloxan-diabetes, starvation, hypophysectomy and adrenalectomy and of fatty acids, ketones and pyruvate on the glycerol output and concentrations of free fatty acids, long chain fatty acyl coenzyme A, glycerol phosphate and citrate cycle intermediates in rat hearts and diaphragm muscles. Biochem J 1964; 93:678-687.

33. Wall SR, Lopaschuk GD. Glucose oxidation rates in fatty acid-perfused isolated working hearts from diabetic rats. Biochim Biophys Acta 1989; 1006:97-103.

34. Triacylglycerol turnover in isolated working hearts of acutely diabetic rats. Can J Physiol Pharmacol 1994; 72:1110-1119.

35. Riebel DK, O-Rourke B, Foster KA. Mechanisms for altered carnitine content in hypertrophied rat hearts. Am J Physiol 1987; 252: H561-H565.

36. Schönekess BO, Allard MF, Lopaschuk GD. Propionyl L-carnitine improvement of hypertrophied heart function is accompanied by an increase in carbohydrate oxidation. Circ Res 1995; 77:726-734.

37. Newgard CB, McGarry JD. Metabolic coupling factors in pancreatic β-cell signal transduction. Annu Rev Biochem 1995; 64:689-719.

38. Cook GA. Differences in the sensitivity of carnitine palmitoyl-transferase to inhibition by malonyl-CoA are due to differences in Ki values. J Biol Chem 1984; 259:12030-12033.

39. Singh B, Stakkestad JA, Bremer J, Borrebaek B. Determination of malonyl-coenzyme A in rat heart, kidney, and liver: A comparison between acetyl-coenzyme A and butyryl-coenzyme A as fatty acid synthase primers in assay procedure. Anal Biochem 1984; 138:107-111.

40. Saddik M, Gamble J, Witters LA, Lopaschuk GD. Acetyl-CoA carboxylase regulation of fatty acid oxidation in the heart. J Biol Chem 1993; 268:25836-25845.

41. Lopaschuk GD, Witters LA, Itoi T, Barr R, Barr A. Acetyl-CoA carboxylase involvement in the rapid maturation of fatty acid oxidation in the newborn rabbit heart. J Biol Chem 1994; 269:25871-25878.

42. Kudo N, Barr AJ, Barr RL, Desai S, Lopaschuk GD. High rates of fatty acid oxidation during reperfusion of ischemic hearts are associated with a decrease in malonyl-CoA levels due to an increase in 5'-AMP-activated protein kinase inhibition of acetyl-CoA carboxylase. J Biol Chem 1995; 270:17513-17520.

43. Lopaschuk GD, Belke DD, Gamble J, Itoi T, Schönekess BO. Regulation of fatty acid oxidation in the mammalian heart in health and disease. Biochim Biophys Acta 1991; 1213:263-276.

44. Mabrouk GM, Helmy IM, Thampy KG, Wakil SJ. Acute hormonal control of acetyl-CoA carboxylase: Roles of insulin, glucagon, and epinephrine. J Biol Chem 1990; 265:6330-6338.
45. Wakil SJ, Titchener EB, Gibson DM. Evidence for the participation of biotin in the enzymatic synthesis of fatty acids. Biochim Biophys Acta 1958; 29:225-226.
46. Bianchi A, Evans JL, Iverson AJ, Nordlund AC, Watts TD, Witters LA. Identification of an isozymic forms of acetyl-CoA carboxylase. J Biol Chem 1990; 265:1502-1509.
47. Thampy KG. Formation of malonyl-CoA in rat heart. J Biol Chem 1989; 264:17631-17634.
48. Iverson AJ, Bianchi A, Nordlund AC, Witters LA. Immunological analysis of acetyl-CoA carboxylase mass, tissue distribution and subunit composition. Biochem J 1990; 269:365-371.
49. Idell-Wenger JA, Grotyohann LW, Neely JR. Coenzyme A and carnitine distribution in normal and ischemic myocardium. J Biol Chem 1978; 253:4310-4318.
50. De Jong JW, Mugelli A, Di Lisa F, Ferrari R. Acute vs. chronic treatment with propionyl-L-carnitine: biochemical, hemodynamic and electrophysiological effects on rabbit heart. In: de Jong JW, Ferrari R, eds. The Carnitine System. Kluwer Academic Publishers: Dordrecht, The Netherlands, 1995; 261-273.
51. Micheletti R, Schiavone A, Bianchi G. Effect of propionyl-L-carnitine on rats with experimentally induced cardiomyopathies. In: de Jong JW, Ferrari R, eds. The Carnitine System. Kluwer Academic Publishers: Dordrecht, The Netherlands, 1995; 307-322.
52. Ciman M, Rossi CR, Siliprandi N. On the mechanism of the antiketogenic action of propionate and succinate in isolated rat liver mitochondria. FEBS Lett 1972; 22:8-10.
53. Tassani V, Catapan F, Magnanimi L, Peschechera A. Anaplerotic effect of propionyl carnitine in rat heart mitochondria. Biochem Biophys Res Commun 1994; 199:949-953.
54. Sundqvist KE, Vuorinen KH, Peuhkurinen KJ, Hassinen IE. Metabolic effects of propionate, hexanoate and propionylcarnitine in normoxia, ischaemia and reperfusion. Eur Heart J 1994; 15:561-570.
55. Paulson DJ, Schmidt MJ, Traxler JS, Shug AL. Improvement of myocardial function in diabetic rats after treatment with L-carnitine. Metabolism 1984; 33:358-363.
56. Siliprandi N, Di Lisa F, Pivetta A, Miotto G, Siliprandi D. Transport and function of L-carnitine and L-propionylcarnitine: relevance to some cardiomyopathies and cardiac ischemia. Z Kardiol 1987; 76(suppl 5.:34-40
57. Paulson DJ, Traxler J, Schmidt M, Noonan J, Shug AL. Protection of the ischemic myocardium by L-propionylcarnitine: effects on the recovery of cardiac output after ischaemia and reperfusion, carnitine transport, and fatty acid oxidation. Card Res 1986; 20:536-541.

58. Liedtke AJ, DeMaison L, Nellis SH. Effects of L-propionylcarnitine on mechanical recovery during reflow in intact hearts. Am J Physiol 1988; 255:H169-176.
59. Motterlini R, Samaja M, Tarantola M, Micheletti R, Bianchi G. Functional and metabolic effects of propionyl-L-carnitine in the isolated perfused hypertrophied rat heart. Mol Cell Biochem 1992; 116: 139-145.
60. Broderick TK, Quinney HA, Lopaschuk GD. L-carnitine increases glucose metabolism and mechanical function following ischaemia in diabetic rat heart. Cardiovas Res 1995; 29:373-378.
61. Hata K, Takasago T, Saeki A, Nishioka T, Goto Y. Stunned myocardium after rapid correction of acidosis. Circ Res 194; 74:794-805.
62. Shönekess BO, Allard MF, Lopaschuk GD. Propionyl L-carnitine improvement of hypertrophied rat heart function is associated with an increase in cardiac efficiency. Eur J Pharmacol 1995:286:155-156.
63. Lopaschuk GD, Spafford MA, Davies NJ, Wall SR. Glucose and palmitate oxidation in isolated working rat hearts reperfused after a period of transient global ischemia. Circ Res 1990; 60:546-553.
64. Renstrom B, Nellis SH, Liedtke AJ. Metabolic oxidation of glucose during early reperfusion. Circ Res 1989; 65:1094-1101.
65. Görge G, Chatelain P, Schaper J, Lerch R. Effect of increasing degrees of ischemic injury on myocardial oxidative metabolism early after reperfusion in isolated rat hearts. Circ Res 1991; 68:1681-1692.
66. Liedtke AJ, DeMaison L, Eggleston AM, Cohen LM, Nellis SH. Changes in substrate metabolism and effects of excess fatty acids in reperfused myocardium. Circ Res 1988; 62:535-542.
67. Lopaschuk GD, Wall SR, Olley PM, Davies NJ. Etomoxir, a carnitine palmitoyltransferase I inhibitor, protects hearts form fatty acid-induced injury independent of changes in long chain acylcarnitine. Circ Res 1988; 63:1036-1043.
68. McVeigh JJ, Lopaschuk GD. Dichloroacetate stimulation of glucose oxidation improves recovery of ischemic rat hearts. Am J Physiol 1990; 259:H1079-H1085.
69. Lopaschuk GD, Wambolt RB, Barr RL. An imbalance between glycolysis and glucose oxidation is a possible explanation for the detrimental effects of high levels of fatty acids during aerobic perfusion of ischemic hearts. J Pharmacol Expt Ther 1993; 264:135-144.
70. Liu B, el Alaoui-Talibi Z, Clanachan AS, Schulz R, Lopaschuk G. Uncoupling of contractile function from mitochondrial TCA cycle activity and $MVO_2$ during reperfusion of ischemic hearts. Am J Physiol 1996; 270:H72-H80.
71. Tani M. Mechanisms of $Ca^{2+}$ overload in reperfused ischemic myocardium. Annu Rev Physiol 1990; 52:543-559.
72. Folts JD, Shug AL, Koke JR, Bittar N. Protection of the ischemic dog myocardium with carnitine. Am J Cardiol 1978; 41:1209-1215.

73. Hulsmann WC, Dubelaar ML, Lamers JMJ, Muccari F. Protection of acyl-carnitine and phenylmethylsulphonyl fluoride in rat heart subjected to ischemia and reperfusion. Biochem Biophys Acta 1985; 847:62-66.

74. Liedtke AJ, Nellis SH. Effect of carnitine in ischaemic and fatty acid supplemented swine hearts. J Clin Invest 1979; 64:440-447.

75. Shug Al, Thomsen JH, Folts JD, Bittar N, Klien MI, Koke JR, Huth PJ. Changes in tissue levels of carnitine and other metabolites during myocardial ischemia and anoxia. Arch Biochem Biophys 1978; 187:25-33.

76. Suzuki Y, Kamikawa T, Kobyashi A, Masumura Y, Yamazaki N. Effects of L-carnitine on tissue levels of acylcarnitine, acyl coenzyme A and high energy phosphate in ischemic dog hearts. Jap Circ J 1981; 45:687-694.

77. Oliver MF, Kurien VA, Greenwood TW. Relation between serum-free fatty acid and arryhthymia and death after myocardial infarction. Lancet 1968; 1:710-715.

78. Saddik M, Lopaschuk GD. Myocardial triglyceride turnover during reperfusion of isolated rat hearts subjected to a transient period of global ischemia. J Biol Chem 1992; 267(6):3825-3831.

# CHAPTER 4

# Carnitine and Mitochondrial Dysfunction

Fabio Di Lisa, Roberta Barbato, Roberta Menabò
and Noris Siliprandi

## MITOCHONDRIAL FUNCTION AND DYSFUNCTION

Since ATP is not cell permeant, a decrease in its content cannot be restored by extracellular sources. Thus, in every cell ATP consumption has to be matched by comparable rates of ATP production. By far mitochondria represent the most relevant site for ATP production. The phosphorylation of ADP into ATP is coupled to oxygen consumption in the process known as oxidative phosphorylation, which occurs at the level of the inner mitochondrial membrane (IMM).[1] The downhill redox gradient created by the flow of the electrons running from NADH to oxygen (redox potential, $\Delta E$) is first utilized to pump $H^+$ out of the matrix space. Since the passive permeability to $H^+$ and to anions and cations is low, $H^+$ ejection results in the establishment of a $\Delta \mu H$ that can be utilized for ATP synthesis via the $F_0F_1$-ATPase. In this process, NADH($H^+$) and $FADH_2$ resulting from cytosolic and mitochondrial oxidative degradation of substrates represent the energy input and ATP the energy output. It must be emphasized that the actual energy currency of mitochondria is $\Delta \mu H$ on which, besides ATP synthesis, other relevant processes depend (i.e. metabolite and ion traffic through IMM).

Pathological conditions, such as anoxia, change mitochondria from ATP producers into active ATP consumers. In fact, ATP is utilized by the reverse operation of $F_0F_1$-ATPase to pump protons maintaining $\Delta \mu H$.[2]

Most of our knowledge on mitochondrial function derives from studies on isolated mitochondria by using selective inhibitors. Indeed, a host of compounds are available to inhibit each single step of the pathway that leads from substrate oxidation to ATP production. In particular, it is possible to

*Carnitine Today*, edited by Claudio De Simone and Giuseppe Famularo.
© 1997 Landes Bioscience.

defect reduces the availability of oxidized coenzymes, resulting in decreased oxidation rates and accumulation of metabolic intermediates. Under these conditions a large proportion of the available carnitine is going to be esterified for the disposal of acetyl CoA no longer degradable by TCA cycle. On the other hand, the reduced rate of β-oxidation is followed by the accumulation of long-chain acyl CoA (LCACoA) and, consequently, of the corresponding carnitine esters.

## CARNITINE, COA AND MITOCHONDRIAL FUNCTION

The importance of free CoA (CoASH) availability for mitochondrial oxidative processes was recognized in the early 1960s, soon after the discovery of CPT and CAT. Hülsmann and Siliprandi[6] demonstrated that the oxygen consumption of mitochondria respiring on α-ketoglutarate was almost blunted by the addition of acetoacetate which traps the available CoASH in the form of acetoacetyl- and acetyl-CoA. Similarly, pyruvate oxidation is inhibited by acetyl-CoA which accumulates when the TCA cycle is blocked by malonate.[7,8] In both conditions, carnitine addition restores mitochondrial function by converting the inhibitory metabolites into their corresponding acylcarnitines.[6-8]

The molecular mechanism underlying the inhibition of pyruvate and α-ketoglutarate oxidation was clarified by Randle et al, who demonstrated that short-chain acyl CoAs stimulate both pyruvate dehydrogenase (PDH) kinase and α-ketoglutarate dehydrogenase kinase leading to the inhibition of the oxidative decarboxylation of these α-keto acids.[9] In addition, CoASH is required for many other relevant processes such as β-oxidation,[10] the catabolism of several amino acids and the detoxification of organic acids and xenobiotics.[11] A reduced availability of carnitine induces a decrease of matrix CoASH and a parallel increase of the acyl-CoA/CoASH ratio, both of which are inhibitory in the aforementioned mitochondrial dehydrogenases. On the other hand, the addition of carnitine to isolated mitochondria induces a profound decrease of the acyl-CoA/CoASH ratio.[12,13]

## CARNITINE AND MITOCHONDRIAL ALTERATIONS INDUCED BY ANOXIA

### ACCUMULATION OF LONG-CHAIN ACYL COA

During the 1970s, the discovery of life-threatening diseases related to carnitine deficiency fuelled a novel interest in carnitine, expanding the research area from biochemistry and physiology to pathophysiology and clinical studies. The major focus was directed toward myocardial ischemia, or more precisely toward the alterations of lipid metabolism which are associated with, or caused by, coronary artery disease. The relationship between carnitine and myocardial ischemia was based on the following observations: (i) an increase in circulating FFA is associated with myocardial ischemia and worsens the prognosis;[14] (ii) intracellular fatty acid oxidation is reduced or inhibited in the ischemic tissue resulting in a large and rapid increase of deleterious intermediates, such as LCACoA;[15-17] and (iii) carnitine administration decreases plasma FFA[18] and reduces the intracellular content of LCACoA.[16]

Profound alterations of mitochondrial physiology are produced by LCACoA [19] which accumulates during ischemia.[15-17] These CoA esters are amphipathic molecules which can insert in the phospholipid bilayer altering both membrane architecture and permeability.[19,20] These changes are more likely to occur at LCACoA concentrations above the CMC (critical micellar concentration) which in the case of palmitoyl CoA is $\cong$ 30 $\mu$M. At lower concentrations, LCACoA are able to specifically affect the activity of various transport systems of the inner mitochondrial membrane without perturbing its permeability.[21] The example of these modifications is the inhibition of adenine nucleotide translocase (ANT).[22] The inhibitory effects of LCACoA are exacerbated by $Ca^{2+}$ and blunted by several cations such as $Mg^{2+}$ and polyamines [21,23] which are present in millimolar concentrations within the matrix space. The protective effect exerted by these cations, which are usually present in mitochondria, may explain the lack of ANT inhibition which was obtained by increasing LCACoA matrix content.[24]

Carnitine addition is able to restore ANT function and, hence, oxidative phosphorylation, by changing LCACoA to LCACars, which are devoid of inhibitory effects. More recently, LCACoA have been added to the long list of promoters of the cyclosporine-sensitive membrane transition pore (MTP).[25,26] Additionally, the abrupt changes of membrane permeability and function brought about by MTP opening can be prevented or partially restored by carnitine.[26,27]

LCACoA accumulation might play a central role in the well-documented free fatty acid (FFA) myocardial toxicity.[14,17,20,28] However, besides the $Mg^{2+}$ effect, it is worthwhile considering that the $K_i$s for transport inhibitions (>5 $\mu$M) are well above the mitochondrial content of total CoA (free + esterified). Furthermore, the concentration of "free" LCACoA is likely to be reduced by the more or less specific binding with various proteins,[29] although it is possible that these esters do not accumulate homogeneously, reaching very high local concentrations within the hydrophobic core of the membranes.

### DECREASED AVAILABILITY OF COASH AND CARNITINE

In isolated mitochondria as well as in the intact heart, LCACoA toxicity could be ascribed, at least in part, to a decreased CoASH availability. The role of CoASH/esterified-CoA and carnitine/esterified carnitine ratios in the evolution of ischemic damage has been investigated in isolated rat

ence of acetoacetate or pyruvate. Biochim Biophys Acta 1964; 93:166-8.

7. Ferri L, Valente M, Ursini F, Gregolin C, Siliprandi N. Acetyl-carnitine formation and pyruvate oxidation in mitochondria from different rat tissues. Bull Mol Biol Med 1981; 6:16-23.

8. Pande S, Parvin R. Characterization of carnitine acylcarnitine translocase system of heart mitochondria. J Biol Chem 1976; 251:6683-91.

9. Kerbey A, Randle P, Cooper R et al. Regulation of pyruvate dehydrogenase in rat heart. Mechanism of regulation of proportions of dephosphorylated and phosphorylated enzyme by oxidation of fatty acids and ketone bodies and of effects of diabetes: role of coenzyme A, acetyl coenzyme A and reduced and oxidized nicotinamide adenine dinucleotide. Biochem J 1976; 154:327-48.

10. Schulz H. Regulation of fatty acid oxidation in heart. J Nutr 1994; 124:165-71.

11. Quistad GB, Staiger LE, Schooley DA. The role of carnitine in the conjugation of acidic xenobiotics. Drug Metab Dispos 1986; 14:521-5.

12. Hansford R, Cohen L. Relative importance of pyruvate dehydrogenase interconversion and feed back inhibition in the effect of fatty acids on pyruvate oxidation by rat heart mitochondria. Arch Biochem Biophys 1978; 191:65-81.

13. Lysiak W, Lilly K, DiLisa F, Toth P, Bieber L. Quantitation of the effect of L carnitine on the levels of acid soluble short chain acyl CoA and CoASH in rat heart and liver mitochondria. J Biol Chem 1988; 263:1151-6.

14. Oliver M, Kurien V, Greenwood T. Relation between serum free fatty acids and arrhythmias and death after acute myocardial infarction. Lancet 1968; 1:710-4.

15. Idell W, Grotyohann L, Neely J. Coenzyme A and carnitine distribution in normal and ischemic hearts. J Biol Chem 1978; 253:4310-8.

16. Shug AL, Thomsen JH, Folts JD. Changes in tissue levels of carnitine and other metabolites during myocardial ischemia and anoxia. Arch Biochem Biophys 1978; 260:14748-55.

17. Van Der Vusse G, Glatz J, Stam H, Reneman R. Fatty acid homeostasis in the normoxic and ischemic heart. Physiol Rev 1992; 72:881-940.

18. Ferrari R, Cucchini F, Visioli O. The metabolical effects of L carnitine in angina pectoris. Int J Cardiol 1984; 5:213-6.

19. Brecher P. The interaction of long chain acyl CoA with membranes. Mol Cell Biochem 1983; 57:3-15.

20. Katz A, Messineo F. Lipid membrane interactions and the pathogenesis of ischemic damage in the myocardium. Circ Res 1981; 48:1-16.

21. Siliprandi N, Di Lisa F, Sartorelli L. Transport and function of carnitine in cardiac muscle. In: Berman M, Gevers W, Opie L, eds. Membranes and muscle. Oxford: IRL Press, 1985:105-119.

22. Pande S, Blanchaer M. Reversible inhibition of mitochondrial adenosine diphosphate phosphorylation by long chain acyl coenzyme A esters. J Biol Chem 1971; 246:402-11.

23. Toninello A, Dalla V, Testa S, Siliprandi D, Siliprandi N. Transport and action of spermine in rat heart mitochondria. Cardioscience 1990; 1:287-94.

24. LaNoue KF, Watts JA, Koch CD. Adenine nucleotide transport during cardiac ischemia. Am J Physiol 1981; 241:H663-671.

25. Gunter T, Pfeiffer D. Mechanisms by which mitochondria transport calcium. Am J Physiol 1990; 258:C755-86.

26. Siliprandi D, Biban C, Testa S, Toninello A, Siliprandi N. Effects of palmitoyl CoA and palmitoyl carnitine on the membrane potential and Mg2+ content of rat heart mitochondria. Mol Cell Biochem 1992; 116:117-23.

27. Pastorino JG, Snyder JW, Serroni A, Hoek JB, Farber JL. Cyclosporin and carnitine prevent the anoxic death of cultured hepatocytes by inhibiting the mitochondrial permeability transition. J Biol Chem 1993; 268:13791-8.

28. Opie L. Effect of fatty acids on contractility and rhythm of the heart. Nature 1970; 227:1055-6.

29. Glatz J, Van DG. Cellular fatty acid binding proteins: current concepts and future directions. Mol Cell Biochem 1990; 98:237-51.

30. Di Lisa F, Menabò R, Barbato R, Siliprandi N. Contrasting effects of propionate and propionylcarnitine on metabolic and energy-linked processes in the ischemic heart. Am J Physiol 1994; 267:H455-H461.

31. Bolukoglu H, Nellis SH, Liedtke AJ. Effects of propionate on mechanical and metabolic performance in aerobic rat hearts. Cardiovasc Drug Ther 1991; 5:37-44.

32. Russell RR III, Taegtmeyer H. Coenzyme A sequestration in rat hearts oxidizing ketone bodies. J Clin Invest 1992; 89:968-73.

33. Brevetti G, Chiariello M, Ferulano G, Policicchio A, Nevola E, Rossini A, Attisano T, Ambrosio G, Siliprandi N, Angelini C. Increases in walking distance in patients with peripheral vascular disease treated with L-carnitine: a double-blind, cross-over study. Circulation 1988; 77:767-73.

34. Siliprandi N, Di Lisa F, Pieralisi G, Ripari P, Maccari F, Menabò R, Giamberardino MA, Vecchiet L. Metabolic changes induced by maximal exercise in human subjects following L-carnitine administration. Biochim Biophys Acta 1990; 1034:17-21.

35. Hultman E, Cederblad G, Harper P. Carnitine administration as a tool of modify energy metabolism during exercise. Eur J Appl Physiol 1991; 62:450.

36. Sartorelli L, Ciman M, Siliprandi N. Carnitine transport in rat heart slices: I° The action of thiol reagents on the acetylcarnitine/carnitine exchange. Ital J Biochem 1985; 34:275-81.
37. Siliprandi N, Di Lisa F, Vecchiet L. Effect of exogenous carnitine on muscle metabolism: a reply to Hultman et al. Eur J Appl Physiol 1992; 64:278.
38. Roe CR, Millington DS, Maltby DA, Kahler SG, Bohan TP. L-carnitine therapy in isovaleric acidemia. J Clin Invest 1984; 74:2290-5.
39. Salamino F, Di L, Burlina A, Menabò R, Barbato R, De T, Siliprandi N. Involvement of erythrocyte calpain in glycine and carnitine treated isovaleric acidemia. Pediatr Res 1994; 36:182-6.

# Effect of L-Carnitine on Fas-Induced Apoptosis and Sphingomyelinase Activity in Human T Cell Lines

Edoardo Alesse, Luisa Di Marzio, Paola Roncaioli, Francesca Zazzeroni,
Adriano Angelucci, Barbara Ruggeri, Italo Trotta, Paola Muzi
and Grazia Cifone

## INTRODUCTION

Fas is a 45 kDa type-I membrane protein and belongs to the tumor necrosis factor (TNF) receptor/nerve growth factor receptor family.[1-3] The Fas ligand (FasL) is a membrane-bound cytokine and a member of the TNF family.[4] The binding of FasL or agonist anti-Fas to Fas induces apoptosis,[1,5] indicating that FasL is a death factor and that Fas is its receptor.[4] The Fas system is involved in the development of T cells, in particular activation-induced suicide of T cells or peripheral clonal deletion.[6] A high expression of the Fas/FasL system in peripheral blood mononuclear cells from HIV-positive subjects has been reported and could be responsible for the observed relevant apoptosis of both infected and uninfected cells.[7-8] It has also been noted that expression of Fas by CD4+ T cells of HIV-infected patients negatively correlated with their CD4+ T cell count.[9] Moreover, it has been reported that Fas stimulation by crosslinking with monoclonal antibodies induced peripheral blood T cell apoptosis in HIV-infected individuals.[10] In contrast, antibodies against other members of the TNF/NGF receptor family, such as CD27, CD30, CD40, 4-1BB, p55 TNF receptor, p75 TNF receptor, and TNF receptor-related protein all failed to induce apoptosis. In addition, the Fas system may be involved in the relative abilities of Th1 and Th2 cells to undergo apoptosis since Th1 clones express high levels of Fas

*Carnitine Today,* edited by Claudio De Simone and Giuseppe Famularo.
© 1997 Landes Bioscience.

ligand, whereas its expression on Th2 is low.[11] This differential Fas ligand expression could explain the selective Th1 depletion observed during HIV infection.[12] Other investigators using an in vitro model have shown that the effect of viral Tat protein on T cell apoptosis is mediated by increased Fas ligand expression at concentrations of Tat similar to that observed in the sera of HIV infected patients.[13] The apoptotic signal through Fas seems to involve the activation of an acidic sphingomyelinase, sphingomyelin breakdown and ceramide production.[14] Ceramide acts as an endogenous mediator of apoptosis in several cell lines[14-16] and its potential role in the pathogenesis of HIV infection has been suggested. Ceramide has indeed been reported to increase and has been shown to potently induce HIV replication in HIV-chronically infected CEM cell line[17] and HL60 cells,[18] $U-1_{IIIB}$ and OM-10.1 cells[19] respectively. Moreover, the ceramide treatment of HIV-LTR transfected cells strongly increases reporter CAT expression, and Rb hypophosphorylation induced by ceramide might remove the E2F-imposed transcriptional inhibition of the viral genome.[20,21]

Our group has recently reported that AIDS patients have significantly higher lymphocyte-associated ceramide levels than healthy controls and that HIV-infected long-term non-progressors have less elevated lymphocyte-associated levels of ceramide than subjects with progressive disease.[22] Remarkably, this is paralleled by a lower frequency of CD4 and CD8 undergoing apoptosis in long-term survivors than in AIDS patients. This background suggests that therapies directed at the downmodulation of ceramide generation have the potential to slow the progression of the disease through reducing the apoptotic cell death.

To better characterize the results obtained after carnitine administration to AIDS patients, we investigated its effects in vitro on apoptosis and ceramide production of Fas-sensitive cell lines (HuT 78 and U937) after Fas crosslinking. Our data indicate that carnitine was able to reduce Fas-induced apoptosis of these cells, likely by preventing sphingomyelin (SM) breakdown and consequent ceramide synthesis.

To assess whether the effects of this drug were specific on SMases, we analyzed its influence on purified neutral and acidic SMase in vitro.

## MATERIALS AND METHODS

### Cell Lines

The human T cell lymphoma Hut78 and the human promyelocytic leukemia U937 cell lines were grown in RPMI 1640 supplemented with 10% FCS, 1 mM glutamine and antibiotics.

## DNA Agarose Gel Elecrophoresis and Klenow Polymerase Labeling

Hut78 and U937 cells ($5 \times 10^6$) were treated with anti-Fas mAb (200 ng/ml; UBI, Lake Placid, NY; clone CH-11) for 8 hrs at 37°C in the presence or absence of L-carnitine (100 µg/ml; C7H16NO3, Mr 161.20, Sigma Tau, Pomezia, Italy) which was added 1 hr before stimulus. The cells were then centrifuged and incubated in 0.5 ml of 50 mM Tris-HCl pH 8.0 containing 1 mM EDTA, 0.25% NP40 (Sigma) and 0.1% RNase A (Sigma) at 37°C for 30 min. 50 ml of 10 mg/ml proteinase K (Boehringer Mannheim, Mannheim, Germany) were then added and the incubation was continued for an additional 2 hrs.[23] After phenol-chloroform extraction the DNA was ethanol precipitated and resuspended in TE (10 mM Tris-HCl pH 7.6 and EDTA 1 mM). Cellular DNA (1.0 mg) was treated with 5 U of Klenow polymerase using 0.5 mCi of $^{32}$P-labeled dCTP in the presence of 10 mM Tris/HCl pH 7.5, 5 mM MgCl$_2$. The reaction was incubated for 10 min at room temperature and terminated by addition of 10 mM EDTA. After removing the unincorporated nucleotides, the labeled DNA was resuspended in 10 mM Tris/HCl pH 7.6 and 1 mM EDTA. Between 3000-5000 Cerenkov counts were applied on a 1.8% agarose gel, and the probes were electrophoresed for 2 hr at 100 V. After drying the gel on 3 MM Wathman paper, the filter was exposed for autoradiography.

## Ceramide Mass Measurement (Diacylglycerol Kinase Assay)

Hut78 and U937 ($5 \times 10^6$ cells/ml) were pre-stimulated with anti-Fas mAb (200 ng/ml) for different times (5-60 min). Where indicated, L-carnitine (100 µg/ml) was added to cell cultures 1 hr before stimulation. Incubation was stopped by immersion of samples in methanol/dry ice (-70°C) for 10 sec followed by centrifugation at 4°C in a microfuge. Lipids were extracted and then incubated with *Escherichia coli* diacylglycerol kinase.[24] DAG kinase assay kit and $^{32}$P-ATPγ (specific activity 3 Ci/mmol) were obtained from Amersham (Buckinghamshire, England). Ceramide phosphate was then isolated by TLC using CHCl$_3$/CH$_3$OH/CH$_3$COOH (65/15/5, vol/vol/vol) as solvent. Authentic ceramide (type III; from bovine brain; Sigma Chemical Co. St. Louis, MO) was identified by autoradiography at Rf 0.25. Quantitative results for ceramide production are expressed as pmoles of ceramide-1-phosphate/mg protein.

## In Vitro Sphingomyelinase Assay

U937 and Hut78 cells were treated with anti-Fas mAb (200 ng/ml) for 10 min at 37°C. Where indicated, L-carnitine (100 µg/ml) was added to cell cultures 1 hr before stimulation. After incubation, the cells were washed, and then, to measure neutral SMase, resuspended in a buffer containing 20 mM HEPES, pH 7.4, 10 mM MgCl$_2$, 2 mM EDTA, 5 mM DTT, 0.1 mM

Na$_3$VO$_4$, 0.1 mM Na$_2$MoO$_4$, 30 mM p-nitrophenylphosphate, 10 mM β-glycerophosphate, 750 mM ATP, 1 μM PMSF, 10 μM leupeptin, 10 μM pepstatin (Sigma Chemical Co.), and 0.2% Triton X-100. After incubation for 5 min at 4°C, cells were lysed by sonication with a cell sonifier (Vibracell, Sonic and Materials Inc., Danbury, CT). Protein concentrations were determined using a protein assay (Bio-Rad Laboratories, Richmond, CA). 50-100 μg of the whole cell lysate were incubated for 2 hrs at 37°C in a buffer (50 μl final volume) containing 20 mM HEPES, 1 mM MgCl$_2$, pH 7.4 and 2.25 μl of [N-methyl-$^{14}$C]sphingomyelin (SM) (0.2 μCi/ml, specific activity 56.6 mCi/mmol, Amersham). To measure acidic SMase, after treatment the cells were washed and the pellet was resuspended in 200 μl of 0.2% Triton X-100 and incubated for 15 min at 4°C. The cells were sonicated and the protein concentration assayed. 50-100 μg of protein were incubated for 2 hrs at 37°C in a buffer (50 μl final volume) containing 250 mM sodium acetate, 1 mM EDTA, pH 5.0, and 2.25 μl of [N-methyl-$^{14}$C]SM. The reaction was stopped by the addition of 250 μl of chloroform:methanol:acetic acid (4:2:1). Phospholipids were extracted, analyzed on TLC plates and SM hydrolysis quantitated by autoradiography and liquid scintillation. SMase activation was expressed as pmol SM hydrolyzed/mg protein.

To assess the effects of L-carnitine directly on aSMase (Sigma; purified from human placenta; activity: 150 units per mg protein; one unit hydrolyzes 1.0 nmole of SM to N-acylsphingosine and choline phosphate per hr at pH 5.O at 37°C) and nSMase (Sigma; purified from *Staphylococcus aureus*; activity 100-300 units per mg protein; one unit hydrolyzes 1 μmole of sphingomyelin per min at pH 7.4 at 37°C), different amounts of enzymes were added to the above described assay system in substitution of cellular sonicates in the presence or absence of different concentrations of L-carnitine.

### STATISTICAL ANALYSIS

For data analysis the Student's t test was performed by the STATPAC Computerized Program and a P value of less than 0.05 was used as the significance criterion.

## EFFECT OF CARNITINE ON FAS-INDUCED APOPTOSIS IN HUT78 AND U937 CELLS

Experiments were performed to investigate the effects in vitro of L-carnitine on Fas crosslinking-induced apoptosis in Hut78 and U937 cells. DNA agarose gel electrophoresis revealed that a 8-hr exposure of Hut78 or U937 cells to anti-Fas mAb caused DNA fragmentation with a pattern characteristic of internucleosomal fragmentation (Fig. 5.1). The addition of L-carnitine (100 μg/ml), 60 min before stimulus, strongly reduced apoptosis-associated DNA fragmentation either in Hut78 or U937 cells. Interestingly, L-carnitine did not influence apoptosis induced by exogenous C2-ceramide (50 μM) in both Hut78 and U937 cells (not shown).

## EFFECT OF L-CARNITINE ON FAS CROSSLINKING-INDUCED CERAMIDE GENERATION IN HUT78 AND U937 CELLS

Full-time courses of ceramide generation to Fas activation with or without L-carnitine are shown in Fig. 5.2. The ceramide levels are reported as pmol/$10^6$ cells. Fas-engagement with anti-Fas mAb resulted in significant ceramide generation, as detected by TLC analysis of phospholipids extracted from cells and subjected to DAG kinase assay. Ceramide reached maximal levels by 10-15 min and was completed within 60 min after stimulus addition. In both cell lines, L-carnitine treatment (100 μg/ml) was able to prevent Fas crosslinking-induced ceramide generation in a time-dependent manner. Indeed, its addition to cell cultures led to a significant inhibition of Fas-crosslinking-induced ceramide release at 5-10 min, whereas the ceramide generation observed 30 min after stimulus was less affected by the presence of the drug. The time-dependence of ceramide generation inhibition induced by L-carnitine could be due to a different effect of the drug on the enzymes responsible for Fas-induced ceramide generation, i.e. acidic SMase and neutral SMase. In Figure 5.3 are reported two representative experiments assessed to analyze ceramide-1-phosphate levels in both Hut78 (A) or U937 (B) after incubation with anti-Fas mAb in the presence or absence of L-carnitine (100 μg/ml). The inhibitory effect of the drug on Fas

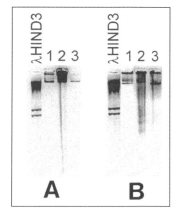

Fig. 5.1. Effect in vitro of L-carnitine on Fas-induced apoptosis in Hut78 (A) or U937 cells (B). DNA fragmentation is shown. Hut78 cells were treated with anti-Fas mAb (200 ng/ml) for 8 hr, in the presence or absence of L-carnitine (100 mg/ml). DNA was then isolated and electrophoresed as described in Materials and Methods section.

λ-HIND3 digest = markers; lane 1: DNA from untreated cells; lane 2: DNA treated with anti-Fas mAb for 8 hr; lane 3: DNA from cells treated with anti-Fas Ab for 8 hr in the presence of L-carnitine which was added to cell culture 1 hr before the addition of stimulus.

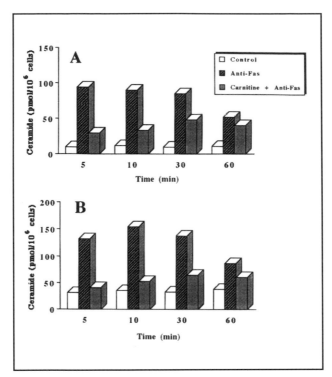

Fig. 5.2. Effect of L-carnitine treatment in vitro on ceramide generation induced by anti-Fas mAb. Hut78 (A) or U937 (B) cells were stimulated with anti-Fas mAb (200 ng/ml) for the inticated times in the presence or absence of L-Carnitine (100 mg/ml). Lipids were extracted, subjected to DAG kinase assay and separated by TLC. Radioactive spots corresponding to ceramide-1-phosphate were visualized by autoradiography, scraped and quantitated by liquid scintillation. Results are expressed as pmoles/10⁶ cells. Two different experiments gave similar results.

crosslinking-induced ceramide generation in both cell lines is evident. Figure 5.4 shows the dose-response of the L-carnitine effect on ceramide generation either in Hut78 or U937 cells induced after 10 minutes from addition of anti-Fas mAb.

## EFFECT OF L-CARNITINE ON FAS CROSSLINKING-INDUCED ACIDIC AND NEUTRAL SMASES

Ceramide may be generated:[25] (a) through activation of ceramide synthase, also known as sphinganine N-acyl transferase, which catalyzes the condensation of sphinganine and fatty acyl-coenzyme A to form dihydroceramide, which is rapidly oxidized to form ceramide; (b) by hydrolysis of sphingomyelin, catalized by sphingomyelinase, a sphingomyelin-specific phospholipase C, yielding ceramide and phosphorylcholine. Two classes of sphingomyelinase, defined by their optimal pHs, have been iden-

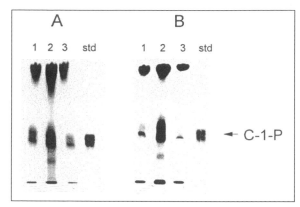

Fig. 5.3. TLC analysis of labelled reaction products of DAG-kinase assay. One representative out of three experiments is shown. Lane 1: untreated cells; lane 2: cells treated with anti-Fas mAb; lane 3: cells treated with anti-Fas mAb in the presence of L-carnitine which was added to cell culture 1 hr before the addition of stimulus; Std: ceramide authentic standard.

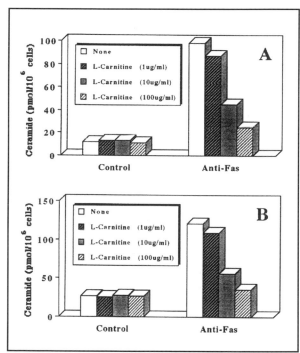

Fig. 5.4. Effect of L-carnitine at the indicated doses on ceramide generation from Hut78 (A) and U937 (B) cells after Fas crosslinking. The cells were treated with L-carnitine 1 hr before addition of anti-Fas mAb (200 ng/ml). The results are expressed as pmol/$10^6$ cells. One representative out of two experiments is shown.

tified: an acidic isoform (pH optimum about pH 5), and two forms with neutral pH optima. Our previous observations (unpublished) indicated that no ceramide synthase activity was induced after Fas-crosslinking. Therefore, we investigated the effect of L-carnitine on acidic and neutral SMase activation which followed Fas-crosslinking in Hut78 or U937 cells (Fig. 5.5). Cellular extracts from Hut78 or U937 cells, stimulated for indicated times

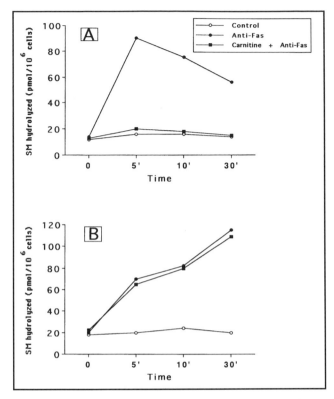

Fig. 5.5. Effect of L-carnitine treatment in vitro on acidic and neutral SMases induced by anti-Fas mAb. Hut78 or U937 cells were stimulated with anti-Fas mAb for different times and cell lysates were then reacted at pH 5.5 or 7.4 with labelled SM vesicles to assay acidic SMase (A), or neutral SMase (B), respectively. After reaction of cell lysates with labeled SM vesicles in the proper buffer, phospholipids were extracted, separated by TLC, and visualized by autoradiography. Radioactive spots (SM) were scraped from the plate and counted by liquid scintillation. Data are expressed as pmoles of SM hydrolyzed/$10^6$ cells. Two different experiments gave similar results.

with anti-Fas mAb were reacted with radiolabeled SM vesicles to detect aSMase or nSMase activation. Both SMases could be detected in extracts from Fas-stimulated cells, as previously shown.[26] Importantly, 60-min pretreatment of cells with L-carnitine (100 μg/ml) prevented Fas-induced SM hydrolysis by aSMase (Fig. 5.5A) but not by nSMase (Fig. 5.5B).

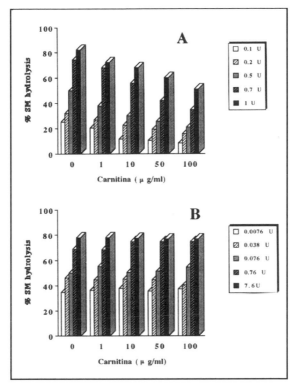

Fig. 5.6. Effect of L carnitine on purified acidic (A) or neutral (B) SMases. Different doses of L-carnitine were added to the SMase assay system in the presence of various amounts of enzymes, as described in Materials and Methods section. Data are expressed as % SM hydrolyzed. Two different experiments gave similar results.

## EFFECTS OF L-CARNITINE ON PURIFIED ACIDIC AND NEUTRAL SMASES IN VITRO

To establish whether L-carnitine was able to directly influence acidic or neutral SMases, we tested both enzyme activities in the presence of the drug. Different amounts of enzymes were added to the SMase assay system in substitution of cellular sonicates in the presence or absence of different concentrations of L-carnitine. Surprisingly, acidic SMase was inhibited in a dose dependent way by L-carnitine, as reported in Fig. 5.6A. Under our experimental conditions, no loss of nSMase activity was detected in the presence of L-carnitine up to 100 µg/ml (Fig. 5.6B), supporting the results obtained in the cell systems. Concerning the inhibition of aSMase, the residual

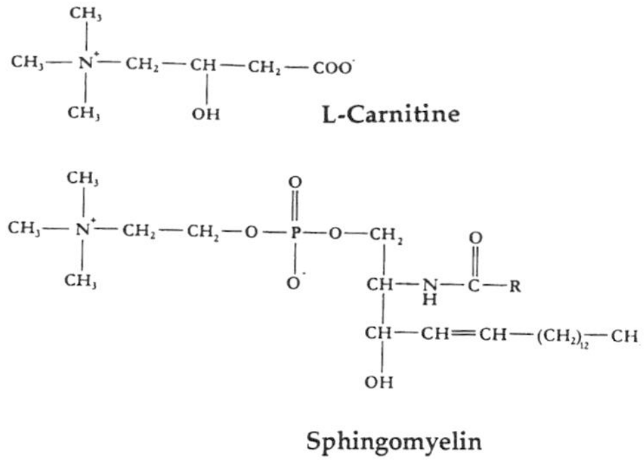

Fig. 5.7. Chemical structures of L-carnitine and sphingomyelin. The identity between the left parts of molecules is evident.

activity decreased proportionally to the added L-carnitine, thus indicating a probable competition between substrate and drug.

## DISCUSSION

Ceramide generation from sphingomyelin hydrolysis occurs via the action of a sphingomyelin-specific form of phospholipase C, a sphingomyelinase, which might initiate signaling leading to programmed cell death in response to ionizing radiation, activation of Fas or TNF receptor or antineoplastic drugs.[14-16,26-28] Sphingomyelinase exists in two forms: a membrane-bound or a cytosolic variant of the neutral sphingomyelinase with a neutral pH optimum and a lysosomal acidic form.[29,30] Nevertheless, the acidic sphingomyelinase, rather than nSMase, has been implicated in generating ceramide relevant to mediation of Fas-induced apoptosis, even if both these enzymes are activated after Fas-crosslinking.[14,26] Deficiences in acidic enzyme are the underlying causes for Niemann-Pick disease A and B.[31,32]

We have previously shown that short-term treatment of AIDS patients with high-dosage L-carnitine via the intravenous route resulted in a substantial reduction of the frequency of CD4 and CD8 cells undergoing apoptosis, as well as the levels of cell-associated ceramide (submitted). In the present work we investigated the effects of L-carnitine in vitro on apoptosis and ceramide production of Fas-sensitive cell lines (Hut78 and U937) after Fas cross linking. Our data indicate that L-carnitine was able to inhibit Fas-induced apoptosis of these cells, likely by preventing in a dose-dependent way the ceramide generation through the inhibition of the aSMase, whereas Fas-activated nSMase did not seem to be significantly influenced by L-carnitine treatment. The mechanisms underlying the inhibitory effect of L-carnitine on aSMase activity have been investigated. In vitro data support the possibility that L-carnitine interferes with the Fas-induced apoptotic event by inhibiting the enzymatic activity of acidic SMase. To assess whether the effects of this drug were specific on SMases, we analyzed its influence on purified acidic and neutral SMase activities in vitro. Experiments designed to assay the effects of L-carnitine on purified SMases indeed show evidence that this drug, which did not affect neutral SMase activity, was able to directly inhibit acidic enzyme in a dose-dependent manner. The inhibitory effect of L-carnitine on purified aSMase was maximally 30-40% even at drug doses which were able to totally inhibit enzymatic activity in the cells. This apparent discrepancy could be explained with the possible transformation of L-carnitine in acyl-carnitines inside the cell.[33] Indeed, our preliminary experiments designed to assess the effects of several carnitine analogs and derivates, suggest that acyl-carnitines are most effective in inhibiting aSMase both in the cells and in the purified enzyme system (manuscript in preparation). The structural basis for the L-carnitine inhibition is still unknown; however, one can speculate that similarities between the carnitine and sphingomyelin (see Fig. 5.7) allow it to be recognized as substrate (or transition state or product) analog by acidic sphingomyelinase. With regard to the inability of L-carnitine to affect neutral SMase either in the cellular extracts or in a purified enzyme system, the different ionization state of the drug depending on pH (inner salt at pH 7.0; positively charged at pH 5.0) could be responsible for the obtained results. The presence at acidic pH of the $(CH_3)_3N^+$ group (present also in the sphingomyelin structure) could facilitate the interaction of L-carnitine with acidic SMase. Computer molecular modeling studies and different kinds of probes are needed to support our hypothesis.

REFERENCES

1. Itoh N, Nagata S. A novel protein domain required for apoptosis: mutational analysis of human Fas antigen. J Biol Chem 1993; 268: 10932-10937.
2. Oehm A, Behrmann I, Falk W, Pawlita M, Maier G, Klas C, Li-Weber M, Richards S, Dhein J, Trauth BC, Ponstingl H, Krammer PH. Purification and molecular cloning of the APO-1 cell surface antigen, a member of the tumor-necrosis factor/nerve growth factor receptor superfamily: sequence identity with the Fas antigen. J Biol Chem 267:10709-10715.
3. Watanabe-Fukunaga R, Brannan CI, Itoh N et al. The cDNA structure, expression and chromosomal assignment of the mouse Fas antigen. J Immunol 148:1274-1279.
4. Nagata S, Golstein P. The Fas death factor. Science 1995; 267: 1449-1456.
5. Suda T, Takahashi T, Golstein P, Nagata S. Molecular cloning and expression of the Fas ligand: a novel member of the tumor necrosis factor family. Cell 1993; 75:1169-1178.

6. Gill BM, Nishikata H, Chan G et al. Fas antigen and sphingomyelin-ceramide turnover-mediated signaling: Role in life and death of T lymphocytes. Immunol Rev 1994; 142:113-125.

7. Clerici M, Hakim FT, Venzon DJ et al. Changes in interleukin-2 and interleukin-4 production in asymptomatic, human immunodeficiency virus-seropositive individuals. J Clin Invest 1993; 91:759-765.

8. Katsikis PD, Wunderlich ES, Smith CA et al. Fas antigen stimulation induces marked apoptosis of T lymphocytes in human immunodeficiency virus-infected individuals. J Exp Med 1995; 181: 2029-2036.

9. Andrieu J-M, Lu W. Viro-immunopathogenesis of HIV disease: implications for therapy. Immunol Today 1995; 16:5-7.

10. Debatin K-M, Fahrig-Faissner A, Enenkel-Stoodt S et al. High expression of APO-1 (CD95) on T lymphocytes from human immunodeficiency virus-1-infected children. Blood 1994; 83:3101-3103.

11. Ramsdell F, Seaman SM, Miller RE et al. Differential ability of T(h)1 and T(h)2 T cells to express fas ligand and to undergo activation-induced cell death. Int Immunol 1994; 6:1545-1553.

12. Clerici M, Shearer GM. The Th1-Th2 hypothesis of HIV infection: new insights. Immunol. Today 1994; 15:575-581.

13. Westerndorp MO, Frank R, Ochsenbauer C et al. Sensitization of T cells to CD95-mediated apoptosis by HIV-1 Tat and gp120. Nature 1995; 375:497-500.

14. Cifone MG, De Maria R, Roncaioli P et al. Apoptotic signaling through CD95 (Fas/Apo-1) activates an acidic sphingomyelinase. J Exp Med 1994; 177:1547-1552.

15. Obeid LM, Linardic CM, Karolak LA, Hannun YA. Programmed cell death induced by ceramide. Science 1993; 259:1769-1771.

16. Jarvis WD, Kolesnick RN, Fornari FA et al. Induction of apoptotic damage and cell death by activation of the sphingomyelin pathway. Proc Natl Acad Sci USA 1994; 91:73-77.

17. Van Veldhoven PP, Matthews JJ, Bolognesi DP, Bell RM. Changes in bioactive in lipids alkylacylglycerol and ceramide, occur in HIV-infected cells. Biochem Biophys Res Commun 1992; 187:209-216.

18. Rivas CI, Golde DW, Vera JC, Kolesnick RN. Involvement of the sphingomyelin pathway in TNF signaling for HIV production in chronically infected HL-60 cells. Blood 1993; 83:2191-2197.

19. Papp B, Zhang D, Groopman JE, Byrn RA. Stimulation of human immunodeficiency virus type 1 expression ceramide. AIDS Res Human Retrov 1994; 10:775-780.

20. Venable ME, Lee JY, Smyth MJ et al. Obeid role of ceramide in cellular senescence. J Biol Chem 1995; 270:30701-30708.

21. Kundu M, Srinivasan A, Pomerantz RJ, Khalili K. Evidence that a cell cycle regulator, E2F1, down-regulates transcriptional activity of the human immunodeficiency virus type 1 promoter. J Virol 1995; 69:6940-6946.

22. De Simone C, Cifone MG, Roncaioli P et al. Ceramide, AIDS and long-term survivors. Immunol Today 1996; 17:48.

23. Rosl F. A simple and rapid method for detection of apoptosis in human cells. Nucleic Acids Res 1992; 20:5243.

24. Preiss J, Loomis CR, Bishop WR et al. Quantitative measurement of sn-1,2-diacylglycerols present in platelets, hepatocytes and ras- and sis-transformed normal rat kidney cells. J Biol Chem 1986; 261: 8597-8600.

25. Spiegel S, Foster D, Kolesnick R. Signal transduction through lipid second messengers. Curr Op Biol 1996; 8:159-167.

26. Cifone MG, Roncaioli P, De Maria R et al. Multiple pathways originate at the Fas/APO-1 (CD95) receptor: sequential involvement of phosphatidylcholine-specific phospholipase C and acidic sphingomyelinase in the propagation of the apoptotic signal. EMBO J 1995; 14:5859-5868.

27. Kolesnick R, Fuks Z. Ceramide: A signal for apoptosis or mitogenesis. J Exp Med 1995; 181:1949-1952.

28. Bose R, Verheij M, Haimovitz-Friedman A et al. Ceramide synthase mediates daunorubicin-induced apoptosis: an alternative mechanism for generating death signals. Cell 1995; 82:405-414.

29. Wiegmann K, Schtzen S, Machleidt T et al. Functional dichotomy of neutral and acidic sphingomyelinases in tumor necrosis factor signaling. Cell, 1994; 78:1005-1015.

30. Schuchman EH, Suchi M, Takahahi T et al. Human acid sphingomyelinase. J Biol Chem 1991; 266:8531-8539.

31. Otterbach B, Stoeffel W. Acid sphingomyelinase-deficient mice mimic the neurovisceral form of human lysosomal storage disease (Niemann-Pick disease). Cell 1995; 81:1053-1061.

32. Horinouchi K, Erlich S, Perl DP et al. Acid sphingomyelinase deficient mice: A model of types A and B Niemann-Pick disease. Nature Genet 1995; 10:288-293.

33. Hoppel C. The physiological role of carnitine. In: Ferrari R, DiMauro S, Sherwood G, eds. L-Carnitine and its role in medicine. Academic Press, 1992: 5-19.

# CHAPTER 6

# Carnitine Deficiency: Primary and Secondary Syndromes

Giuseppe Famularo, Franco Matricardi, Eleonora Nucera,
Gino Santini, Claudio De Simone

## INTRODUCTION

Emerging literature has shown that carnitine deficiency may be frequently recognized in human and the list of disorders associated with carnitine deficiency is growing.

A considerable expansion in our understanding of the molecular metabolism of carnitine has led to the unequivocal demonstration that carnitine loss is the central pathogenic mechanism in the rare syndromes of primary carnitine deficiency, fully explaining the metabolic abnormalities and the clinical course of these subjects. Low levels of carnitine have been shown to be associated with many other acquired disorders, but whether the changes in carnitine levels observed in these subjects are impressive clinically remains to be fully established. It is attractive to speculate that carnitine supplementation may have significant implications for therapy in many diseases, including those recently recognized such as AIDS or chronic fatigue syndrome. However, progress toward these goals awaits the complete elucidation of the function of this molecule in the cellular metabolism under both normal conditions and in diseases.

## CARNITINE METABOLISM

Carnitine, 3-hydroxy-4-N-trimethyl-aminobutyric acid, is present in all tissues and acts as an essential cofactor in the system that transports long-chain fatty acids across the inner mitochondrial membrane, where they undergo $\beta$-oxidation and energy production[1,2]

Carnitine is obtained mainly from the diet, the major sources being red meat, poultry, fish and dairy products. Variable amounts, ranging from

*Carnitine Today,* edited by Claudio De Simone and Giuseppe Famularo.
© 1997 Landes Bioscience.

15 to 87% of ingested carnitine, are actively transported through the small intestine to systemic circulation.[1,2] However, carnitine is also synthesized in liver, brain, and kidney from protein-bound lysine and methionine, the final synthetic step occurring in the liver.[1,2] Remarkably, the amount of absorbed carnitine may modify the extent of synthesis of carnitine. Skeletal muscles and myocardium cannot synthesize carnitine and are, therefore, entirely dependent on carnitine uptake from the blood.[1,2]

The transport of carnitine into tissues is against a concentration gradient, which allows tissue carnitine concentrations to be 20- to 50-fold higher than plasma levels.[1,2] This active uptake is performed by specific transporters; additionally, different functional systems for carnitine uptake, with varying affinity for carnitine, have been described.[1,2]

Normal values for plasma carnitine levels have been established for all age groups (approximately 25 μmol/L during infancy and 54 μmol/L in old age) but females have lower levels than males.[1,2]

Carnitine distribution in major tissues is shown in Table 6.1. Several factors, such as sex hormones and the glucagon to insulin ratio, may impact on carnitine distribution and levels in tissues.[1,2] Skeletal muscles contain more than 90% of total body carnitine, whereas only 1.6% of total body carnitine is contained in liver and kidney and 0.6% in extracellular fluids.[1,2] Carnitine concentration in the brain is relatively low (approximately 10% of the heart, skeletal muscle and liver concentrations), though brain is one of the few tissues capable of endogenous biosynthesis.[1,2] Interestingly, neuromediators may affect both uptake and distribution of carnitine in the brain.[3]

Carnitine in tissues and extracellular fluids is present as either free carnitine or carnitine esters (acylcarnitines).[1,2] In plasma, acylcarnitines account for approximately 10 to 15% of the total pool and most plasma acylcarnitines are present as acetyl-carnitine.[1,2] Remarkably, the proportion of esterified carnitines may vary greatly with nutritional conditions, exercise and disease states.

Carnitine is not degraded except by some type of intestinal bacteria and is excreted in the urine as either free carnitine or acylcarnitin.[1,2] The proximal renal tubule reabsorbs more than 90% of filtered carnitine at normal plasma concentrations.[1,2] In urine, free carnitine generally accounts for approximately 75% of the total carnitine and acylcarnitines are represented by a relatively large amount of acetyl-carnitine and small amounts of other acylcarnitines.[1,2] However, the reported urinary levels of carnitine are highly variable, though this variability may be due in part to the circadian nature of excretion.[1,2]

**Table 6.1. Carnitine concentrations in human tissues**

| Tissue | Carnitine Level (nmol/g wet weight) |
| --- | --- |
| Skeletal muscle | 1140 -3940 |
| Myocardium | 610 -1300 |
| Kidney | 330 - 600 |
| Liver | 500 -1000 |
| Brain | 500 -1000 |

## FUNCTIONS OF CARNITINE

Carnitine is crucial to the shuttle of long-chain fatty acids across the inner mitochondrial membrane and controls the rates of beta-oxidation of long-chain fatty acids, thus playing a pivotal role in energy metabolism. As a consequence, alterations in carnitine metabolism or levels may substantially affect energy production in mitochondria.[1,2]

Normally, long-chain fatty acids are released by lipolysis and cross into the mitochondria through a series of steps. The initial step is the activation of the fatty acid to coenzyme A (CoA) in the cytosol to form fatty acyl-CoA. Once activated, the fatty acyl-CoA cannot cross into the mitochondria until transferred by carnitine. It is now recognized that the transport of activated long-chain fatty acids into the mitochondria is under the control of at least three different proteins: carnitine palmitoyltransferase I, acylcarnitine translocase, and carnitine palmitoyltransferase II.[1,2] Carnitine palmitoyltransferase I catalyzes the transfer of the fatty acid moiety from long-chain fatty acyl-CoA to carnitine and this is the rate-limiting step for beta-oxidation of fatty acids. The second step is the transport of long-chain acylcarnitine from the outside to the inside of the mitochondrial membrane. This is catalyzed by the mitochondrial acylcarnitine translocase that allows the transfer of one long-chain acylcarnitine molecule into the mitochondria and the export of one molecule of free carnitine or acylcarnitine out of the mitochondria. Once the long-chain acylcarnitine molecule reaches the mitochondrial matrix, it is again transferred to CoA via carnitine palmitoyltransferase II. The long-chain acyl-CoA molecule that is formed is then ready to undergo beta oxidation and coupling of beta-oxidation, with the electron transport pathway within the mitochondria leads to the formation of chemical energy. Carnitine released in the matrix of the mitochondria can return to the cytosol via carnitine acyltranslocase.

Due to the reversible transesterification of the acyl-CoAs with carnitine and the fact that acylcarnitine can cross the mitochondrial membrane, the intramitochondrial relationship between acyl-CoA and free CoA is reflected in the extramitochondrial acylcarnitine to free carnitine ratio.[1,2] This acylcarnitine to free carnitine ratio is very sensitive to changes in mitochondrial metabolism. It is considered normal when it is 0.25 and abnormal when it is greater than 0.4; this state is referred to as carnitine insufficiency, and indicates that more carnitine is needed to handle any increased need for the production of acylcarnitines.[1,2]

Carnitine also has other functions which involve the following areas: 1) carnitine provides a route for removal of poorly metabolized, potentially toxic acyl-CoAs to prevent CoA sequestration, thus maintaining adequate cellular concentrations of free and esterified CoA; 2) acetyl-carnitine is probably a storage form of energy for the cell, at least in sperm and macrophages; 3) peroxisomes contain a carnitine acetyltransferase and a carnitine octanoyltransferase that use long-chain fatty acids and these two transferases seem to be involved in the oxidation of fatty acids by these organelles in addition, there is a long-chain carnitine transferase located in the endoplasmic reticulum whose function is still unknown; and 4) carnitine stabilizes cell membranes and enhances calcium transport.[1,2]

The influences of carnitine on fatty acid and intermediary metabolism have been shown to be mediated, either directly or indirectly, by reactions catalyzed by specific carnitine acyltransferases that are under exquisite forms of regulation.[1,2] This regulation is not completely understood; for example, the inhibition of carnitine palmitoyltransferase by malonyl CoA is being actively investigated. To understand the basis for the therapeutic aspects of carnitine actions, it is important that this area be fully elucidated.

## CARNITINE DEFICIENCY IN HUMANS

Carnitine deficiency was first recognized as a cause of human disease in the early 1970s.[4,5] Since then, many different kinds of carnitine deficiency syndromes, impairments in fatty acid oxidation and lipid storage myopathy have been discovered. In patients suffering from impaired carnitine transport, cardiac myopathy has proven particularly responsive to carnitine therapy. In other types of carnitine deficiency, carnitine has sometimes been beneficial as a therapeutic agent, but further progress in this area is needed to fully understand the role of endogenous carnitine in the pathogenesis of various disorders and the role of exogenous carnitine in the therapy of those conditions.

Carnitine deficiency is defined as a state of carnitine concentration in plasma or tissues that is below the requirement for the normal function of the organism. In clinical practice, plasma levels are commonly used to diagnose carnitine deficiency and levels less than 2 $\mu$mol/L, in all age groups, are usually considered deficient.[4,5] These values, though, do not closely mirror the carnitine concentrations in tissues.[1,2]

Carnitine requirements depend on many factors, such as age, diet, tissue dependence on beta-oxidation of fatty acids for energy metabolism, and metabolic conditions (stress, fed versus fasting and rest versus exercise) and the balance between requirements and levels in tissues determines the metabolic and clinical impact of reduced concentrations of carnitine. Remarkably, in most conditions tissue carnitine levels may have to fall to less than 10% to 20% of the normal range before the metabolic effects can be recognized under clinical standards.[4,5]

Both primary carnitine deficiencies and secondary carnitine deficiencies have been identified (Table 6.2).

## PRIMARY CARNITINE DEFICIENCIES

These disorders are characterized by a decrease of intracellular carnitine content that impairs fatty acid oxidation and that is not associated with another identifiable systemic illness that might deplete tissue carnitine.[4,5]

Even though earlier reports have been somewhat conflicting and many cases have been reclassified, there is now consensus about the criteria to define primary carnitine deficiency: a) the metabolic disorder is caused directly by inadequate carnitine levels, as shown by reduced concentrations in plasma or tissues or both; b) fatty acid oxidation is impaired; c) the metabolic disorder is corrected when normal carnitine concentrations are restored; d) there is no evidence of other primary defects in intramitochondrial beta-oxidation (Table 6.3).

The exclusion of other defects in fatty acid oxidation is essential for the diagnosis of primary carnitine deficiency and is supported by the absence of an abnormal dicarboxylic aciduria characteristically seen in defects of fatty acid oxidation with secondary carnitine deficiency. The relevance of an early recognition of this potentially lethal disorder is highlighted by the exquisite response to carnitine therapy that in most cases results in a favorable outcome of an otherwise lethal disorder.

Depending on tissue distribution of low carnitine levels, primary carnitine deficiencies have been subdivided into systemic and myopathic forms.[4,5] In the systemic form, there is a profound reduction of carnitine levels in plasma and even in most tissues, whereas in the myopathic form the low content is usually restricted to the skeletal muscles.[4,5] In addition, a subset of subjects with primary systemic carnitine deficiency have a severe progressive cardiomyopathy leading to life-threatening heart failure.[4,5] The clinical and biochemical criteria to fit a patient in the category of primary carnitine deficiencies are shown in Table 6.4.

**Table 6.2. Primary and secondary carnitine deficiency: causes**

Primary Carnitine Deficiency
  Systemic carnitine deficiency
  Myopathic carnitine deficiency
  Progressive cardiomyopathy with systemic
  carnitine deficiency

Secondary Carnitine Deficiency
  Genetically determined metabolic errors
    Fatty acid oxidation disorders
      Carnitine cycle
        Carnitine palmitoyltransferase I
        Translocase
        Carnitine palmitoyltransferase II
        (infantile and adult form)
      Beta-oxidation cycle
        Acyl-CoA dehydrogenases
          Short-chain acyl-CoA dehydrogenase
          Medium-Chain acyl-CoA dehydrogenase
          Long-chain acyl-CoA dehydrogenase
          Very-long chain acyl-CoA dehydrogenase
          Multiple acyl-CoA dehydrogenases
          (Severe, mild, and riboflavin-responsive)
        Short-chain 3-hydroxyacyl-CoA dehydrogenase
        Trifunctional protein
        2,4-dienoyl-CoA reductase
    Branched-chain amino acid disorders
      Isovaleric acidemia
      Propionic acidemia
      Methylmalonic acidemia
      3-Methylcrotonyl-CoA carboxylase deficiency
      3-Methyl-glutaconic aciduria
      3-Hydroxymethylglutaryl-CoA lyase deficiency
      2-Methylacetoacetyl-CoA thiolase deficiency
    Glutaric aciduria I
    Mitochondrial disorders
      Multiple and isolated respiratory chain deficiencies
    Other genetic defects
      5-Methylene tetrahydrofolate reductase deficiency
      Adenosine deaminase deficiency
      Ornithine transcarbamilase deficiency
      Carbamoylphosphate synthase I deficiency
    Dysgenetic syndromes
      Williams-Beuren syndrome
      Ruvalcaba-Myhre-Smith syndrome

**Table 6.2. Primary and secondary carnitine deficiency: causes (continued)**

Acquired conditions
    Decreased synthesis
        Cirrhosis
        Chronic renal disease
        Extreme prematurity
    Decreased intake
        Chronic total parenteral nutrition
        Malnutrition
        Lacto-ovovegetarians and strict vegetarians
        Soy protein infant formula without added L-carnitine
        Malabsorption (cystic fibrosis, short-gut syndrome,
            celiac disease)
    Decreased body stores/increased requirements
        Pregnant and lactating women
            Extreme prematurity
            Intrauterine growth retardation
            Infant of carnitine-deficient mother
            Critically ill patients (increased catabolism)
            (cachexia, cancer, surgery, trauma, burns, thermal
                injury, starvation, overexcretion)
            Sepsis
    Increased loss
        Fanconi Syndrome
        Renal tubular acidosis
        Hemodialysis and peritoneal dialysis
        Hyperthyroidism
    Adaptative mechanism
        Heart failure
            Dilated cardiomyopathy
            Ischemic heart disease
            Myocarditis
            Diptheria
            Valvular heart disease
            Hypertension
            Diabetes
    Mitochondrial dysfunctions
        AIDS
        Chronic fatigue syndrome
        Idiopathic inflammatory myopathies
        Drugs

Pathophysiology

Intracellular carnitine deficiency hinders the entry of long-chain fatty acids into the mitochondrial matrix and less or no long-chain substrates are available for beta-oxidation and energy production. The modulation of intramitochondrial free CoA is also impaired, causing increased acyl-CoA esters in the mitochondria and affecting pathways of intermediary metabolism that require CoA (Krebs cycle, pyruvate oxidation, amino acid oxidation, and mitochondrial and peroxisomal beta oxidation). In addition, due to the low carnitine content in the liver, reduced ketone body production during fasting and hypoglycemia frequently occur, as energy utilization depends almost completely on carbohydrates.

A defect involving the transport of carnitine from plasma to cells in affected tissues appears to play a pivotal pathogenic role.[4,5] It has been demonstrated in cultured fibroblasts from these subjects and, although conclusive data are not available, this defect probably affects most tissues.[4,5] The excessive urinary excretion of carnitine also suggests a defect in the renal transport of carnitine and the low and delayed plasma response to orally administered carnitine observed in one patient indicates an intestinal transport defect as well.[4,5] In contrast, carnitine uptake in liver is not affected. No evidence of defective biosynthesis or excessive degradation has so far been reported in these patients.[4,5]

Animal models, such as mice with juvenile visceral steatosis, are now being developed to provide highly reductive data for investigating the biochemical and metabolic features, even at the molecular level, of systemic carnitine deficiency.[6] These mice have microvesicular liver steatosis, hypoglycemia, hyperammonemia, cardiac hypertrophy, and growth retardation that show a good response to carnitine therapy. Carnitine levels are

---

*Table 6.3. Criteria defining syndromes of primary carnitine deficiency*

- The disorder is caused directly by inadequate carnitine levels in plasma or tissues or both

- Subjects have impaired fatty acid oxidation

- The metabolic abnormalities are corrected when carnitine concentrations are restored to the normal values

- Primary defects of intramitrochondrial beta-oxidation have been ruled out

low in blood and tissues and a strongly reduced transport of carnitine has been shown in the kidney. Furthermore, a generalized mitochondrial abnormality parallels the degree of carnitine deficiency.[6]

## Clinical manifestations

Failure to thrive, recurrent respiratory infections, and recurrent attacks resembling hypoglycemia are commonly observed. The mean age of onset is 2 years, with onset ranging from 1 month to 7 years of age, and no sex predominance has been recognized. However, these subjects are normal at birth and may appear healthy for many years.

Three different types of presentations have been reported: progressive cardiomyopahy, hypoketotic hypoglycemic encephalopathy, and skeletal myopathy, but all forms of presentation can be observed in the same family.[4,5]

Progressive cardiomyopathy is the most common form of onset and usually develops at an older age. The resulting heart failure poorly responds to general treatment and, if carnitine deficiency is not early recognized and carnitine supplementation not administered, irreversible heart failure ensues, leading to death.[4,5] In a few patients, myocardial carnitine concentrations have been measured with levels below 5% of normal range.[4,5]

Acute encephalopathy with hypoketotic hypoglycemia and reduced consciousness is more commonly seen in younger infants but these subjects also have cardiac involvement. The acute metabolic episodes are triggered by viral illnesses associated with vomiting or reduced oral intake or change to a diet poor in carnitine. If no carnitine replacement is given, patients suffer recurrent episodes of encephalopathy.[4,5]

Hepatomegaly is common and liver biopsy demonstrates fatty infiltration and low carnitine content. Glucose and ketone bodies are inappropriately low; transaminases and ammonia are moderately elevated and

---

*Table 6.4. Criteria to classify a patient in the primary carnitine deficiencies*

Clinical data
- Muscle weakness
- Episodes of hypoketotic coma
- Cardiomyopathy
- Hepatomegaly

Biochemical data
- Low carnitine concentrations in plasma, liver and skeletal muscle
- Impaired carnitine uptake by fibroblasts

metabolic acidosis, prolonged prothrombin time, and elevated creatine kinase may be found.[4,5]

Skeletal myopathy is also observed in these patients, with mild motor delay, hypotonia, or slowly progressive proximal weakness. The biopsy of skeletal muscles shows very low carnitine concentrations and fatty infiltration.[4,5]

Cognitive delay and dysfunction of the central nervous system may develop, probably resulting from the hypoglycemia due to the reduced glucose consumption in the later stages of fasting, when ketone bodies generated from hepatic fatty acid oxidation become limited as a source of energy. Peripheral nerve dysfunction can also occur in these patients.[4,5]

Gastrointestinal manifestations, including recurrent abdominal pain, vomiting, diarrhea and gastro oesophageal reflux, have been observed; remarkably, carnitine deficiency has been recently shown to cause gastrointestinal dysmotility.[7] Pyloric stenosis has also been observed.[4,5]

A few patients may have a mild to moderate hypochromic anemia, but red cell features are variable.[4,5] The pathogenesis remains to be fully established even though it has been suggested that carnitine regulates the lipid metabolism in red blood cells and may protect them from membrane damage by toxic fatty acyl-CoA derivatives.[4,5]

## Diagnosis

The levels of carnitine are exceedingly low (usually less than 10% of the normal concentrations) in plasma, skeletal muscle, liver, and myocardium, and acylcarnitines are proportionately reduced, thus explaining the normal acylcarnitine to free carnitine ratio.[4,5] However, a few patients may have acylcarnitines in the normal or even the high range and the acylcarnitine to free carnitine ratio is high.[4,5] The urinary excretion of carnitine is increased in most cases, with fractional excretion of free carnitine exceeding 100% of the filtered load.[4,5] No abnormal organic acids are found in the urine and this is crucial to the differential diagnosis with intramitochondrial fatty acid disorders.[4,5]

The diagnosis is easy when laboratory evidence of carnitine deficiency in plasma and tissues parallels the clinical presentation. The assay of carnitine uptake shows negligible transport in cultured fibroblasts, allowing definitive diagnosis.[4,5] Interestingly, the parents of these patients have moderately low or normal plasma carnitine levels and, when carnitine transport is investigated in fibroblasts, they show intermediate values of uptake, suggesting an autosomal recessive pattern of inheritance.[4,5] A symptomatic heterozygote with myocardial and skeletal muscle involvement has been described.[4,5]

The family history is also useful in order to focus on this disorder. Several patients have an antecedent of a sibling deceased because of cardiac disease or sudden death. When tissues of these siblings have been investigated, fatty infiltration of liver and myocardium and reduced levels of carnitine have frequently been found. Furthermore, consanguinity has been reported in some families.[4,5]

## Treatment

Most patients improve significantly with L-carnitine therapy.[4,5] The mainstay of treatment is oral carnitine at daily doses of 100 to 200 mg/kg. At this dose carnitine is able to reach the systemic circulation by passive diffusion through the intestine. Variable plasma levels are achieved and carnitine concentrations increase slightly in the skeletal muscles, whereas they return to normal values in the liver.[4,5] However, the evaluation of therapy efficacy should be based on clinical parameters rather than on carnitine levels, since improvement in expected characteristics of the patients is generally more important than simply achieving a certain level of carnitine or a specific ratio of acylcarnitine to free carnitine in plasma or tissues. The intravenous route may have advantages in initiating treatment when high peak concentrations are required in order for carnitine to reach tissues other than the liver, or when oral carnitine therapy is not feasible due to poor compliance or tolerance. On carnitine treatment metabolic crises disappear, fasting ketogenesis is recovered and skeletal muscle strength, myocardial function and growth significantly improve.[4,5] No severe side effects related to carnitine therapy have been observed, but a few patients may have intermittent diarrhea and fishy body odor.[4,5] However, as a rule a short-term reduction in the dosage of carnitine dispels these inconveniences. Carnitine supplementation of these subjects should be considered under stress conditions such as viral illnesses, fasting and vomiting, even in the absence of clinical symptoms of carnitine deficiency.

MYOPATHIC CARNITINE DEFICIENCY

## Pathophysiology

No definitive biochemical defect has been recognized. Investigations of cultured skeletal myocytes at different stages of differentiation have shown changes in the kinetic properties of carnitine transport system, suggesting the existence of a skeletal muscle-specific carnitine transporter that gradually develops during myogenesis and is eventually fully expressed in the adult tissue.[4] It has been speculated that a defect in this developmentally regulated carrier is the cause of primary myopathic carnitine deficiency.[4,5] Other studies failed to show any defect of carnitine uptake in cultured myoblasts, demonstrating instead a faster rate of carnitine efflux.[4]

Myocardium and skeletal muscles may be affected together, but isolated myocardial carnitine deficiency has been reported in a family with
normal carnitine levels in plasma and skeletal muscles,[4,5] probably reflecting an inborn myocardium-specific defect in the transport for carnitine.

The existence of a primary carnitine deficiency syndrome affecting
only the skeletal muscle has been somewhat questioned. In fact, it may be
exceedingly difficult to discriminate between myopathic and systemic carnitine deficiency syndrome because in most cases tissues other than the
skeletal muscle, such as liver or myocardium, are not available for measurement of carnitine levels. In addition, the genetic defects of beta-oxidation
often closely resemble primary myopathic carnitine deficiency under clinical
standpoints. Short-chain acyl-CoA dehydrogenase deficiency has been found
in cultured fibroblasts from one patient with the myopathic form of carnitine deficiency and this has suggested that other fatty acid oxidation defects, either generalized or tissue-specific, may contribute to the pathogenesis of this disorder.[4] Several factors support this view: a) fatty acid oxidation defects have not been definitively ruled out in many cases reported in
the literature; b) carnitine concentrations in liver and myocardium have
not been measured in several patients described in the literature; c) a few
patients have little or no response to carnitine therapy; d) many patients
have elevated acyl carnitines in either plasma or skeletal muscles and this
suggests a secondary carnitine deficiency; e) in one patient an increased
urinary excretion of the dicarboxylic acid adipic acid has been found, and
this alteration may be present in several defects of fatty acid oxidation.[4,5]

## Clinical manifestations

Symptoms may appear early in the life but usually they occur during
the 2nd or 3rd decade.[4,5] Patients have progressive weakness of proximal
skeletal muscles of variable degree, paralleled by exercise intolerance, wasting, myalgias, and myoglobinuria.[4,5] Usually, there is no evidence of liver or
heart involvement even though a few patients may present with a
cardiomyopathy leading to heart failure.[4,5] Peripheral nerve involvement
has been also reported.[4,5]

## Diagnosis

Low levels of carnitine are measured in skeletal muscles and accumulation of lipid droplets (skeletal muscle fat infiltration, however, is rare in
infancy) and abnormal mitochondria are found.[4,5] In contrast, the levels of
carnitine are in the normal or even the high range in plasma and other
tissues, such as liver or myocardium.[4,5] Carnitine esters are normal, with no
abnormal excretion of either carnitine or organic acids in the urine.[4,5] The
finding of intermediate levels of carnitine in skeletal muscles of some par-

ents suggests autosomal recessive inheritance.[4,5] A symptomatic heterozygote for systemic carnitine deficiency with low concentrations in the skeletal muscles has been described; this supports the view that a few patients with myopathic carnitine deficiency may actually be heterozygous for the systemic form.[4,5]

## Therapy

The clinical course may improve following carnitine or acetyl-carnitine supplementation.[4,5] However, the response is variable, ranging from moderate improvement to normalization of skeletal muscle strength. Even the increases of carnitine levels in skeletal muscles are variable but, in general, normal concentrations are not completely achieved.[4,5] Relapses are frequent and can be managed by modulating the supplementation therapy.

Patients may profit more from combined therapy with carnitine and corticosteroids.[4,5] It is likely that corticosteroids, in addition to their ability to decrease lipogenesis and promote fatty acid mobilization, have a more specific effect on carnitine transport. Low-fat diet and oils containing medium-chain triglycerides are also useful in the therapeutic strategy.[4,5]

### PROGRESSIVE CARDIOMYOPATHY WITH SYSTEMIC CARNITINE DEFICIENCY

A life-threatening dilated cardiomyopathy which, untreated, has a progressive course eventfully leading to death may be the clinical hallmark of a few patients with systemic carnitine deficiency.[4,5] This is not surprising once it is considered that the impairment of energy production induced by carnitine deficiency has significant consequences for myocardial functioning, as myocardium chiefly relies on aerobic breakdown for energy supply.

In these subjects carnitine levels are markedly low in plasma, myocardium, skeletal muscles and liver, but skeletal muscle and liver dysfunctions are usually subtle.[4,5] Familiar clusters have been observed; in most cases, there is an autosomal recessive inheritance and obligate heterozygotes usually have intermediate levels of carnitine in plasma and skeletal muscle.[4,5]

Models of inherited carnitine deficiency with cardiomyopathy have been described in dogs and Syrian hamsters.[4,5,8] Animals have severe congestive heart failure with severely reduced myocardial carnitine content, and high-dose carnitine therapy improves myocardial function and clinical outcome, paralleling the increase in carnitine levels.[4,5,8] Remarkably, in these models withdrawal of carnitine therapy causes myocardial dysfunction, and clinical signs of heart failure recur.

In humans, the clinical response to carnitine is dramatic and most patients soon recover a normal myocardial function.[4,5]

## SECONDARY CARNITINE DEFICIENCIES

Secondary carnitine deficiencies are much more common than the primary forms and include both genetic and acquired conditions which are associated with a decrease of carnitine levels in plasma or tissues or both (Table 6.2).

### GENETICALLY DETERMINED METABOLIC ERRORS

Carnitine deficiency has been reported in several metabolic disorders, but the most characteristic causes of genetically determined metabolic errors associated with secondary carnitine deficiency are the defects of fatty acid oxidation.[4,5,9]

### Pathophysiology

As fat is the primary source of fuel during prolonged fasting, a defect in this pathway has consequences for virtually all tissues. Tissues which normally use fat, including liver and skeletal muscle, cannot use this fuel effectively and other sources of energy are warranted. Since ketones are not being produced, the only other source of fuel is glucose. As a consequence, glucose cannot be reserved for those tissues strictly dependent on it for energy metabolism, such as brain.

Since fat is mobilized during fasting but cannot be used for energy production, fats enter a variety of alternative pathways, such as storage as intracellular triglyceride, conjugation and excretion as carnitine or glycine esters. Intracellular fatty acyl-CoA compounds that accumulate at or near the site of the metabolic block interfere with many critical pathways, particularly those requiring CoA as a cofactor, and may also interfere with transport systems, including those requiring carnitine as a cofactor. Taken together, all these mechanisms contribute to multiple dysfunctions of tissues requiring fats for their energy metabolism and result in both the accumulation of intracellular fat within these tissues and failure of energy-requiring metabolic pathways.[4,5,9]

Table 6.5 shows the clinical and biochemical abnormalities shared by patients with these enzyme defects. Hypoketotic hypoglycemia is one of the more consistent features, reflecting the impaired fat utilization for fuel metabolism and the accelerated rate of glucose utilization. Increased free fatty acids in the serum provide further evidence of the abnormal fat metabolism and make it possible to rule out other abnormalities, such as hyperinsulinism.

Plasma levels of carnitine are usually reduced to concentrations between 10 and 50% of the normal range; tissue levels have been far less frequently reported but are generally reduced.[4,5,9] In addition, regardless of

---

**Table 6.5. Clinical and biochemical abnormalities in patients with fatty acid oxidation defects**

Clinical data
- Metabolic crises usually following fasting
- Cardiomyopathy
- Skeletal myopathy
- Encephalopathy

Biochemical data
- Hypoketotic hypoplycemia
- Increased serum levels of free fatty acids
- Low levels of tissue and plasma carnitine with increased esterified carnitine
- Dicarboxylic aciduria

---

carnitine concentrations, patients have increased levels of acylcarnitines and a consequent shift in the esterified/free carnitine ratio.[4,5,9]

Accumulated acyl-CoA intermediates react with matrix carnitine to form acylcarnitines that can leave mitochondria through the action of the inner membrane carnitine acylcarnitine translocase and, in contrast to their corresponding acyl-CoAs, are eventually lost from the cell and excreted in the urine. The presence of an intramitochondrial carnitine acetyltransferase, an enzyme with broad specificity for short-chain acyl-CoAs, ensures the formation of the corresponding acylcarnitines and the release of free CoA in these subjects.

The initial loss of intracellular carnitine, in the form of acylcarnitine, would be buffered by free carnitine in plasma. However, due to the continuous formation of acyl-CoAs, when chronic acylcarnitine excretion exceeds the amounts of dietary and endogenously synthesized carnitine, the balance would become negative and ultimately lead to the depletion of carnitine stores in tissues.[4,5,9] Even the low renal threshold for carnitine excretion demonstrated in these subjects contributes to the pathogenesis of carnitine deficiency.[4,5,9] Furthermore, the increased plasma levels of acylcarnitines have been proposed to impair carnitine transport in the tubular cells, further enhancing the urinary loss.[4,5,9]

Specific patterns of urinary acylcarnitines matching the corresponding acyl-CoAs are usually observed in these subjects and this can be a useful tool for the diagnosis of the primary genetic defect.[4,5,9] Even the presence of dicarboxylic acids, the microsomal omega-oxidation products of non-metabolized acyl-CoAs specific for the enzyme defect, is a consistent finding in the urine of affected children during metabolic crises.[4,5,9] Since dicarboxylic acids are also recognized when subjects are fed certain formulas, such as those containing medium-chain triglycerides, or in diabetes, the amounts of these intermediates must be evaluated in relation to the amount of ketones. In these subjects, dicarboxylic acids as a rule significantly exceed the amount of ketones.[4,5,9] Remarkably, the presence of dicarboxylic acids strongly supports the diagnosis of enzyme defect of the beta-oxidation spiral and, in most cases, rules out a defect in fatty acid or carnitine transport.

### Clinical presentation

These disorders have specific clinical and metabolic signatures and appear to be inherited in an autosomal recessive fashion.[4,5,9] The age of onset is variable. Acute metabolic decompensation usually occurs in infancy. Cardiomyopathy and lipid storage skeletal myopathy develop later.

Given the central role of fats in fuel homeostasis during fasting, it is not surprising that children with inborn errors of these pathways are most prone to clinically evident dysfunction during fasting; hence, patients are more likely to be found comatose or unresponsive in the morning after an overnight fast.[4,5,9] Factors which decrease oral intake, such as intercurrent viral illnesses, and increased energy expenditures, such as fever and physical exercise, may result in severe metabolic decompensation. Patients have altered consciousness, sometimes complicated by seizures, apnea or cardiorespiratory arrest. The acute encephalopathy can be accompanied by liver involvement, hypotonia and cardiac dysfunction. Hypoketotic hypoglycemia is characteristic, often paralleled by increased transaminases and ammonia. Metabolic acidosis, elevated serum creatine kinase levels, hyperuricemia, and impaired coagulation may be found. Liver biopsy, if performed during the metabolic crisis, usually shows microvesicular and macrovesicular steatosis. Abnormal organic acids are found in the urine of subjects with defects in the beta-oxidation spiral, but not in patients with carnitine cycle defects.[4,5,9] Failure to thrive and developmental delay may be recognized before the onset of the acute encephalopathy. Less frequent clinical manifestations include cardiac arrythmias, neuropathy, recurrent myo globinuria, pigmentary retinopathy, and renal abnormalities.[4,5,9]

### Carnitine treatment

The role of carnitine therapy in the management of subjects with secondary carnitine deficiency associated with genetically determined metabolic errors has not been so far investigated systematically. However, exogenously administered carnitine buffers the excess of acyl-CoAs which accumulate in the mitochondria as a consequence of the metabolic defects.[4,5,9] Carnitine supplementation may improve the clinical course and reduce both the frequency and severity of metabolic attacks.[4,5,9] In contrast, a few patients continue to suffer acute metabolic attacks despite replacement therapy. Probably these patients require an accurate and meticulous dietary treatment in conjunction with carnitine supplementation.

Most patients treated with carnitine have enhanced excretion of relevant carnitine esters, but whether this reflects increased production through enhanced acyl-CoA oxidation or increased elimination of toxic acyl-CoA intermediates remains to be established. Furthermore, concern has been raised about the use of carnitine replacement therapy in patients with long-chain fatty acid oxidation defects because it promotes long-chain acylcarnitine formation, may result in ventricular arrythmogenesis and membrane dysfunction.[8]

It remains unclear whether carnitine therapy should be started in all cases of secondary carnitine deficiency syndromes associated with inborn metabolic errors, but the insidious nature of the symptoms associated with carnitine insufficiency suggests that replacement therapy should be considered in all subjects with documented low plasma or tissue concentrations. Avoidance of fasting, intake of low-fat meals enriched in carboydrates, and supplementation of riboflavin and glycine are also useful in the management of these patients.[4,5,9]

## Fatty acid oxidation defects

These are the most frequent causes of carnitine deficiency among genetically determined metabolic errors that cause secondary carnitine deficiency. The fatty acid oxidation defects are subdivided into defects of the carnitine cycle for the transport of long-chain fatty acids into the mitochondria and defects of the beta-oxidation spiral that occurs within the mitochondria.[4,5,9] In the next sections, we will discuss in detail the most frequent defects of enzymes of the carnitine cycle and beta-oxidation spiral, the defects of carnitine palmitoyltransferase II and medium-chain acyl-CoA dehydrogenase (MCAD), respectively.

## Carnitine palmitoyltransferase II defect

More than 50 subjects with this defect have been reported.[4,5,9] These subjects usually present in late childhood or early adulthood with recurrent episodes of muscle cramping or myoglobinuria triggered by fasting, exercise or stress; the ketone response to fasting may be delayed.

Carnitine levels in plasma and tissues are commonly in the normal range in these patients.[4,5,9] In contrast, subjects presenting with the severe infantile or neonatal form have low plasma and tissue carnitine levels, paralleled by elevated long chain acylcarnitines.[4,5,9] The outcome is very poor and acute metabolic encephalopathy, cardiomyopathy, arrythmias and renal dysplasias are the most frequent presenting features.[4,5,9]

Carnitine palmitoyltransferase II activity is deficient in fibroblasts, liver, and skeletal muscle. A more severe degree of enzyme deficiency has been reported in subjects with the infantile form compared with the adult form.[4,5,9]

## MCAD defect

More than 100 cases of MCAD defects have been reported.[4,5,9] In Caucasian populations of Northern European origin its frequency has been estimated to be of the order of 1 in 100,00 to 1 in 20,000, but no Japanese or Afroamerican patients with MCAD deficiency have been reported.[4,5,9] In contrast, the other enzyme defects of the beta-oxidation spiral appear not to be related to specific ethnic groups.

These patients have recurrent episodes of hypoglycemic hypoketotic encephalopathy without skeletal muscle or myocardial involvement. Developmental abnormalities, failure to thrive, seizures and cerebral palsy have also been reported. A silent phenotype has been observed, as several asymptomatic cases have been described in families where other individuals had severe symptoms.

Medium-chain dicarboxylic acids are recognized during acute episodes and glycine conjugates (hexanoylglycine, suberylglycine and phenylpropionylglycine) in urine, even when patients are asymptomatic, are found.[4,5,9]

Low levels of plasma and tissue carnitine are measured in more than 90% of patients in the fed state, and the presence in plasma and urine of 6- to 10-carbon saturated and unsaturated acylcarnitines, mainly octanoyl-carnitine, is specific for MCAD deficiency.[4,5,9]

The enzyme deficiency may be demonstrated in cultured fibroblasts, leukocytes, and other tissues (liver, skeletal muscle and myocardium). A point mutation at codon 985 that causes a substitution of a lysine for a glutamate is found in most of the patients.[4,5,9]

## Other genetically determined metabolic errors associated with secondary carnitine deficiency

In addition to defects of the carnitine cycle and defects of the beta-oxidation spiral, yet other genetically determined metabolic errors may be associated with carnitine deficiency.

Subjects with branched-chain amino acid disorders share some metabolic abnormalities with fatty acid oxidation defects due to the block of acyl-CoA oxidation, and low plasma and tissue total carnitine levels, increased acylcarnitine to free carnitine ratios, and excretion of acylcarnitines specifically mirroring the abnormal acyl-CoA species that accumulate at or near the site of the metabolic block are observed.[4,5,9]

In other genetically determined metabolic errors different mechanisms cause carnitine deficiency. For example, subjects with cytochrome c oxidase deficiency leading to impairment of the mitochondrial respiratory chain have an impaired energy-dependent carnitine uptake.[9] This would interfere with carnitine transport, including renal reabsorption in tissues, and may explain the low plasma and tissue levels commonly seen in these patients.

ACQUIRED CONDITIONS

Acquired metabolic conditions, particularly those affecting the liver and kidney, may secondarily affect carnitine homeostasis[4,5] (Table 6.2). Multiple mechanisms may be involved in secondary carnitine deficiency.[4,5] Reduced carnitine synthesis may be associated with extreme prematurity, liver cirrhosis, and chronic renal disease. Decreased carnitine intake due to diets with low carnitine content or parenteral nutrition or decreased reabsorption in malabsorption syndromes, such as celiac disease, may also cause carnitine deficiency. Reduced body stores and increased requirements for carnitine may accompany several clinical conditions, such as pregnancy, prematurity, or increased catabolism in critically ill patients. Excessive renal losses have been associated with Fanconi syndrome and renal tubular acidosis.

In the next sections, we will focus on carnitine deficiency associated with myocardial diseases and heart failure, diabetes, renal failure and hemodialysis, sepsis and drugs.

## MYOCARDIAL DISEASES AND SECONDARY CARNITINE DEFICIENCY

Myocardial carnitine deficiency with metabolic abnormalities in the utilization of long-chain fatty acids has been documented in heart failure, in both experimental models and humans.[8,10,11] Low total and free myocardial carnitine concentrations have been found in myocardial tissue obtained at autopsy, cardiac surgery and right ventricular endomyocardial biopsy in patients with heart failure, regardless of the underlying disease (dilated cardiomyopathy, myocarditis, coronary heart disease, valvular heart disease and hypertension).[8,10,11] Carnitine deficiency appears to represent a non-specific indicator of metabolic stress on the myocardium and should be regarded as a secondary defect or a compensatory mechanism that follows pressure or volume overload. Accordingly, no correlation has been established between the degree of myocardial carnitine loss and the etiology of end-stage heart failure, as subjects with dilated cardiomyopathy and heart failure due to coronary or valvular heart disease or myocarditis do show a comparable degree of myocardial carnitine loss.[8,10,11]

Carnitine loss is homogeneously distributed in the myocardium of the failing heart, even though the reduction of carnitine levels is frequently more pronounced in the left than in the right ventricle.[8,10,11] In an autopsy study of myocardial infarction, severely reduced levels were found in the infarcted zone, intermediate levels in the border zone, and normal concentrations in the remaining healthy myocardial tissue.[8,10,11]

Conversely, the levels of carnitine esters are increased in the myocardium of failing heart and this could have a relevant pathogenetic role, as long-chain acylcarnitines appear to be directly implicated in ventricular arrythmogenesis.[8,10,11]

Changes in the myocardial content of carnitine may be found early in the course of heart failure, as patients with mild impairment of left-ventricular function, with ejection fractions from 30 to 55%, already exhibit significant reductions in myocardial carnitine content.[8,10,11] Furthermore, the lowest myocardial carnitine concentrations are associated with the most severely decreased ejection fraction and the most severe hemodynamic abnormalities,[8,10,11] supporting the view that a greater degree of myocardial carnitine loss implies a worse prognosis in these patients.[8,10,11]

Interestingly, the correlation between myocardial carnitine deficiency and clinical severity of heart failure proved most significant in patients with dilated cardiomyopathy in comparison to subjects with other underlying disorders.[8,10,11] However, a high interindividual variability in the myocardial levels of carnitine has been found in subjects with heart failure and this suggests that many factors, such as the duration and clinical severity of myocardial injury, genetic background, nutritional status, availability of substrates, hormonal regulation and the activation of other compensatory mechanisms, may significantly impact on the degree of carnitine loss. It is likely that either functional or structural injury to the carrier system for myocardial transmembrane carnitine transport leads to the inability to maintain adequate myocardial concentrations. Several factors, such as ischemia, oxidant stress and the unregulated production of cytokines (tumor necrosis factor [TNF]-alpha) may trigger this damage. In turn, since carnitine and its esters take part in the heart antioxidant network and protect myocardium from injury due to ischemia or oxidant stress,[12] a vicious cycle ensues, as carnitine loss may increase the susceptibility of myocardium to injury and this further increases the loss of carnitine. In addition, carnitine and carnitine palmitoyltransferase are integral components of the cell membrane phospholipid fatty acid turnover, probably through a specific interaction with one or more cytoskeletal protein(s) and this pathway appears involved in the antioxidant network of cell membranes. Interestingly, recent studies have demonstrated that the reduced activity of carnitine palmitoyltransferase could have a crucial role in the pathogenesis of heart failure.[8,10,11]

Leakage of carnitine from tissues with high carnitine concentrations, such as skeletal muscles and myocardium itself, as well as impaired renal function, explain the common finding of elevated plasma concentrations of carnitine, regardless of myocardial levels, in most patients with heart failure.[8,10,11] Furthermore, an association has been claimed linking this with poor outcome, as the highest plasma carnitine concentrations are measured in subjects with end-stage heart failure.[8]

The reduced carnitine content may substantially limit the oxidation of fatty acids and the fuel metabolism of myocardium, as fatty acids provide about 70% of the energy needs of the human myocardium whereas the remaining 30% are covered by glucose and lactate, and this is probably critical to the impaired mechanical function of myocardium. Even though increased glucose and lactate utilization occurs in subjects with heart failure, paralleling the myocardial loss of carnitine to compensate for the impaired fatty acid oxidation, these mechanisms can cover only in part the total myocardial energy demand.[8,10,11]

CARNITINE THERAPY OF SUBJECTS WITH HEART FAILURE

Carnitine therapy may be of value in the management of subjects with heart failure.[8,10,11,13,14] Improvement in cardiopulmonary exercise capacity and peak oxygen consumption has been observed in treated subjects. In some experimental models of myocardial carnitine deficiency, the benefit of carnitine therapy on myocardial mechanical function has been ascribed to the increase of overall glucose utilization rather than the normalization of fatty acid metabolism.[15] Even the elevated plasma renin activity observed in patients with heart failure may be strongly reduced following carnitine therapy.[16] An additional mechanism contributing to this effect of carnitine and its esters is the down-modulation of TNF-alpha,[17] which is thought to be implicated in the pathogenesis of heart failure as well.[18,19]

Carnitine therapy appears particularly effective in correcting the exertional fatigue and shortness of breath that many subjects continue to experience despite optimal treatment of heart failure. Exertional symptoms do not simply result from underperfusion of skeletal muscles, but muscle deconditioning and impaired energy metabolism have a central role. In this respect, therapy with propionyl carnitine has several advantages over carnitine.[20,21] Carnitine transferases of skeletal muscle indeed have a higher affinity for propionyl-carnitine than for carnitine or other derivatives, thus accounting for the high specificity of propionyl-carnitine for skeletal muscle. Furthermore, propionyl-carnitine, while sharing with carnitine the same mechanism of action, carries the propionyl group and enhances the uptake of this agent by myocardium. This has a great relevance since propionate can be used by mitochondria as an anaplerotic substrate, thus providing energy in the absence of oxygen consumption. In the failing myocardium, mitochondria are progressively damaged, but propionyl carnitine may protect mitochondria upon free radical-mediated damage more effectively than carnitine or other acylcarnitines[20,21] Finally, due to the particular structure of the molecule, with a long lateral tail, propionyl carnitine has a specific pharmacological effect independent of its effect on energy metabolism, resulting in peripheral dilation and positive inotropism.[20,21] It should be noted that propionate alone cannot be administered because of its toxicity.[22]

CARNITINE THERAPY OF SUBJECTS WITH ISCHEMIC HEART DISEASE
Carnitine therapy does protect myocardium towards ischemia, even though there are some inconsistencies in the literature.[23-25]

Carnitine therapy has been demonstrated to improve the impaired lipid metabolism in viable myocardium in patients with ischemic heart disease,[23-25] but the mechanisms responsible for the protective effects of carnitine are not completely understood. It appears unlikely that these effects are entirely mediated by direct actions on lipid metabolism, eventhough complex derangements in fatty acid metabolism, including a fall in the levels of phospholipids and an increase in the levels of lysolecithin, free arachidonic acid, and long-chain and acylcarnitine derivatives (mostly propionyl-carnitine), occur in myocardium subjected to hypoxia and are thought to contribute significantly to the disturbances of cardiac functions during ischemia[26] and elicit many pharmacologic effects, such as an increase in the number of of alpha-1 adrenoceptors in cardiomyocytes and an increase in the electrical instability of membranes because of alterations of the voltage-dependent L-type $Ca^{2+}$ current in myocardial cells.[26]

It has been suggested that any intervention directed at inhibiting fatty acid degradation has the potential to decrease the extent of damage in myocardium subjected to hypoxia and reperfusion.[26] Therefore, it seems paradoxical that carnitine, which increases the rate of fatty acid oxidation by the synthesis of long-chain acylcarnitines, can exert beneficial effects. Recently, the stimulation of glucose metabolism and, especially the antioxidant activity of carnitines, has been regarded as central for the mechanical recovery of ischemic hearts resulting from carnitine therapy.[12,25,27] In experimental models, the administration of carnitine or its derivatives before ischemia is induced has been reported to protect myocardium from dysfunctions associated with oxidant stress[26] and these effects appear dose-dependent but independent of direct influences on coronary flow or on the electrophysiological properties of Purkinje fibers. Available data suggest that carnitine and its esters may protect myocardial cells from oxidant stress by stabilizing cell membranes, rendering them more resistant to free radicals, perhaps by facilitating the repair of phospholipid bilayers damaged by oxidant stress, rather than acting as direct scavengers of free radicals or decreasing their generation.[26] The influences of carnitine and its derivatives

**Table 6.6. Effects of carnitines on cellular membranes**

| Carnitine or derivative | Membrane function |
|---|---|
| Carnitine | Stabilization of erythrocyte membranes<br>Stabilization of liver mitochondrial membranes |
| Carnitine; propionylcarnitine | Protection of membranes against oxidant stress and free radicals |
| Palmitoylcarnitine | Alteration of erythrocyte membrane functions<br>Induction of electrical instability of cardiomyocyte membranes; alterations in voltage-dependent Ca++ current in cardiac and smooth muscle cells<br>Increase of alpha-1 adrenoceptors in cardiomyocytes<br>Reduction in surface negative charge and erythrocyte electrophoretic mobility<br>Inhibition of sodium pump current<br>Inhibition of gap junction conductance in cardiac cells<br>Constriction of coronary blood vessels |
| Ethylester of palmitoylcarnitine | Vasodilation of coronary blood vessels |

on cell membranes are summarized in Table 6.6. These effects of carnitine are believed to be mediated by mechanisms related to their ability to intercalate readily into lipid bilayers and affect surface charges on ion channels or on gap junction proteins. Remarkably, these are independent of reactions catalyzed by carnitine acyltransferases.[26]

The efficacy of carnitine therapy in subjects with myocardial ischemia may be limited by the slow rate of carnitine uptake. Since short-chain carnitine esters are taken up with greater affinity than carnitine by the myocardium, it is reasonable that these compounds, such as propionyl carnitine and acetyl carnitine, may have a greater clinical efficacy. Preliminary basic and preliminary work supports this hypothesis.[23-25] Furthermore, it is conceivable that the greatest beneficial effect may be obtained with pretreatment in order to sustain elevated intracellular levels before myocardial ischemia ensues. Furthermore, changes in carnitine metabolism take place during even short periods of mild myocardial ischemia; this indicates that carnitine supplementation may be also useful in patients with transient mild myocardial ischemia.[99]

Recent reports have demonstrated that a significant improvement in exercise tolerance and capacity as well as reductions in angina, use of cardioactive drugs, electrocardiographic manifestations of ischemia, dysrythmias and perhaps even mortality may be obtained with carnitine supplementation of subjects with ischemic heart disease.[28-30] Early carnitine treatment of patients with acute myocardial infarct has been shown to significantly reduce the mean infarct size as assessed by cardiac enzymes and QRS-score.[31] In the CEDIM trial, carnitine therapy had a significant impact on left ventricular remodeling after acute anterior myocardial infarction, as carnitine treatment started early after acute myocardial infarction and continued for 12 months significantly reduced the left ventricular dilation during the first year after infarction, resulting in smaller left ventricular volumes at 3, 6 and 12 months after the emergent event.[32]

The role of inhibitors of carnitine palmitoyltransferase, such as etoximir and oxfenicine, in the treatment of ischemic heart disease is being actively investigated. Preliminary data suggest that these compounds improve postischemic myocardial function either through oxidation of alternate substrates, such as glucose, during reperfusion or decreasing the myocardial levels of long-chain acylcarnitines during ischemia.[33] The prevention of increased long-chain acylcarnitines during ischemia by inhibitors of carnitine palmitoyltransferases results in decreased cardiac disturbances as well as decreased levels of alpha-1-adrenoceptors[26] and may well support the potential of these compounds as antiarrythmic drugs. In this regard, it has been suggested that even the antiarrythmic properties of lidocaine and propranolol may be partially linked to the downmodulation of long-chain acylcarnitine through the inhibition of carnitine palmitoyltransferase activity.[33]

## DIABETES AND SECONDARY CARNITINE DEFICIENCY

The levels of carnitine are reduced in the myocardium of diabetic animals depending upon the severity and duration of the disease and this probably contributes to the impaired myocardial contractility frequently seen throughout the course of diabetes.[8,34,35] In streptozotocin-treated diabetic rats carnitine deficiency and mechanical impairment of myocardium are associated with increased myocardial levels of long-chain acyl-CoA esters.[8,34,35] Preliminary reports in humans have suggested an association between myocardial carnitine deficiency and the depressed pump performance of the diabetic heart,[8,35] but further studies are required to better investigate this issue.

Most diabetic patients have low total and free plasma levels even in the blood; the low levels of myocardial concentrations have been proposed to result from reduced uptake secondary to the low blood content.[8,35,36]

However, there is also evidence for a defective myocardial transport and/or decreased renal reabsorption. The finding that the sulfonylureas glibenclamide and tolbutamide affect the metabolism of carnitine through inhibiting acyltransferase activity in liver microsomes indicates the potential of these drugs to contribute to the pathogenesis of carnitine deficiency in diabetic subjects.[8,37,38]

Taking all things into account, carnitine supplementation should be considered for the therapy of the diabetes-related cardiomyopathy. Interestingly, even inhibitors of carnitine palmitoyltransferase may improve the performance of diabetic heart, probably through reducing the levels of long-chain acylcarnitines in the myocardium. For example, a recent report has demonstrated that the inhibitor of carnitine palmitoyltransferase etoximir significantly improved and almost normalized the impaired mechanical function of myocardium in chronic diabetic rats and also ameliorated the alterations in the conducting system of the diabetic heart.[38] These effects were paralleled by the restoration of carnitine content in myocardium and liver. In addition, etoximir appears to act as both antidiabetic and lipid-lowering agent.[38] However, a long-term evaluation of the metabolic consequences of strategies directed at blocking the activity of carnitine palmitoyltransferase is warranted in diabetic subjects.

RENAL FAILURE, HEMODIALYSIS, KIDNEY TRANSPLANTATION

Carnitine levels largely depend on renal handling. With declining glomerular filtration rate, even carnitine filtration decreases and this leads to elevated plasma concentrations and the tubular handling of carnitine and its esters becomes abnormal as well.[39] The preferential reabsorption of free carnitine and rejection of acylcarnitines by tubules is impaired, thus explaining the marked increase in plasma concentrations of carnitine esters.

With the advent of hemodialysis overtly low levels of carnitine in plasma and tissues have been, in contrast, frequently measured.[39] About 10% of patients undergoing chronic hemodialysis have low carnitine concentrations and often they report weakness of skeletal muscles as a major complain.[39,40]

Carnitine is very readily dialysable and an elevated fraction, up to 90%, of the blood carnitine pool is lost during a dialysis session. Remarkably, the degree of carnitine loss during hemodialysis is strongly affected by membrane-dialyzers since losses are much greater (>30%) with high-permeability membranes than with cellulose ones.[40,41] A low protein supply may further contribute to the negative carnitine balance.[39,40] In these patients the altered carnitine status correlates with anemia.[42]

Available studies urgently recommend carnitine supplementation during or immediately after the hemodialysis procedure.[39,43-46] Both the short-term (intra- and post-dialytic) side effects (arrythmias, asthenia, skeletal muscle cramps and weakness, erythrocyte damage) and the chronic side-effects of hemodialysis (skeletal myopathy, cardiomyopathy, changes in skeletal muscle morphology and altered fat metabolism) may be successfully prevented or treated by intravenous or oral carnitine administration following each hemodialysis session and significantly more carnitine-receiving patients improve clinically than those receiving placebo.[39,43-46] Carnitine therapy also reduces the requirements for erythropoietin treatment in these subjects, probably through increasing red blood cell survival by stabilizing their cell membrane.[47] In turn, other studies failed to demonstrate a clear-cut benefit of carnitine therapy side-effects of hemodialysis.[47]

There is recent evidence that carnitine therapy even improves the depressed chemotaxis of neutrophils in subjects undergoing hemodialysis, a crucial factor predisposing these patients to bacterial infections.[49]

In contrast, the addition of carnitine to the dialysate does not reduce the side-effects of hemodialysis nor prevents reduction in carnitine concentrations in the skeletal muscle.[39]

Subjects undergoing continous ambulatory peritoneal dialysis and intermittent peritoneal dialysis have an abnormal profile of carnitines.[39] Most of them have normal levels of total and free plasma carnitine but elevated acylcarnitines, probably due to the differential loss of free carnitine in comparison to acylcarnitines across the peritoneal cavity.[39] However, a few reports have demonstrated a progressive decline in plasma carnitine levels in patients undergoing peritoneal dialysis over a 2 year period;[39,50] this suggests that even patients undergoing long-term peritoneal dialysis may be at risk for carnitine deficiency.

Little is known about carnitine status in subjects undergoing kidney transplantation. Most studies have demonstrated a complete normalization of plasma carnitine levels in subjects with normally functioning graft, as assessed by normal serum levels of creatinine.[39] In contrast, subjects with impaired function of the renal graft have elevated plasma carnitine concentrations comparable to those found in patients with uremia undergoing conservative management.[39] Even an abnormal ratio of acyl to free carnitine has been reported.[39]

A recent report has demonstrated that carnitine deficiency may be a cause of acute tubular necrosis after renal transplantation.[51] Ischemic injury to an allograft from a cadaveric donor can lead to delayed graft function, which has been associated with acute rejection and decreased graft survival. Extensive local release of cytokines, including TNF-alpha, further enhances the injury due to ischemia.[52] Taken together, these data, as well as the ability of carnitine to down-modulate TNF-alpha, suggest a potential role for carnitine therapy in the management of ischemic acute renal failure in transplant recipients. In addition, carnitine supplementation has been

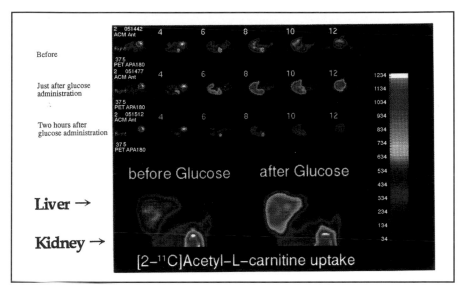

Fig. 10.7. [2-¹¹C]acetyl-L-carnitine uptake in the liver and kidney of rhesus monkey before and after glucose administration. Reprinted with permission from Yamaguti K, Kuratsune H et al. Biochem Biophys Res Commun 1996; 225:740-746.

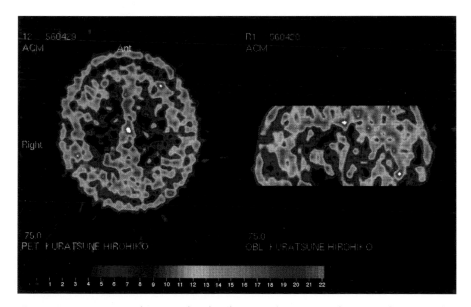

Fig. 10.10. PET scans showing the distribution of ACM in a horizontal section (left image) and sagittal section (right image) of the human brain. These images were constructed from 30 min to 45 min after injection of the radioactive tracer. ACM, [2-¹¹C]acetyl-L-carnitine.

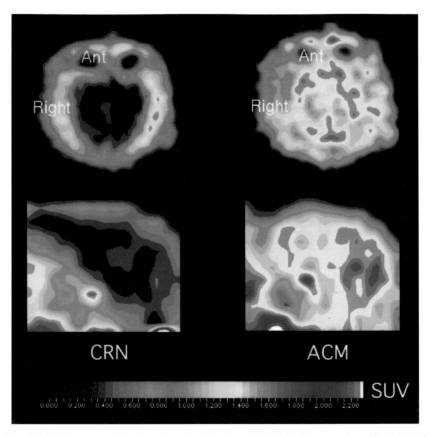

Fig. 10.9. PET scans showing the distribution of CRN (left images) and ACM (right images) in a horizontal section (upper images) and sagittal section (lower images) of the head of rhesus monkeys. These images were constructed from 30 min to 45 min after injection of the radioactive tracer. CRN, L-[methyl-[11]C]carnitine; ACM, [2-[11]C]acetyl-L-carnitine.

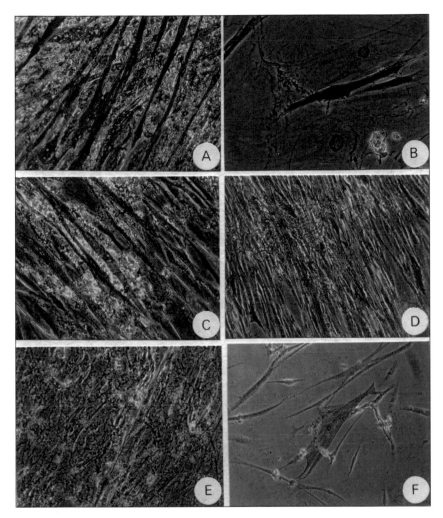

Fig. 12.2 A-F. Effect of AZT on human myotubes in culture. Representative flasks from each of cultures were immunoreacted with N-CAM antibodies. Cultures treated with 250 µM AZT, (B) show a reduction of myotubes compared with the untreated control cultures (A). C: cultures treated simultaneously with 5 mM L-carnitine and 250 µM AZT demonstrate significant prevention of the myotoxic effect of AZT, as shown by the increase in the number of myotubes. D: cultures treated for 3 weeks with 250 µM AZT followed by 3 weeks with L-carnitine also show an increment in the number of myotubes when compared to cultures treated only with AZT (B). E: cultures treated with AZT for 3 weeks, followed by no drugs (only medium) for 3 more weeks note a decreased number of myotubes when compared to cultures which received L-carnitine (D). F: cultures treated with AZT (for 6 weeks) and L-carnitine (from 3rd to 6th week) also show an increased number of the myotubes (X 200).

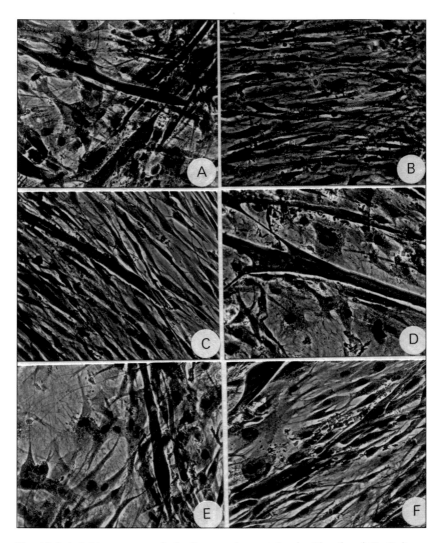

Fig. 12.3 A-F. Human muscle in tissue culture stained with oil-red-O. Cultures treated with 250 µM demonstrate a remarkable increase of lipid droplets (B) compared to the untreated control cultures (A). C: cultures treated with 5 mM L-carnitine together with 250 µM AZT resulted in substantial reduction of lipid droplets. Observe the significant reduction in the lipid droplets in cultures treated with carnitine (3 weeks) after AZT treatment (3 weeks) (D) and in cultures treated with complete medium after AZT treatment (3 weeks) (E). F: cultures treated with AZT for 6 weeks and carnitine (from 3rd to 6th week) demonstrate also a reduction in the lipid droplets (X 200).

shown to result in elevated plasma levels of insulin-like growth factor I (IGF-I) (C. De Simone et al, unpublished results) and IGF-I, when administered to animals subjected to renal ischemia, does reduce the extent of renal dysfunction and accelerate the recovery of the kidney.[53,54] Therefore, it is conceivable that carnitine therapy could have beneficial effects on ischemic renal failure through locally enhancing the levels of IGF-I. Clinical trials evaluating the effectiveness of IGF-I treatment in ischemic acute renal failure are under way, but this approach may be substan tiallylimited by the toxic effects associated with IGF-I administration.[55] In contrast, carnitine therapy is safe, and toxic effects thta might reasonably be expected due to carnitine administration have not been reported even in subjects receiving high-dose carnitine.[56,57]

Even the regimen of immunosuppression could significantly impact on carnitine metabolism in recipients of renal allograft. Patients treated with cyclosporin have been shown to have higher plasma concentrations of total free carnitine and acylcarnitines than subjects treated with azathioprine.[39]

## IDIOPATHIC INFLAMMATORY MYOPATHIES

Mitochondrial dysfunction has been shown in skeletal muscles from subjects with inflammatory myositis.[58] This appears associated in a few patients with carnitine deficiency, abnormal carnitine distribution, and defects of mitochondrial respiratory chain enzyme complexes in the skeletal muscle.[58] The view that carnitine therapy may have value in the management of inflammatory myositis is being actively investigated.

### Septic Shock

Most patients with sepsis have decreased carnitine levels in the liver, heart, skeletal muscles and renal cortex.[59]

In contrast, plasma levels are elevated and this may reflect the redistribution of carnitine from tissues to the peripheral blood.[56] However, the increase of plasma levels of carnitine may be transient and followed by a significant reduction. The impairment of the active process of carnitine transport, as shown in myocardium, appears central to the reduced content of carnitine in tissues during sepsis,[59] even though the effects of sepsis on carnitine carriers in tissues are largely unknown.

Studies of both humans and experimental animals have shown that the urinary excretion of carnitine is significantly increased during sepsis.[59] This is also commonly observed in conditions at high risk for sepsis, such as burns, starvation or surgical trauma.[59] In these conditions, the urinary loss of carnitine is negatively related to nitrogen balance and indicates that the elimination of carnitine mirrors the increased body catabolism of

Although many questions exist concerning the ultimate molecular mechanisms of action of carnitine and its congeners in endotoxemia, and the optimal kinetics and dosage schedules are yet to be demonstrated, it is envisaged that these compounds may be helpful, when associated with conventional therapy, in that they can effectively down-modulate inflammatory cytokines and ameliorate the host's metabolic processes. Clinical trials with carnitine and its congeners in the treatment and prophylaxis of septic shock syndrome in humans are justified.

## DRUGS AND CARNITINE DEFICIENCY

Several drugs have been reported to alter the profile of carnitines in both humans and experimental animals (Table 6.7). In most cases, low levels of carnitines in either blood or tissues or both have been found, resulting from various toxic mechanisms. The clinical relevance of these abnormalities requires to be further investigated, but now it is well known that carnitine deficiency may substantially contribute to the toxicity of such drugs as anthracyclines, valproate, and pivaloyl-antibiotics. In turn, the deficiency of vitamin C (ascorbic acid) could also lead to carnitine loss. In the next sections, we will focus on these issues.

### ANTHRACYCLINES

Treatment with anthracyclines, particularly adriamycin (doxorubicin), which are especially used as highly effective cancerostatic agents in leukemia patients as well as other cancer patients, may be severely cardiotoxic.[64] Patients receiving a total cumulated dose of 400-500 mg/m$^2$ may have irreversible heart failure leading to death in 30-40% of cases.

Myocardial carnitine deficiency, and the consequent impairment in mitochondrial energy metabolism, appear involved in the pathogenesis of adriamycin cardiotoxicity. Low myocardial levels of carnitine are commonly observed in the myocardium of subjects taking adriamycin, but overt carnitine deficiency is otherwise found only in those patients with severe cardiomyopathy or chronic heart failure.[8,65] In contrast, these patients have elevated plasma levels of carnitine, probably reflecting the leakage of carnitine from myocardium injured by adriamycin.[8,65] Furthermore, adriamycin directly damages mitochondria and interferes with fatty acid oxidation[66] and inhibits the activity of carnitine palmitoyltransferase.[67]

These phenomena, as well as the myocardial accumulation of adriamycin, may be competitively inhibited by carnitine under in vitro conditions.[65] Remarkably, carnitine does not appear to reduce the cytotoxicity of adriamycin towards cancer cells.[65]

In experimental animals the severe adriamycin-related cardiomyopathy may be prevented by concomitant administration of carnitine.[65]

Carnitine therapy did reduce the anthracycline-induced myocardial accumulation of long-chain acyl-CoA and improve as well oxygen consumption, energy metabolism, and ATP levels in the myocardium.[65]

In humans, several studies have reported encouraging results with carnitine therapy in order to protect cancer subjects from the cardiotoxicity of adriamycin[65] so that the dose of adriamycin could be increased above 400-500 mg/m², resulting in more effective anticancer treatment.

Finally, preliminary reports highlight the potential of carnitine therapy in reducing the cellular toxicity of ifosfamide.[68]

VALPROATE

This is an anticonvulsant drug commonly used in many different types of seizure disorders. Chronic therapy is associated with decreased plasma carnitine levels [4,69,70] However, these patients may have tissue carnitine deficiency, such as in the skeletal muscle, irrespective of plasma levels.[4,69] Most studies showing low carnitine levels in patients treated with valproate have investigated children, but significantly low levels have also been reported in treated adults.[4,69] The prevalence of carnitine deficiency in treated subjects varies from 4 to 76% in various studies.[4,69] The reasons for this wide variation in prevalence of plasma carnitine deficiency are unclear but presumably reflect differences in the study groups investigated.

Specific risk factors for the onset of carnitine deficiency have been identified:[4,69] a) high-dosage valproate is administered long-term; b) valproate is administered in combination with other anticonvulsant drugs (valproate polypharmacy). Remarkably, carnitine deficiency has been reported even in patients not treated with valproate but taking other anticonvulsants (carbamazepine, phenytoin, phenobarbital); c) valproate is given to very young subjects, especially to infants; d) valproate is given in the presence of further carnitine-consuming illnesses or other carnitine-consuming therapies; e) low levels of carnitine are already present when valproate treatment is started; f) patients have multiple disabilities; g) valproate is given to heterozygotes for plasmalemmal carnitine transporter defect[71] or other inborn errors potentially causing carnitine deficiency.

Subjects with valproate-related carnitine deficiency may have a severe or fatal hepatotoxicity, Reye-like syndrome or pancreatitis.[4,69] Microvesicular peripheral steatosis and abnormalities of mitochondria are found in the liver, and these changes are associated with reduced intracellular levels of free CoA and increased concentrations of medium-chain acyl-CoA compounds.[4,69]

The pathogenesis of carnitine loss in these patients has been extensively investigated. Valproate forms CoA thioesters and carnitine esters (valproyl-carnitine) and this is a relevant detoxifying mechanism of both valproate and some of its unsaturated toxic metabolites.[4,69,70] In turn, this causes a secondary disturbance of intermediary metabolism, and the inhibition of fatty acid oxidation.[4,69,70]

Most subjects treated with valproate have an increased acylcarnitine to total carnitine ratio in the urine, and decreased renal tubular reabsorption of free carnitine has been reported.[4,69] Remarkably, valproate impairs carnitine uptake by cells through inhibiting the activity of the membrane carnitine transporter, and there is a direct relationship linking this effect with the duration of exposure and concentration of valproate.[4,69] This mechanism through decreasing the carnitine uptake may explain the decreased renal tubular reabsorption as well as the tissue depletion. Even therapy with other anticonvulsants (carbamazepine, phenytoin, phenobarbital) is associated with increased urinary excretion of free carnitine but the effect of these drugs upon carnitine transport across cell membrane has so far not been investigated.

Carnitine therapy protects the host with respect to valproate hepatotoxicity.[4,69] The clinical course significantly improves and carnitine levels return to the normal range following carnitine therapy. Other studies, in turn, have shown that carnitine treatment does not always prevent the emergence of hepatotoxicity,[4,69] but it does alleviate valproate-induced hyperammonemia, particularly the transient hyperammonemia observed in valproate-treated children following ingestion of protein-enriched meals.[72] Carnitine treatment may improve skeletal muscle weakness and failure to thrive, but other reports failed to show any benefit in this regard.

These effects of carnitine therapy depend on decreased membrane carnitine transport inhibition and greater buffering capacity for the excess of potentially toxic acyl-CoA. As a consequence, intramitochondrial free CoA increases, thereby reducing mitochondrial dysfunction.

Carnitine should be administered prophylactically to all children under 2 years of age during treatment with valproate, and selectively when there is clinical or laboratory evidence of carnitine deficiency. For example, if the patients complain of fatigue during prolonged valproate treatment, it is advised to supplement carnitine. Preliminary data suggest that carnitine treatment may benefit high-risk, symptomatic patients and those with overt carnitine deficiency, but it is unlikely that low-risk, asymptomatic patients and those with normal carnitine levels may gain any advantage from carnitine therapy.[4,69] In addition, the thrombocytopenia associated with high valproate dose is not corrected by carnitine therapy.[73] Remarkably, carnitine does not adversely impact on either the anticonvulsant properties of valproate or its pharmacokinetics.[4,69]

PIVALOYL-ANTIBIOTICS

The detoxification and elimination of pivalic acid from pivaloyl-antibiotics (pivampicillin, pivmecillinam, pivcephalexin, cefditoren-pivoxil, cefetamet, pivaloxylmethylcephem) may lead to severe carnitine deficiency in plasma and tissues. Indeed, pivalic acid is eliminated almost exclusively (>95-99%) in the form of pivaloyl-carnitine.[74-77] Depending on the dosage of the antibiotic, even short-term treatment may cause carnitine deficiency and all subjects taking pivaloyl-antibiotics are at risk for carnitine deficiency irrespective of age.[78]

Subjects concomitantly taking clofibrate have an even greater risk of becoming carnitine-depleted, as clofibrate has been shown to significantly increase the concentrations of pivaloyl-carnitine.[79]

There is also evidence of low carnitine levels in plasma, myocardium and liver from pups of lactating rats treated with sodium pivalate, which indicates that pivaloyl antibiotics should not be administered to lactating women due to the risk of carnitine deficiency in their newborns.[80]

As a consequence of pivalate-induced carnitine deficiency, impaired myocardial mechanical performance and severe abnormalities of fatty acid oxidation and ketone body production have been observed in animal models.[81] A recent clinical study has demonstrated that treatment with these antibiotics may lead to reduction in left ventricular mass and interventricular septum thickness, paralleling the carnitine depletion.[82] In contrast, in experiments performed on rats sodium pivalate treatment significantly reduced the myocardial carnitine content and shifted substrate utilization towards increased glucose utilization, but the myocardial mechanical performance was not compromized.[83] However, it is likely that longer treatment duration and higher pivalate dosages may impair myocardial function even in this model.

Based on relevant clinical studies, researchers urgently recommend that carnitine supplementation should be prescribed in order to prevent the development of carnitine deficiency in all subjects taking pivaloyl-antibiotics. However, whether carnitine therapy can be impressive clinically in the management of these subjects remains to be conclusively established.[65]

CEPHALOSPORINS

Some cephalosporin antibiotics (cephaloridine, ceftazidim, cefsulodin) have a betain structure that is chemically related to carnitine.[65] Because of the similarity of their structure to carnitine, these antibiotics may inhibit several carnitine-dependent mitochondrial metabolic pathways, such as pyruvate and palmitoyl carnitine oxidation and acetyl/carnitine exchange.[65] Furthermore, cephaloridine specifically inhibits the tubular reabsorption of carnitine and acylcarnitines,[84] thus resulting in a strong increase of free and acylated carnitines excreted by the kidneys. The increased urinary excretion of carnitines is paralleled by a fall in the blood levels of carnitine. It is reasonable that the carnitine loss observed during treatment with cephalosporins may further contribute to the mitochondrial nephrotoxicity of cephalosporins,[65] possibly through altering the normal lipid metabolism.[85]

OTHER ANTI-INFECTIOUS AGENTS

Pyrimethamine and sulphadiazine, commonly used in the treatment of toxoplasmosis, may cause severe carnitine deficiency in rats and humans.[86] The increased urinary excretion of carnitine appears central to the pathogenesis of carnitine loss in treated subjects. The proportion of acylcarnitines in the total carnitine pool markedly increases and this is thought to reflect the abnormal mitochondrial metabolism of fatty acids related to the carnitine deficiency.[86]

Chronic emetine administration has been shown to cause an approximate 90% loss of carnitine from skeletal muscles in a female patient, resulting in a severe myopathy with mitochondrial damage and atrophy of type 2 muscle fibers.[87]

BENZOIC ACID

Benzoic acid may be used for the treatment of hyperammonemia and is added as a conservation agent to many pharmaceutical preparations. Benzoic acid is also detoxified and excreted facultatively in humans as benzoylcarnitine.[88] There is evidence that, following the administration of benzoic acid, carnitine deficiency may occur in both experimental animals and humans, and this is paralleled by a marked increase in the amount of benzoylcarnitine excreted in the urine.[89-92] Furthermore, even the urinary excretion of other acylcarnitines is strongly increased, probably reflecting the impaired mitochondrial energy metabolism.[91]

IMMUNOGLOBULIN G (IgG)

A case report has demonstrated that one patient with non-Hodgkin's lymphoma developed a severe myopathic carnitine deficiency and early heart failure.[93] More detailed investigations demonstrated that IgG inhibits the active myocardial transport of long-chain fatty acids in the myocardium, probably through specific blockade of the carnitine carrier, resulting in an impaired uptake and enrichment of carnitine by the myocardium.[93] In this patient, the inhibition of carnitine uptake proved to take place competitively with L-carnitine and to be dependent on the activity of the underlying lymphoma.[93] In fact, the impaired fatty acid metabolism in the myocardium was overcome by raising the carnitine level with exogenous supplementation, as well as by inhibiting the production of IgG by lymphoma cells with steroid therapy.[93] However, carnitine deficiency so far has not been demonstrated upon receipt of intravenous immunoglobulin.

### LIDOCAINE

Experiments in rats have shown that lidocaine administration, even at a single dose, may result in a strong reduction of plasma carnitine levels.[95] Evidence of injury to the skeletal muscles and mitochondria resembling those of carnitine deficiency has been observed after administration of lidocaine as well as bupivacaine, which is structurally related to lidocaine.[95] Interestingly, both catabolic urinary nitrogen loss and stress-induced increase in plasma free fatty acids were markedly reduced by the administration of carnitine.[95]

The mechanisms explaining the carnitine loss in this model are not as yet elucidated, but the potential risk caused by the induction of carnitine deficiency in the severely ill subjects treated with these drugs should not be underestimated. Remarkably, these drugs can themselves be the cause of arrythmias and worsen preexisting arrythmias. The hypothesis that arrythmias occurring during treatment with these substances may be due to the reduction or depletion of myocardial carnitine reserves should be tested.

### QUATERNARY NITROGEN COMPOUNDS

Edrophonium has been shown to acutely modify carnitine levels in different rat tissues, as shown by increased hepatic and reduced blood and renal levels.[96] In this model, the impact on carnitine levels was neither accompanied by significant variations of serum parameters of carbohydra te, fat, and protein metabolism nor of insulin levels.[96] Compounds structurally similar to edrophonium had a comparable effect on carnitine levels, but this was not related to cholinergic action, as physostigmine and ambenonium at concentrations known to increase cholinergic activity did not modify carnitine distri bution in tissues.[96] In addition, atropine, an acetylcholine antagonist, affected carnitine distribution in a way similar to edrophonium.[96] It is likely that quaternary nitrogen compounds affect intercellular carnitine transport through direct action on plasma membrane.

### ASCORBIC ACID

Hyperexcretion of carnitine in experimental scurvy has been correlated with a lower rate of carnitine transport into the renal brush-border membrane vesicles.[97,98] In guinea pigs, experimental vitamin C deficiency is associated with low carnitine concentrations in blood and some tissues, and with elevated rates of free and total carnitine excretion.[97,98] Even though ascorbic acid is a cofactor for two enzymes in the pathway of endogenous carnitine biosynthesis, ascorbate-deficient animals do not have abnormalities in carnitine biosynthesis, pointing to excessive urinary excretion as the crucial factor in the pathogenesis of carnitine deficiency associated with vitamin C deficiency. Subjects with scurvy should be considered at risk for carnitine deficiency, but no studies have so far investigated the carnitine metabolism in these patients.

REFERENCES

1. Carter L, Abney TO, Lapp DF. Biosynthesis and metabolism of carnitine. J Child Neurol 1995; 10 (Suppl):2S3-2S7.
2. Bremer J. The role of carnitine in intracellular metabolism. J Clin Chem Clin Biochem 1990; 28:297-301.
3. Virmani MA, Conti R, Spadoni A, Rossi S, Arrigoni Martelli E. Inhibition of L-carnitine uptake into primary rat cortical cell cultures by GABA and GABA uptake blockers. Pharmacol Res 1995; 31:211-215.
4. Pons R, De Vivo DC. Primary and secondary carnitine deficiency syndromes. J Child Neurol 1995; 10 (Suppl):2S8-2S21.
5. Di Donato S, Garavaglia B, Rimoldi M, Carrara F. Clinical and biomedical phenotypes of carnitine deficiencies. In:Ferrari R, Di Mauro S, Sherwood G, eds. L-Carnitine and Its Role in Medicine: from Function to Therapy. London: Academic Press, 1992:81-98.
6. Miyagawa J, Kuwajima M, Hanafusa T et al. Mitochondrial abnormalities of muscle tissue in mice with juvenile visceral steatosis associated with systemic carnitine deficiency. Virchows Arch 1995; 426:271-279.
7. Weaver LT, Rosenthal SR, Gladstone W, Winter HS. Carnitine deficiency: A possible cause of gastrointestinal dysmotility. Acta Pediatr 1992; 81:79-81.
8. Regitz-Zagrosek V, Fleck E. Myocardial carnitine deficiency in human cardiomyopathy. In: De Jong JW, Ferrari R, eds. The Carnitine System. A New Therapeutical Approach to Cardiovascular Diseases. Dordrecht: Kluwer Academic Publishers, 1995:145-166.
9. Bennett MJ, Hale DE. Defects of mitochondrial beta-oxidation enzymes. In: Ferrari R, Di Mauro S, Sherwood G, eds. L-Carnitine and Its Role in Medicine: from Function to Therapy. London: Academic Press, 1992:187-206.
10. Regitz V, Fleck E. Role of carnitine in heart failure. In: Ferrari R, Di Mauro S, Sherwood G, eds. L-Carnitine and Its Role in Medicine: from Function to Therapy. London: Academic Press, 1992:295-323.
11. Patel AK, Thomsen JH, Kosolcharoen PK, Shug AL. Myocardial carnitine status: clinical, prognostic and therapeutic significance. In: Ferrari R, Di Mauro S, Sherwood G, eds. L-Carnitine and Its Role in Medicine: from Function to Therapy. London: Academic Press, 1992:325-335.

12. Arduini A, Dottori S, Molajoni F, Kirk R, Arrigoni Martelli E. Is the carnitine system part of the heart antioxidant network? In: De Jong JW, Ferrari R, eds. The Carnitine System. A New Therapeutic Approach to Cardiovascular Diseases. Dordrecht: Kluwer Academic Publishers, 1995:169-181.

13. Fernandez C. Profile of long-term L-carnitine therapy in cardiopathic patients. In: Ferrari R, Di Mauro S, Sherwood G, eds. L-Carnitine and Its Role in Medicine: from Function to Therapy. London: Academic Press, 1992:337-341.

14. Rizos I, Primikiropoulos A, Hadjinikolau L et al. Hemodynamical effects of L-carnitine on patients with congestive heart failure due to dilated cardiomyopathy. Eur Heart J 1995; 16:181.

15. Broderick TL, Panagakis P, Di Domenico et al. L-carnitine improvement of cardiac function is associated with a stimulation in glucose but not fatty acid metabolism in carnitine-deficient rats. Cardiovasc Res 1995; 30: 815-820.

16. Rizos I, Primikiropoulos A, Hadjinikolau L et al. Effect of L-carnitine on plasma renin activity on patients with severe and moderate heart failure. European Society of Cardiology, Amsterdam, The Netherlands, August 20-24th, 1995. (Abstract)

17. Famularo G, De Simone C. A new era for carnitine? Immunol Today 1995.

18. Levine B, Kalman J, Mayer L, Fillit HM, Packer M. Elevated circulating levels of tumor necrosis factor in severe chronic heart failure. N Engl J Med 1991; 323:236-240.

19. Colucci WS, Braunwald E. Pathophysiology of heart failure. In: Braunwald E, ed. Heart Disease (5th edition). Philadelphia: W.B. Saunders, 1997: 394-420.

20. Ferrari R, Anand I. Utilization of propionyl-L-carnitine for the treatment of heart failure. In: De Jong JW, Ferrari R, eds. The Carnitine System. A New Therapeutical Approach to Cardiovascular Diseases. Dordrecht: Kluwer Academic Publishers, 1995: 323-335.

21. Caponnetto S, Brunelli C. Hemodynamic and metabolic effect of propionyl-L-carnitine in patients with heart failure. In: De Jong JW, Ferrari R, eds. The Carnitine System. A New Therapeutical Approach to Cardiovascular Diseases. Dordrecht: Kluwer Academic Publishers, 1995:337-351.

22. Ferrari R, Pasini E, Condorelli E et al. Effect of propionyl-L-carnitine on mechanical function of isolated rabbit heart. Cardiovasc Drugs Ther 1991; 5 (Suppl 1):17-23.

23. Paulson DJ, Shug AL. Experimental evidence of the anti-ischemic effect of L-carnitine. In: De Jong JW, Ferrari R, eds. The Carnitine System. A New Therapeutical Approach to Cardiovascular Diseases. Dordrecht: Kluwer Academic Publishers, 1995:183-197.

24. Pepine CJ, Welsch MA. Therapeutic potential of L-carnitine in patients with angina pectoris. In: De Jong JW, Ferrari R, eds. The Car-

nitine System. A New Therapeutical Approach to Cardiovascular Diseases. Dordrecht: Kluwer Academic Publishers, 1995:225-243.

25. Rizzon P, Di Biase M, Biasco G, Pitzalis MV. Carnitine and myocardial infarction. In: De Jong RW, Ferrari R, eds. The Carnitine System. A New Therapeutical Approach to Cardiovascular Diseases. Dordrecht: Kluwer Academic Publishers, 1995:245-249.

26. Fritz IB, Arrigoni Martelli E. Sites of action of carnitine and its derivatives on the cardiovascular system: interactions with membranes. Trends Pharmacol Sci 1995; 14:355-360.

27. Broderick TL, Quinney HA, Lopaschuk GD. L-carnitine increases glucose metabolism and mechanical function following ischemia in diabetic rat heart. Cardiovasc Res 1995; 29:373-378.

28. Kressig R. L-carnitine in the treatment of stable angina pectoris. Ars Med 1995; 85:200-202.

29. Watanabe S, Ajisaka R, Masuoka T et al. Effects of L- and DL-carnitine on patients with impaired exercise tolerance. Jpn Heart J 1995; 36:319-331.

30. Watanabe S, Ajisaka R, Eda K et al. Effects of L-carnitine on patients with ischemic heart disease evaluated by myocardial SPECT with 123I-beta-methyl iodophenyl pentadecanoic acid (BMIPP). J Nucl Cardiol 1995; 2:S47 (Abstract).

31. Singh RB, Niaz MA, Agarwal P, Beegum R, Rastogi SS, Sachan DS. A randomised, double-blind, placebo-controlled trial of L-carnitine in suspected acute myocardial infarction. Postgrad Med J 1996; 72:45-50.

32. Iliceto S, Scrutinio D, Bruzzi P et al. Effects of L-carnitine administration on left ventricular remodeling after acute anterior myocardial infarction: the L-carnitine Ecografia Digitalizzata Infarto Miocardico (CEDIM) trial. J Am Coll Cardiol 1995; 26:380-387.

33. Madden MC, Wolkowicz PE, Pohost GM, McMillin JB, Pike MM. Acylcarnitine accumulation does not correlate with reperfusion recovery in palmitate-perfused rat hearts. Am J Physiol 1995; 268:2505-2512.

34. Knabb MT, Russell BA. Inhibition of cardiac carnitine palmitoyltransferase I activity with antiarrythmic drugs. J Pennsylvania Acad Sci 1995; 69:49-52.

35. Paulson DJ, Sanjak M, Shug AL. Carnitine deficiency and the diabetic heart. In: Lee Carter A, ed. Current Concepts in Carnitine Research. Boca Raton: CRC Press, 1992; 215-230.

36. Feuvray D. Carnitine metabolism during diabetes and hyperthyroidism. In: De Jong JW, Ferrari R, eds. The Carnitine System. A New Therapeutical Approach to Cardiovascular Diseases. Dordrecht: Kluwer Academic Publishers, 1995:199-208.

37. Broadway NM, Saggerson ED. Inhibition of liver microsomal carnitine acyltransferases by sulphonylurea drugs. FEBS Lett 1995; 371:137-139.

38. Schmitz FJ, Rosen R, Reinauer H. Improvement of myocardial function and metabolsim in diabetic rats by the carnitine palmitoyltransferase inhibitor etoximir. Horm Metab Res 1995; 27:515-522.
39. Ahmad S. Carnitine, kidney and renal dialysis. In: Ferari R, Di Mauro S, Sherwood G, eds. L-Carnitine and Its Role in Medicine: from Function to Therapy. London: Academic Press, 1992; 381-400.
40. Ayer SB, Montemeyer L, Delauder D. Incidence and pattern of carnitine deficiency in a free standing dialysis unit. J Am Soc Nephrol 1995; 6:572 (Abstract).
41. Lago M, Perez Garcia R, Arenas J et al. Carnitine losses in hemodialysis: influence of different membrane-dialyzers and relationship with nutritional status. Nefrologia 1995; 15:55-61.
42. Borum P, Ross E. Altered plasma and red-cell carnitine status in hemodialysis-patients correlates with anemia. FASEB J 1995; 9:156 (Abstract).
43. De Los Reyes B, Garcia RP. Effects of low intravenous dose of L-carnitine in patients on hemodialysis. Kidney Int 1995; 48:284 (Abstract).
44. Kandemir EG, Evrenkaya TR, Cebeci BS, Ozcan A, Tulbek MY. Effect of L-carnitine on lipid abnormalities and cardiac dysfunctions in chronic hemodialysis patients. Bull Gulhane Mil Med Acad 1995; 37:441-447.
45. Labonia WD. L-carnitine effects on anemia in hemodialyzed patients treated with erythropoietin Am J Kidney Dis 1995; 26:757 764.
46. Brass EP. Pharmacokinetic considerations for the therapeutic use of carnitine in hemodialysis-patients. Clin Ther 1995; 17:176-185.
47. Kavadias D, Fourtounas C, Tsouchnikas J, Vlachonasios T, Barboutis K. Reduction of the cost of erythropoietin therapy by coadministration of L-carnitine in hemodialysis patients. Nephrol Dial Transplant 1995; 10:1047 (Abstract).
48. Sloan RS, Smith B, Golper TA. The intradialytic effects of oral L-carnitine: results of a double-blind, placebo-controlled trial. J Am Soc Nephrol 1995; 6:588 (Abstract).
49. Suleymaniar G, Yilmaz H, Coskun M, Ersoy F, Yegin O, Yakupoglu G. The beneficial effect of L-carnitine on neutrophil chemotaxis in chronic renal failure patients on hemodialysis (HD). Nephrol Dial Transplant 1995; 10:1025 (Abstract).
50. Kirby DPJ, Constantin Teodosiu D, Short AH et al. Free and total carnitine concentrations in continuous ambulatory peritoneal dialysis patients. Proceedings of the Nutrition Society 1995; 54:4 (Abstract).
51. Bakker SJL, Yin M, Koostra G. Tissue thiamine and carnitine deficiency as a possible cause of acute tubular necrosis after renal transplantation. Transplant Proc 1996; 28:314-315.

52. Goes N, Urmson J, Ramassar V, Halloran PF. Ischemic acute tubular necrosis induces an extensive local cytokine response: evidence for induction of interferon-gamma, transforming growth factor-beta 1, granulocyte-macrophage colony-stimulating factor, interleukin-2, and interleukin-10. Transplantation 1995; 59:565-572.

53. Hammerman MR, Miller SB. Therapeutic use of growth factors in renal failure. J Am Soc Nephrol 1994; 5:1-11.

54. Safirstein RL, Bonventre JV. Molecular response to ischemic and nephrotoxic acute renal failure. In: Schlondorff D, Bonventre JV, eds. Molecular Nephrology: Kidney Function in Health and Disease. New York: Marcel Dekker, 1995, 839-854.

55. Waters D, Danska J, Hardy K et al. Recombinant human growth hormone, insulin-like growth factor 1, and combination therapy in AIDS-associated wasting. Ann Intern Med 1996; 125:865-872.

56. De Simone C, Tzantzoglou S, Famularo G et al. High dose L-carnitine improves immunologic and metabolic parameters in AIDS patients. Immunopharmacol Immunotoxicol 1993; 15:1-12.

57. De Simone C, Famularo G, Tzantzoglou S et al. Carnitine depletion in peripheral blood mononuclear cells from patients with AIDS: effect of oral L-carnitine. AIDS 1994; 8:655-660.

58. Gonzalez-Crespo M, Arenas J, Cabello A et al. Free carnitine and carnitine esters levels in muscle of patients with idiopathic inflammatory myositis. Arthritis Rheum 1995; 38:9 (Abstract).

59. Famularo G, De Simone C, Arrigoni Martelli E, Jirillo E. Carnitine and septic shock: a review. J Endotoxin Res 1995; 2:141-147.

60. Winter BK, Fiskum G, Gallo LL. Effects of L-carnitine on serum triglyceride and cytokine levels in rat models of cachexia and septic shock. Br J Cancer 1995; 72:1173-1179.

61. Delogu G, De Simone C, Famularo G, Fegiz A, Paoletti F, Jirillo E. Anaesthetics modulate tumour necrosis factor alpha: effects of L-carnitine supplementation in surgical patients. Preliminary results. Med Inflamm 1993; 2 (Suppl):S33-S36.

62. Hayashi N, Yoshihara D, Kashiwabara N, Takeshita Y, Handa H, Yamakawa M. Effect of carnitine on decrease of branched chain amino acids and glutamine in serum of septic rats. Biol Pharm Bull 1996; 19:157-159.

63. Linz DN, Garcia VF, Arya G et al. Weanling and adult rats differ in fatty acid and carnitine metabolism during sepsis. J Pediatr Sur 1995; 30:959-966.

64. Aviles A, Arevila N, Diaz-Maquero JC, Gomez T, Garcia R, Nambo MJ. Late cardiac toxicity of doxorubicin, epirubicin, and mitoxantrone therapy for Hodgkin's disease in adults. Leuk Lymphomas 1993; 11:275-279.

65. Cierpka D. Carnitene (Sigma Tau) in acquired carnitine deficiency. Sigma-Tau Pharma Ltd., Pomezia (Italy), 1994.

66. Lee Carter A, Pierce R, Culbreath C, Howard E. Conjunctive enhancement of adriamycin by carnitine. In: Lee Carter A, ed. Current Concepts in Carnitine Research. Boca Raton: CRC Press, 1992, 245-251.

67. Battelli D, Bobyleva V, Ballei M, Arrigoni Martelli E, Muscatello U. Interaction of carnitine with mitochondrial cardiolipin. Biochim Bophys Acta 1992; 1117:33-36.

68. Schlenzig JS, Charpentier C, Rabier D, Kamoun P, Sewell AC, Harpey JP. L-carnitine: a way to decrease cellular toxicity of ifosfamide? Eur J Pediatr 1995:154:686-687.

69. Coulter DL. Carnitine deficiency in epilepsy: risk factors and treatment. J Child Neurol 1995; 10 (Suppl):2S32-2S39.

70. Van Wouwe JP. Carnitine deficiency during valproic acid treatment. Int J Vitamin Nutr Res 1995; 65:211-214.

71. Tein I, Di Mauro S, Xie ZW, De Vivo DC. Heterozygotes for plasmalemmal carnitine transporter defect are at increased risk for valproic acid-associated impairment of carnitine uptake in cultured human skin fibroblasts. J Inherit Metab Dis 1995; 18:313-322.

72. Gidal B, Rust RS, Inglese CM et al. Effect of carnitine supplementation on valproate-mediated transient hyperammonemia in children. Epilepsia 1995; 36:533 (Abstract).

73. Delgado MR, Liu H, Mills J, Browne R. Effect of L-carnitine supplementation on the platelet count of children with epilepsy with high valproate dose and/or serum levels. Epilepsia 1995; 36:68 (Abstract).

74. Holme E, Jodal U, Lindstedt S, Nordin I. Effects of pivalic acid-containing prodrugs on carnitine homeostasis and on response to fasting in children. Scand J Clin Lab Invest 1992; 52:361-372.

75. Nakashima M, Uematsu T, Oguma T et al. Phase I clinical studies of S-1108: safety and pharmacokinetics in a multiple administration study with special emphasis on the influence on carnitine body stores. Antimicrob Agents Chemother 1992; 36:762-768.

76. Shimizu K, Saito A, Yamamoto S. Carnitine status and safety after administration of S-1108, a new oral cephem to patients. Antimicrob Agents Chemother 1993; 37:1043-1049.

77. Rose SJ, Stokes TC, Patel S, Cooper MB, Betteridge DJ, Payne JE. Carnitine deficiency associated with long-term pivampicillin treatment: the effect of a replacement therapy regimen. Postgrad Med J 1992; 68:932-934.

78. Abrahamsson K, Holme E, Jodal U, Lindstedt S, Nordin I. Effect of short-term treatment with pivalic acid containing antibiotics on serum carnitine concentration: a risk irrespective of age. Bioch Mol Med 1995; 55:77-79.

79. Diep QN, Bohmer T. Increased pivaloylcarnitine in the liver of the sodium pivalate-treated rat exposed to clofibrate. Biochim Biophys Acta 1995; 1256:245-247.

80. Davis AT. Carnitine depletion in rat pups of lactating mothers given sodium pivalate. Biol Neonate 1995; 68:211-220.
81. Broderick TL, Christos SC, Wolf BA, Di Domenico D, Shug AL, Paulson DJ. Fatty acid oxidation and cardiac function in the sodium pivalate model of secondary carnitine deficiency. Metab Clin Exp 1995; 44:499-505.
82. Abrahamsson K, Mellaner M, Eriksson BO et al. Transient reduction of human left ventricular mass in carnitine depletion induced by antibiotics containing pivalic acid. Br Heart J 1995; 74:656-659.
83. Morris GS, Zhou Q, Wolf BA et al. Sodium pivalate reduces cardiac carnitine content and increases glucose oxidation without affecting cardiac functional capacity. Life Sci 1995; 57:2237-2244.
84. Tune BM, Hsu CY. Toxicity of cephaloridine to carnitine transport and fatty acid metabolism in rabbit renal cortical mitochondria: structure-activity relationships. J Pharmacol Exp Ther 1994; 270:873-880.
85. Tune BM, Hsu CY. Toxicity of cephalosporins to fatty acid metabolism in rabbit renal cortical mitochondria. Biochem Pharmacol 1995; 49:727-734.
86. Sekas G, Paul HS. Hyperammonemia and carnitine deficiency in a patient receiving sulfadiazine and pyrimethamine. Am J Nutr 1995; 95:112-113.
87. Kuntzer T, Reichmann H, Bogousslavsky J. Emetine-induced myopathy and carnitine deficiency. J Neurol 1990; 237:495-496.
88. Sakuma T, Asai K, Ichiki T, Sugiyama N, Kidouchi K, Wada Y. Identification of benzoylcarnitine in the urine of a patient of hyperammonemia. Tohoku J Exp Med 1989; 159:147-151.
89. Ratnakumari L, Quershi IA, Butterworth RF. Effect of L-carnitine on cerebral and hepatic energy metabolites in congenitally hyperammonemic mice and its role during benzoate therapy. Metabolism 1993; 42:1039-1046.
90. Ali A, Qureshi IA. Benzoyl-CoA ligase activity in the liver and kidney cortex of weaning guinea-pigs treated with various inducers - relationship with hippurate synthesis and carnitine levels. Dev Pharmacol Ther 1992; 18:55-64.
91. Sakuma T. Alteration of urinary carnitine profile induced by benzoate administration. Arch Dis Child 1991; 66:873-875.
92. Michalak A, Qureshi IA. Tissue acylcarnitine and acylcoenzyme A profiles in chronically hyperammonemic mice treated with sodium benzoate and supplementary L-carnitine. Biomed Pharmacother 1995; 49:350-357.
93. Deufel TH, Siegert W, Pongratz D, Jacob K, Wieland OH. Myopathic carnitine deficiency associated with lymphocytic malignant non-Hodgkin lymphoma and immunoglobulin G-k. Klin Wschr 1984; 62:669-674.

94. Ferrari L, Maccari F, Chiodi P, Ramacci MT, De Angelis C, Angelucci L. Lidocaine-induced reduction in carnitine levels and morphological muscular alterations. Pharmacol Res 1990; 22 (Suppl 2):197 (Abstract).

95. Rossignoli L, Bertini L, Molino FM et al. L-carnitine combined with various anesthesiological techniques: its role in the development of endocrine-metabolic response to surgical stress. Alim Nutr Metab 1992; 13:57-67.

96. Pessotto P, Liberati R, Petrella O, Hulsmann WC. Quaternary nitrogen compounds affect carnitine distribution in rats. Particular emphasis on edrophonium. Biochim Biophys Acta Lipids Lipid Metab 1996; 1299:245-251.

97. Rebouche CJ. The ability of guinea pigs to synthesize carnitine at a normal rate from epsilon-N-trimethyllysine or gamma butyrobetaine in vivo is not compromised by experimental vitamin C deficiency. Metab Clin Exp 1995; 44:624-629.

98. Rebouche CJ. Renal handling of carnitine in experimental vitamin C deficiency. Metab Clin Exp 1995; 44:1639-1643.

99. Bartels GL, Remme WJ, Scholte HR. Acute myocardial ischemia induces cardiac carnitine release in man. Eur Heart J 1997; 18:84-90.

# CHAPTER 7

# Carnitine Against Ischemia and Lipopolysaccharide Toxicity

W.C. Hülsmann

## INTRODUCTION

Cytokines, such as tumor necrosis factor (TNF) and interleukin-1 (IL-1), have been found in infectious and degenerative diseases in response to the reaction of membrane lipopolysaccharides with macrophages.[1-3] Some cytokines react with cell walls of capillary endothelium, resulting in contraction. This generates edema, which affects the microcirculation. We have used lipopolysaccharide from *E.coli* in studies on edema of rat hearts and found that during Langendorff perfusion a considerable increase of interstitial fluid production.[4] This increase causes loss of proteins such as lipoprotein lipase and non-protein compounds such as carnitine, part of which are stored in interstitium.[5,6] Loss of interstitial compounds also occurs through the lack of oxygen in tissues due to increased capillary permeability.[7] The presence of carnitine in interstitium is important for exchange-diffusion of long-chain acylcarnitine (LCAC), which accumulates in ischemic cells.[8,9] The exchange may be catalyzed by a plasmalemmal translocase. In mitochondria such an exchange was proposed two decades ago[10,11] and has since been identified by Pande and Murthy in other organelles as well.[12] Indirect evidence forecast a similar translocase in plasmalemma.[6] It allows cells to excrete LCAC from myocytes into interstitium, where it may react with endothelial plasmalemma and reduce the $Ca^{2+}$ overload of threatened capillary endothelium,[5,6,13] the basis of edema. The reduction of edema improves (re)perfusion of tissues.[5,6] However, ischemia is also the basis for the loss of carnitine from the interstitial space, so that its supplementation may be required to allow LCAC to be removed from ischemic cells. It should be noted that there is no reason for carnitine administration to enrich intracellular carnitine when acylcarnitine accumulation is a fact. In dogs we found

*Carnitine Today*, edited by Claudio De Simone and Giuseppe Famularo.
© 1997 Landes Bioscience.

that carnitine acutely increased the force of contraction of paced skeletal muscle in the absence of carnitine deficiency, as proven in biopsies.[14,15] Therefore, acute action of carnitine on muscle function should be exterior to cells (in interstitium). We have shown a carnitine stock outside myocytes in heart after injection of rats with [14]C-carnitine prior to isolation of the heart for Langendorff perfusion. Two carnitine pools were found: one which was labeled quickly and rapidly released during reperfusion after a period of ischemia, and the other which retained carnitine under these conditions.[16] We considered the slow-release pool to be present in cardiomyocytes and the fast-release pool in vascular endothelial cells, as we thought the latter cell type to be more fragile.[16] Later, this was found to be incorrect when we showed that carnitine diffuses only slowly from isolated endothelial cells, even during lactic acidosis and generation of oxygen free radicals[17]—conditions known to occur in ischemia. Hence, the compartment which loses carnitine after ischemia is likely to be the interstitium.

That ischemia causes capillaries to leak has been known since 1928,[7] and that LCAC is a membrane stabilizer has been known since we found that micromolar palmitoylcarnitine inhibits the loss of myoglobin and lactate dehydrogenase from Langendorff hearts during reperfusion after a period of ischemia.[18] In that study we found similar effects of another amphiphile, phenylmethylsulfanylfluoride.[18] Indeed, specificity is lacking as numerous amphiphiles are capable of membrane stabilization in ischemic and inflammatory diseases. We have found in paced dog muscle that edrophonium was as efficient as (acyl)carnitine in increasing the force of contraction.[15] The effect of both of these quaternary nitrogen compounds was not additive, suggesting similar action on oxygen supply to ischemic tissue.[15] Recently, a number of quaternary nitrogen compounds have been found to acutely modify the distribution of carnitine in different rat tissues.[19] They lowered carnitine levels in blood and kidney and acutely increased carnitine in liver,[19] suggesting carnitine accumulation in the interstitium of organs. This finding supports our view that the retention of (inter)cellular carnitine in tissues is affected by the changing tightness of inter-endothelial gap junctions. L-carnitine becomes effective as a membrane stabilizer only after conversion to LCAC, as low levels of L-carnitine or short-chain acylcarntine were not active compared to LCAC.[18] Moreover, our studies in dogs showed that L-carnitine could not be replaced by D-carnitine and that the L-isomer had no effect when insulin had been injected.[14] Insulin lowers fatty acid levels and inhibits carnitine-palmitoyl-transferase-1,[20] the enzyme that converts L-carnitine to LCAC. LCAC has a higher affinity for capillary endothelium than short-chain acylcarnitine, as calcium overload may be prevented by millimolar L- or D-propionyl-carnitine[21] compared to micromolar palmitoylcarnitine.[13] That non-physiological amphiphylic quaternary N-compounds may be effective against edema formation follows from the effect of edrophonium as mentioned,[15,19] and by other positively charged drugs that inhibit $Ca^{2+}$ fluxes, such as chloroquine, flunarizine and chlorpromazine. These will not be discussed here, as we shall focus on the potent endogenous quaternary N-compound LCAC, which only accumulates in ischemic areas. Carnitine administration, which mobilizes LCAC in ischemic areas, contrasts that of unnatural cationic amphiphiles, as these will act on non-ischemic areas as well and might create undesirable side-effects.

## L-CARNITINE IN THE TREATMENT OF ISCHEMIC MUSCLES

### PREVENTION OF CARNITINE DEFICIENCY IN CARDIAC INTERSTITIUM

Acidosis, known to occur in ischemia, causes edema by increased access to interstitum,[22] followed by the loss of carnitine and other compounds from interstitium. When carnitine is infused during ischemia, supplementation of FFA for LCAC production is generally not required as lipolysis will be activated in states of stress, when glucagon and catecholamine levels are high and insulin is low. The problem that remains is for L-carnitine to reach the ischemic area; therefore vascular obstructions must be removed, restoring flow and bringing carnitine to the site of ischemia. After the release of obstruction, reflow is facilitated by propionyl-L-carnitine, as shown by Sassen et al for the heart.[23] That the energy charge in the affected area decreased initially must be interpreted by the cost of ATP for functional recovery. Hence in ischemia there is an absolute need to release vascular obstruction, followed by the promotion of reflow in which (acyl)carnitine may play a role. According to Bernouilli's law, higher flow rates cause lower (intracapillary) pressure, causing the dissipation of edema and, therefore, the improvement of $O_2$ diffusion from capillaries to tissues. The fact that, during low flow perfusion of Langendorff hearts, vasoconstriction was as efficient as superoxide dismutase to increase heart function[24] may explain our observation. It may also explain the observation of Snoeckx et al[25] that increase in perfusion pressure promotes recovery after global ischemia of the heart.

The improvement of reflow by promotion of LCAC transport from cells to the interstitium does not harmonize with treatment of ischemia with glucose combined with insulin and potassium.[26] This so-called GIK treatment may be expected to promote (lactic) acidosis by stimulation of glycolysis[27] while inhibiting fatty acid metabolism (including LCAC formation; see McGarry and Foster[20]).

Recently we found in paced rat Langendorff hearts, perfused with media not containing fluorocarbon or erythrocytes as $O_2$ carriers, that insufficient tissue oxygenation resulted in the release of catabolic products such as lactate, urate and lysolecithin.[6] This was found to diminish after the addition of L-carnitine to the perfusion medium whereas LCAC release increased.[6] The inverse behavior of excretion suggests that LCAC indeed reduces tissue ischemia. The release of lysolecithin in ischemia indicates membrane degradation, which in vivo may lead to the release of platelet activating factor (ref. 28) as well as cytokines in myocardial infarction.[2] Therefore, it can be expected that carnitine administration may reduce the release of these factors from hypoperfused tissues undergoing membrane degeneration. Indeed, carnitine has been shown to reduce the loss of phospholipids from ischemic myocardium,[29] explaining its effect on limitation of infarct size.[30] The observation of Spagnoli et al[31] that in myocardial infarction, carnitine is lost, supports the necessity of carnitine treatment.

SKELETAL MUSCLE ISCHEMIA IN RELATION TO CARNITINE TREATMENT

As mentioned in the Introduction, we found that in dogs carnitine acutely increased the force of contraction of paced skeletal muscle in the absence of carnitine deficiency.[14,15] We also observed that chronic carnitine treatment reduced triglyceride accumulation in dog skeletal muscle,[32,33] and Natali et al[34] found that acute hypercarnitinemia increased fatty substrate oxidation in humans. This finding corresponds with our observation Langendorff rat hearts where carnitine was found to diminish lipidosis.[35] Brevetti et al[36] found an increase in the walking distance of patients with peripheral vascular disease treated with carnitine.

DIABETIC PSEUDOHYPOXIA AND CARNITINE TREATMENT

Reduced carnitine levels have been found in diabetes and long-term fasting.[37-40] Williamson et al[41] have used the term "pseudohypoxia" in diabetes. This situation has in common with fasting that low insulin levels are accompanied by fatty acid mobilization and that permeability of capillaries increases, which may lead to a loss of interstitial carnitine. Therefore, treatment with carnitine may be expected to reduce interstitial edema and promote the oxygenation of tissues as described.

## SUMMARY

Capillary endothelial cells may suffer from $Ca^{2+}$ overload by the action of various agents such as fatty acids, products of arachidonic acid metabolism and cytokines. The result is edema formation and increase of lymph production, causing the loss of interstitial components, of which we have studied lipoprotein lipase and carnitine. Multifactorial mechanisms are operative after ischemia followed by reperfusion and after bacterial invasion. The effect of carnitine administration in endotoxemia has recently been reviewed by Famularo et al.[42] The loss of carnitine from interstitium, as proposed in the present paper, may lead to defective release of long-chain acylcarnitine from cells that accumulate this substance in hypoxic tissues.

The cationic amphiphilic nature of long-chain acylcarnitine may abolish endothelial $Ca^{2+}$ overload and restore aerobiosis. This may also be achieved by nonphysiological cationic amphiphiles and gluco-corticoids which, however, may affect the $Ca^{2+}$ level in areas that do not suffer from ischemia and, hence, may cause undesirable side-effects.

REFERENCES

1. Beutler B, Mahoney J, Le Trang N et al. Purification of cachectin, a lipoprotein lipase suppressing hormone secreted by endotoxin induced EAW 264.7 cells. J Exp Med 1985; 161:984-995.
2. Neumann FJ, Ott I, Gawaz M et al. Cardiac release of cytokines and inflammatory reponses in acute myocardial infarction. Circulation 1995; 92:748-755.
3. Filkins JP. Monokines and the metabolic pathophysiology of septic shock. Fed Proc 1985; 44:300-304.
4. Hulsmann WC, Dubelaar ML, DeWit LEA et al. Cardiac lipoprotein lipase: effects of lipopolysaccharide and tumor necrosis factor. Mol Cell Biochem 1988; 79:137-145.
5. Hulsmann WC, Peschechera A, Arrigoni-Martelli E. Carnitine and cardiac interstitium. Cardioscience 1994; 5:67-72.
6. Hulsmann WC, Peschechera A, Serafini F et al. Release of ischemia in paced rat Langendorff hearts by supply of L-carnitine; role of endogenous long-chain acylcarnitine. Mol Cell Biochem 1996; 156:87-91.
7. Landis EM. Micro-injection studies of capillary permeability III: the effect of a lack of oxygen on the permeability of the capillary wall of fluid and to plasma proteins. Am J Physiol 1928; 83:528-543.
8. Shug AL, Thomsen JD, Folts JD et al. Changes in tissue levels of carnitine and other metabolites during myocardial ischemia and anoxia. Arch Biochem Biophys 1978; 187:25-33.
9. Idell-Wenger JA, Grotyohann LW, Neely JR. Coenzyme A and carnitine distribution in normal and ischemic hearts. J Biol Chem 1978; 253:4310-4318.
10. Pande SV. A mitochondrial carnitine acylcarnitine translocase system. Proc Natl Acad Sci USA 1975; 72:883-887.
11. Ramsay RR, Tubbs PK. The mechanism of fatty acid uptake by heart mitochondria: an acylcarnitine-carnitine exchange. FEBS Lett 1975; 54:21-25.
12. Pande SV, Murthy MSR. Carnitine-acylcarnitine translocase deficiency: implications in human pathology. Biochim Biophys Acta 1995; 1226:269-276.
13. Inoue N, Hirata K, Akita H et al. Palmitoyl-L-carnitine modifies the function of vascular endothelium. Cardiovasc Res 1994; 28:129-134.
14. Dubelaar ML, Lucas CMHB, Hulsmann WC. Acute effect of L- carnitine upon skeletal muscle force tests in the dog. Am J Physiol 1991; 260:E189-E193.

15. Dubelaar ML, Lucas CMBH, Hulsmann WC. The effect of L- carnitine on force development of the latissimus dorsi muscle in dogs. J Card Surg 1991; 6(1):270-275.
16. Hulsmann WC, Dubelaar ML. Carnitine requirement of vascular endothelial and smooth muscle cells in imminent ischemia. Mol Cell Biochem 1992; 116:125-129.
17. Peschechera A, Ferrari LE, Arrigoni-Martelli E et al. Uptake and release of carnitine by vascular endothelium in culture; effect of protons and oxygen free radicals. Mol Cell Bioch 1995; 142:99-106.
18. Hulsmann WC, Dubelaar ML, Lamers JMJ et al. Protection by acylcarnitines and phenylmethylsulfanylfluoride of rat heart subjected to ischemia and reperfusion. Biochim Biophys Acta 1985; 847:62-66.
19. Pessotto P, Liberati R, Petrella O et al. Quaternary nitrogen compounds affect carnitine distribution in rats; particular emphasis on edrophonium. Biochim Biophys Acta 1996;1299:245-251.
20. McGarry JD, Foster DW. Regulation of hepatic fatty acid oxidation and ketone body formation. Ann Rev Biochem 1980; 49:395-420.
21. Van Hinsbergh VWM, Scheffer MA. Effect of propionyl-L-carnitine in human endothelial cells. Cardiovasc Drugs and Ther 1991; 5(1):97-105.
22. Chambers R, Zweifach BW. Intercellular cement and capillary permeability. Physiol Rev 1947; 27:436.
23. Sassen LMA, Besztarosti K, VanDerGiessen WJ et al. L-propionylcarnitine increases postischemic blooflow but does not affect recovery of energy charge. Am J Physiol 1991; 261:H172-H180.
24. Hulsmann WC, Dubelaar ML. Early damage of vascular endothelium during cardiac ischemia. Cardiovasc Res 1987; 21:674-677.
25. Snoeckx LH, Van der Vusse GJ, Van der Veen FH et al. Recovery of hypertrophied rat hearts after global ischemia at different perfusion pressures. Pflügers Arch 1989; 413:303-312.
26. Oliver MF, Opie LH. Effects of glucose and fatty acids on myocardial ischemia. Lancet 1994; 343:155-158.
27. Baily IA, Radda GK, Seymour AL et al. The effect of insulin on myocardial metabolism and acidosis in normoxia and ischemia. Biochim Biophys Acta 1982; 720:17-27.
28. Hulsmann WC. Vulnerability of vascular endothelium in lipopolysaccharide toxicity: effect of (acyl)carnitine on endothelial stability. Mediators of Inflammation 1993; 2:S21-23.
29. Nagao B, Kobayashi A, Yamazaki N. Effects of L-carnitine on phospholipids in ischemic myocardium. Jpn Heart J 1987; 28:243-251.
30. Ura K, Hironaka Y, Sakurai I. Effect of carnitine on size limitation of experimental myocardial infarction. Am J Cardiovasc Pathol 1990; 3:131-142.

31. Spagnoli LG, Corsi M, Villaschi S. Myocardial carnitine deficiency in acute myocadial infarction. Lancet 1982; i:1419-1420.
32. Dubelaar ML, Lucas CMBH, Hulsmann WC. On the mechanism of fat accumulation in wrapped latissimus dorsi muscle (cardiomyoplasty) and the effect of chronic L-carnitine administration. Basic Appl Myol 1991; 1:305-310.
33. Dubelaar ML, Glatz JFC, DeJong YF et al. L-carnitine combined with minimal electrical stimulation promotes type transformation of canine latissimus dorsi. J Appl Physiol 1994; 76:1636-1642.
34. Natali A, Santoro D, Brandi LS et al. Effects of acute hypercarnitinemia during increased fatty substrate oxidation in man. Metabolism 1993; 42:594-600.
35. Hulsmann WC, Stam H, Maccari F. The effect of excess (acyl) carnitine on lipid metabolism in rat heart. Biochim Biophys Acta 1982; 713:39-45.
36. Brevetti G, Chiariello M, Ferulano G et al. Increases in walking distance in patients with peripheral vascular disease treated with L-carnitine: A double-blind, crossover study. Circulation 1988; 77:767-773.
37. Choi YR, Fogle PJ, Bieber LL. The effect of long-term fasting on the branched-chain carnitines and branched-chain acyl-transferases. J Nutr 1979; 109:155-161.
38. Pearson DJ, Tubbs PK. Carnitine and derivatives in rat tissues. Biochem J 1967; 105:953-963.
39. Fogle PJ, Bieber LL. Effect of streptozotocin on carnitine and carnitine acyl transferases in rat heart, liver and kidney. Biochem Med 1976; 22:119-126.
40. Feuvray D, Idell-Wenger JA and Neely JR. Effects of ischemia on rat myocardial function and metabolism in diabetes. Circ Res 1979; 44:322-329.
41. Williamson JR, Chang K, Frangos M et al. Hyperglycemic pseudohypoxia and diabetic complications. Diabetes 1993; 801-813.
42. Famularo G, De Simone C, Arrigoni-Martelli E et al. Carnitine and septic shock: a review. J Endotoxin Res 1995; 2:141-147.

# Carnitine and Derivatives in Experimental Infections

Nicola M. Kouttab, Linda L. Gallo, Dwayne Ford,
Chris Galanos, Michael Chirigos

## INTRODUCTION

Energy in humans and higher animals is generated through β-oxidation of long-chain fatty acids, which are transported across the mitochondrial membrane by carnitine (3-hydroxy-4-methyl-ammoniobutanoate). The bulk of body carnitine is found in cardiac and skeletal tissue, and to a lesser extent in various organs such as the liver.[1-3] Thus, generating adequate levels of carnitine is an important factor in maintaining normal metabolic processes.[4,5] Indeed, it has been shown that L-carnitine O-palmitoyltransferase deficiency is accompanied by hypoketoic hypoglycemia and cardiomyopathy,[6] an observation which may indicate a role for carnitine in cardiac disease.[7-9] Metabolic disorders of fatty acids have also been associated with carnitine deficiency. Syndromes and symptoms include liver dysfuction, disorders of the central nervous system, and skeletal muscle weakness.[10] In addition to its classical role in energy metabolism, recent studies have provided evidence for an immunomodulatory role for carnitine, particularly in alleviating pathogenic symptoms induced by infectious agents, as discussed below.

During infection, polymorphonuclear leukocytes (PMN) are mobilized to participate in the control and destruction of pathogens. This is accomplished by extravasation into inflammatory tissue, followed by phagocytosis of pathogens and their destruction by oxidative reactions. During this process cytokines which participate in various immunoregulatory functions are produced. Studies in vitro examined the effect of carnitine on PMN activation and mobilization when incubated with *Staphylococcus aureus*.[11,12] In the presence of 100 mg/ml of carnitine, the expression of the adhesion molecule CD11b was upregulated, the oxidative functions of PMN were maintained and the producton of TNF-α was consistently reduced.[12] These studies did indicate that the activity of carnitine varied with each donor, and that the ultimate effect of carnitine may be dependent upon the "initial status of the cell." Other studies have shown that variations in carnitine levels occur in various disease states. When compared to healthy controls, granulocyte carnitine levels were higher in bacterial infections, and lymphocyte carnitine levels were higher in Crohn's disease. Thus, carnitine levels in lymphocytes or granulocytes may reflect an enhanced metabolic rate of these cells during disease states, which, in turn, may impact immunoglobulin formation or phagocytosis.[13]

Numerous studies have reported that an excessive production of cytokines plays a prominent role in the pathogenesis of disease. In particular, tumor necrosis factor-alpha (TNF-α) has been implicated in the induction of several clinical symptoms. In studies in patients with tuberculosis, excessive TNF-α may participate in the induction of fever, weight loss, necrosis, release of acute phase proteins and intravascular coagulation.[14] In contrast, a moderate production of TNF-α may participate in a protective role in the course of pleuritis in tuberculosis patients.[15] Treatment of patients with tuberculosis with acetyl-L-carnitine (ALC) was observed to enhance the T-dependent anti-bacterial immunity.[16,17] Additionally, in a double-blind study, patients with active tuberculosis infection were either treated orally with 2 gm of ALC per day for 30 days, or received placebo only. The results showed that T cell function increased in patients treated with ALC, but decreased in patients receiving placebo. The immuno-modulatory effect of ALC could be attributed to: (1) its ability to supplement energy needed by lymphocytes to fight infection; (2) its ability to prevent chemotherapeutic impairment of lymphocyte funtion[18] or potentiate lymphocyte antibacterial activity; and (3) the release of immuno-enhancing neurohormones and neuropeptides through its ability to modulate the hypothalamus-pituitary-adrenal axis.[19] Other studies have demonstrated that an excessive production of TNF-α adversely affects HIV disease progression.[20-22] Treatment of patients with ALC enhanced immune reponses in HIV-infected patients.[23-25] Of interest, however, is that in the studies in tuberculosis patients and HIV-infected patients discussed above, no modification of in vivo TNF-α production was observed. Therefore, it appears that the amelioration of symptoms in patients treated with ALC may also involve mechanisms independent of TNF-α modulation.

Studies have also pointed to a central role of TNF-α in the pathogenesis of septic shock.[26-29] It was shown that the sensitivity of mice to lipopolysaccharide (LPS) can be enhanced following bacterial infection. Both gram-positive[30] and gram-negative, killed or live bacteria can induce this sensitivity.[31] It was observed that whereas 200 mg of endotoxin was required to kill C57BL/6 mice before infection, only 1 mg of endotoxin could achieve the same lethality in mice infected for 5 days with *S. typhimurium*.[31] The mechanism for this increased sensitivity was attributed to the enhanced production, as well as enhanced sensitivity to, TNF-α.[32] In experiments where mice were lethally sensitized to LPS by D-galactosamine or by infection with *Propionobacter acnes*, ALC was capable of protecting mice from death, or significantly prolonging survival in both models. Protection was observed whether sensitization was to LPS or TNF-α. In these experiments, protection from lethality was observed when 5 mg of ALC was given 30 minutes, with maximum protection at 1-2 hours, prior to administration of LPS or TNF-α.[33] Similarly, ALC protected mice infected with *P. acnes* against LPS challenge.[32] Other studies reported that carnitine at 500 mg/kg body weight given at 16 hours, and at 30 minutes pre-LPS administration, increased the survival rate of rats.[34]

In studies using Sprague-Dawley rats, it was observed that the administration of LPS induced the pathogenesis observed in septic shock.[35] Treatment of these rats with carnitine or isovalerylcarnitine tartrate (VBT) markedly delayed and decreased the severity of the disease. Rats treated with carnitine and VBT had greater food consumption and less loss of body weight than untreated rats. Treated rats did not show the acute LPS-induced rise in serum triglycerides. Thus, these studies concluded that carnitines may have therapeutic potential in the treatment of sepsis, with one mechanism being to partition fatty acids from esterification to oxidation.[35] Furthermore, the studies indicated that both carnitine and VBT may have decreased the lethality induced by LPS treatment.

Products of LPS toxicity such as TNF and PAF have been shown to affect a variety of cell types including endothelial cells. These cells catalyze carnitine-dependent fatty acid oxidation.[36] It has been shown that during reperfusion of Langendorff rat hearts a loss of carnitine may occur in endothelial cells, which may in part be caused by the generation of oxygen free radicals.[37] Although TNF did not affect lipoprotein lipase activity or interstitial fluid production, PAF did increase permeability of the endothelium. Treatment with carnitine could prevent the loss of flow regulation in endothelial cells—an event which may prevent the early stages of endotoxic shock.[38]

The observations that carnitine can modulate the immune response led to the initiation of studies investigating a potential therapeutic effect of carnitine in bacterial infection, and in particular, infections which can lead to septic shock. These studies utilized animal models which included:

1. Amelioration of lipopolysaccharide (LPS)-induced sepsis by carnitine in male Sprague-Dawley rats.
2. *Klebsiella pneumoniae* infection in C57BL/6 mice.
3. *Salmonella typhimurium* infection in C57BL/6 mice.

The proposed dose and treatment schedules for the bacterial infection models were as follows:

Dose of carnitine:               200 mg/kg body weight
Route of treatment: Intraperitoneal (IP)
Route of Infection:  Intravenous
Treatment Schedule:         Daily starting at day minus 1 (-1)
                                          of infection

Schedule:

Day -1          Sacrifice animals for pretreatment values
Day -1          Start treatment with carnitine
Day 0           Infect animals
Day +1          Sacrifice
Day +3          Sacrifice
Day +5          Sacrifice
Day +8          Sacrifice if surviving

A slight variation of the above models was used for the rat model. In this regard, rats were injected at time zero with LPS 24 mg/kg body weight, followed immediately with L- or D-carnitine injected IP at 100 mg/kg body weight. The carnitine injections were repeated at 2, 8 and 16 hours post LPS administration. For all studies control groups injected with sodium bicarbonate ($NaHCO_3$; carnitine vehicle) were included.

The parameters measured in these studies included the following:

1-          Survival
2-          Delayed death
3-          Body temperature
4-          Body weight
5-          Food consumption
6-          High density and low density lipids (HDL, LDL) in serum
7-          Blood glucose
8-          Cytokines in serum : IL-1, IL-6, TNF-$\alpha$, IFN$\gamma$
9-          Carnitine levels: liver, serum, muscle, spleen
10-        Histology: liver, kidney, lung
11-        Eicosanoids: PGE2, 6-keto PGF$\alpha$, TXB2, LTB4 (measured by Dr. I.L.Bonta, Erasmus Universty Rotterdam, The Netherlands)

The above parameters were selected because of previous reports demonstrating changes in these parameters upon treatment with carnitine.

For the studies using *S.typhimurium* a culture was purchased from the American Type Culture Collection (ATCC) No. 19585, which taxonomically is called *Salmonella cholerasuis*, subspecies cholarasuis, serotype typhimurium. A lyophilized culture was rehydrated in tryptic soy broth (TSB), inoculated in a MacConkey agar plate and incubated overnight at

37°C. The culture used in the studies was established from a single colony. Each subsequent culture was grown overnight at 37°C in TSB and all cultures were resuspended in PBS for optical density (OD) reading. A 10-fold serial diluion of the suspension was executed for visual measurement of colony forming units (CFU), and 2-fold dilutional experiments were used to establish a linear relationship between OD and concentration of overnight cultures. The bacterial strain was biochemically identified on a Vitek apparatus and typed using a DIFCO *Salmonella* typing test. The results were conclusive that the organism used in these studies was *Salmonella* serotype typhimurium.

The lethal dose of the organism that best fit the time course of the experiments was $10^6$ CFU in 0.1 ml of PBS. Lethality began on day 3 or 4 and was complete by day 5-8.

In a typical experiment, Balb/c mice (6 weeks old) were pretreated on day minus 1 with 200 mg/kg body weight with L-carnitine. On day zero the animals wre infected intravenously with 1 x $10^6$ CFUs. The groups were as follows: *S.typhimurium* alone, *S.typhimurium* + L-carnitine; L-carnitine alone. The mice were sacrificed at days 1, 3 and 5 post-infection with *S.typhimurium,* and tissue and blood were collected for the various parameters to be examined. Additional groups of mice were used to determine the ability of carnitine to increase survival. All experimental procedures used were established in our laboratories.

## RESULTS OF MURINE STUDIES

### CHEMISTRY

The studies in the murine systems yielded similar results and representative data are given.

Serum chemistry assays revealed little or no differences between treated and untreated mice. L-carnitine increased HDL and triglycerides and lowered LDL on day 3. No effect was observed for glucose and cholesterol. Body weight and temperature did not show significant differences between treated and untreated groups, nor was a difference observed in food consumption. Flow cytometry data revealed no differences in the spleen cell populations of the various groups examined. This phenotypic characterization included expression of CD3, CD4, CD8, B220 and CD11b (Becton-Dickinson, San Jose, CA.).

### TISSUE PATHOLOGY

Tissue pathology was observed mainly in the liver and spleen, but not in the lung or kidney. In the liver, sections revealed multifocal neutrophilic micro-abesses with necrosis of adjacent hepatocytes, indicative of sepsis induced by *S. typhimurium.* In the spleen, there was reactive lymphoid hyperplasia and extramedullary hematopoiesis. Occasional megakaryocytes were noted. Focal neutrophilic aggregates were present with admixed apoptotoic debris. Again, no differences were observed between carnitine-treated or untreated *S. typhimurium* infected mice.

CYTOKINES AND EICOSANOIDS

Treatment with L-carnitine was capable of modulating cytokine levels, in particular on day 3 post infection; see Figure 8.1, Table 8.1. Although serum levels of IL-1α, IFNγ, and IL-6 did not change with L-carnitine treatment, there was a significant decrease in TNF-α and, to some extent, in IL-1β. All cytokines were measured using ELISA (R&D Systems, Minneapolis, MN.). The decrease in the production of TNF-α was further investigated by examining the mRNA using RT-PCR. The RT-PCR was performed on purified total RNA using Clonetech kits (Clonetech Laboratories, Inc, San Diego, CA.) as described by the manufacturer. As a control for sample amount and quality, GAPDH was amplified in parallel with the sample. The results, (Fig. 8.2) clearly show that the mRNA for TNF-α is reduced in mice infected with *S. typhimurium* and treated with L-carnitine as compared to infected untreated mice.

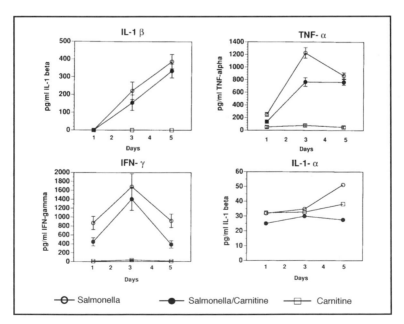

Fig. 8.1. Graphic representation of cytokine levels in mice infected with *S. typhimurium* and treated or untreated with L-carnitine. Cytokine levels were determined by ELISA on sera obtained at day 3 post infection.

Results for eicosanoid levels are presented in Table 8.2. Treatment of *S. typhimurium* infected mice with L-carnitine did not appear to influence levels of 6K-PGE2. However, there was a significant decrease (approximately 50%) in levels of TXB2.

### DELAYED DEATH OF L-CARNITINE TREATED MICE

Results from three separate experiments showed that treatment of infected mice can delay death in some animals. Table 8.3 presents data from three experiments which show that 30% of the mice treated with 200 mg/kg body weight of L-carnitine survived for 11, 12 and 23 days. Untreated mice died within 8 days post-infection with *S. typhimurium*.

## RESULTS OF RAT STUDIES

The results of studies using the rat model (L.L.G.) are summarized below:

### ANIMAL HEALTH AND SURVIVAL

There were some moderate effects of L-carnitine and D-carnitine treated animals as compared to the untreated group. At 15 hours post LPS administration, the majority of animals had died. During this time, there were 12 deaths among the LPS injected animal, whereas there were 9 deaths in the L-carnitine treated group and 11 deaths in the D-carnitine treated group.

Changes in body temperature were also observed. At 1 hour post LPS administration the average temperature in all groups dropped 2.4 to 2.6°C. However, by 4 hours post-LPS, the temperature began to recover in both L-carnitine and D-carnitine treated groups, but not in the LPS administered group. Furthermore, by 15 hours post-LPS administration the temperature was at or near normal in both carnitine treated groups.

*Table 8.1. Cytokine levels in mice infected with* S. typhimurium *and treated or untreated with L-carnitine\**

| Cytokine | Day | Normal | Salmonella | Salm/Carn | Carnitine |
|----------|-----|--------|------------|-----------|-----------|
| IL-1β | 3 | 8.5 | 221.7 ±49.5 | 154.8 ±43.7 | 8.5 ±8.4 |
| IL-1α | 3 | 9.9 | 34.9 ±6.5 | 30.0 ±5.8 | 32.8 ±6.2 |
| TFN-α | 3 | 65.7 | 1227.4 ±83.7 | 764.5 ±69.6 | 78.3 ±22.4 |
| IFN-γ | 3 | 291 | 1682.5 ±288.8 | 1402.8 ±253.6 | 35.2 ±14.9 |
| IL-6 | 3 | 91 | 350.6 ±38.1 | 325.6 ±36.9 | 7.8 ±13.0 |

\*Values are in pg/ml. Mean ± SEM; n=3

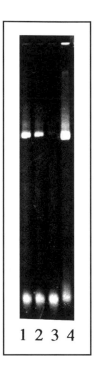

Fig. 8.2. Analysis of mRNA for TFNα showing reduction of TNFα mRNA in mice treated with L-carnitine. Total RNA was obtained from spleen cells of mice infected with *S. typhimurium* at day 3 post infection, and mRNA for TNFa was measured after amplification by polymerase chain reaction. Lanes 1, *S.typhimurium*; 2, *S. typhimurium* + L=carnitine; 3, L-carnitine alone; 4, positive control.

No significant differences in body weight or food intake were observed among carnitine treated or untreated groups.

SERUM CYTOKINES AND PLASMA EICOSANOIDS

All cytokines (TNF-α, IL-1, IL-6, IFNγ) as measured by chemiluminescence ELISA, were elevated post-LPS administration (Table 8.4). At 3 hours post-LPS, TNF-α levels in the L-carnitine and D-carnitine treated rats were markedly lowered. Similarly, at 15 hours post-LPS TNF-α remained lowered in both carnitine treated groups. Similar results were observed for the other cytokines.

The eicosanoids measured were 6-keto PGF-α, TXB2, PGE2, and LTB4. It was clear (Table 8.5) that LPS administration increased LTB4 levels and 6k-PGF-α and appeared to lower PGE2 levels. However, there was no evidence that the carnitine isomers had any effect on eicosanoid levels.

SERUM GLUCOSE AND LACTATE

Serum glucose was lowered significantly while serum lactate was elevated significantly by LPS. However, neither of the carnitine isomers modulated these LPS-induced changes.

**Table 8.2. Eicosanoid levels in mice infected with** S. **typhimurium** *and treated or untreated with L-carnitine\**

| Eicosanoid | Day | Normal | Salmonella | Salm/Carn | Carnitine |
|---|---|---|---|---|---|
| 6K-PGF1α | 3 | 331 | 1034 | 1199 | 1255 |
| PGE2 | 3 | 500 | 1071 | 1043 | 1002 |
| TXB2 | 3 | 870 | 2531 | 1322 | 3526 |

\*Values are in pg/ml. Measured by Dr.IL Bonta, Erasmus University Rotterdam, Rotterdam, The Netherlands

**Table 8.3. Survival time of mice infected with** S. **typhimurium** *and treated with L-carnitine\**

| Group survival | No. Survived | Survival Time | % |
|---|---|---|---|
| **Exp. 1** | | | |
| Infected | 0/10 | 5-7 days | 0% |
| Treated | 3/10 | 9 days | 33% |
| **Exp. 2** | | | |
| Infected | 0/10 | 3-5 days | 0% |
| Treated | 2/10 | 10-12 days | 20% |
| **Exp. 3** | | | |
| Infected | 0/10 | 5-9 days | 0% |
| Treated | 3/10 | 11-23 days | 30% |

\*L-carnitine was given intraperitoneally at 200 mg/kg body weight

TISSUE PATHOLOGY

As described for the murine systems, rats given LPS demonstrated pathologic processes consistent with sepsis in liver tissue, but not in kidney or lung. No differences in tissue pathology were observed between carnitine treated or untreated rats.

## DISCUSSION

The present studies provide evidence that carnitine can improve the course of sepsis in animal models infected with bacteria or injected with LPS. The main effects observed in these studies are the ability of carnitine to modulate the production of several cytokines and, in particular, to significantly decrease the production of TNF-α, a cytokine implicated in the pathogenesis of septic shock. In addition, at least 30% of animals treated with carnitine showed increased survival.

**Table 8.4. Cytokine levels in sera of rats given LPS and treated with carnitine\***

| Sera | 15 hrs post LPS |
|---|---|
| **IL-1 Levels** | |
| LPS only | 502 (74) |
| LPS + L-carnitine | 303 (13)** |
| LPS + D-carnitine | 322 (86) |
| **IL-6 levels** | |
| LPS only | 369 (61) |
| LPS + L-carnitine | 267 (29) |
| LPS + D-carnitine | 190 (65) |
| **IFN-γ** | |
| LPS only | 387 (60) |
| LPS + L-carnitine | 342 (20) |
| LPS + D-carnitine | 304 (107) |
| **TNF** | |
| LPS only | 571 (152) |
| LPS + L-carnitine | 316 (57) |
| LPS + D-carnitine | 339 (111) |

*Cytokine levels were measured by a chemiluminescence assay, see reference 53. Cytokine levels were also measured at 3 hours post LPS treatment; similar results were obtained as presented above for 15 hours, see ref. 53. Values are in pg/ml, Mean plus/minus SEM
**Significantly less than "LPS only" IL-1 $p < 0.03$; IFN-γ $p < 0.001$; TNF $p < 0.002$.

Other parameters measured such as tissue pathology, cell phenotypic markers, and triglycerides did not show differences between carnitine treated or untreated mice. One explanation for such results is that these experiments were not of long duration, for example all mice dying within eight days and thus not allowing sufficient time for changes to be observed.

Several reasons can be cited for the ability of carnitine to alleviate pathogenic processes during infection. Studies have shown that a consequence of sepsis is the decrease of carnitine in the liver[34] and muscle.[39] Thus treatment with carnitine can replenish carnitine supplies, thereby maintaining normal tissue functions. It is also clear from various studies, as discussed above, that carnitine can decrease the production of TNF-α, to which several pathogenic processes have been attributed. In addition, several studies have pointed to the ability of carnitine or its derivatives to modulate immune responses. It was reported by De Simone and colleagues that an increase in carnitine concentration in the serum can potentiate certain functions such as mixed lymphocyte responses to mitogens.[40,41] Other studies have also shown that treatment of carnitine-depleted post-operative patients with L-

**Table 8.5. Plasma eicosanoid levels in rats given LPS and treated with Carnitine**

| Plasma | | Hours Post LPS | |
|---|---|---|---|
| | 1 | 3 | 15 |
| **6kPGF-1α** | | | |
| Control | 516 (70)# | | |
| LPS only | 1256 (198) | 904 (92)* | 370 (100) |
| LPS + L-carnitine | 1740 (131) | 1194 (21)* | 431 (25) |
| LPS + D-carnitine | 1586 (273) | 934 (109) | 367 (25) |
| | | | |
| **TXB2** | | | |
| Control | 4899 (478) | | |
| LPS only | 2886 (170)** | 1110 (197)** | 2153 (690)** |
| LPS + L-carnitine | 3182 (440)** | 1503 (139)** | 1025 (272)** |
| LPS + D-carnitine | 3868 (330)** | 2010 (599)** | 551 (123)** |
| | | | |
| **PGE2** | | | |
| Control | 723 (83) | | |
| LPS only | 380 (19)** | 128 (37)** | 441 (64)** |
| LPS + L-carnitine | 487 (73) | 231 (26)** | 411 (232)** |
| LPS + D-carnitine | 558 (39) | 203 (61)** | 160 (59)** |
| | | | |
| **LTB4** | | | |
| Control | 168 (54) | | |
| LPS only | 1483 (389)* | 5776 (2030)* | 273 (60) |
| LPS + L-carnitine | 2943 (1430) | 6498 (1933)* | 470 (111)* |
| LPS + D-carnitine | 685 (458) | 4881 (2765) | 4450 (2498) |

\#   pg/ml, Mean plus/minus SEM
\*   Significantly greater than control value p < 0.05
\*\* Significantly less than control value p < 0.05

carnitine enhances lymphocyte mitogenesis.[42] The improvement of immune functions during aging and stress upon carnitine treatment has also been well documented.[43] Our own and other studies have clearly demonstrated that carnitine can modulate cytokine production, as well as other immune functions in humans and animal models.[44,45]

The mechanisms by which carnitine reduces TNF-α is not clear. It is speculated that carnitine increases prostaglandin release from macrophages,[46-49] and increases c-AMP levels, which in turn may act to decrease TNF-α production. Increase in prostaglandin and c-AMP levels may also potentiate IL-6 levels which may participate in reducing TNF levels.[50,51] It should be mentioned however, that while it appears clear that TNF-α may precipitate pathogenic processes during septic shock, other mechanisms may also be involved in inducing the lethality observed in endotoxemia.[52-56]

The results of these studies provide evidence that carnitine and its derivatives can ameliorate the pathogenic symptoms of sepsis. These results justify future studies which should consider the use of carnitine in combination with other agents such as antibiotics or antibodies against certain cytokines or their receptors (IL-1, TNF-α) for a treatment modality in infectious disease, particularly in those leading to septic shock.

## REFERENCES

1. Bieber LL, Farrell S. Carnitine octanolytransferase of mouse liver peroxisomes: properties and effect of hypolepidemic drugs. Arch Biochem 1983; 222:123-132.
2. Demaugre F, Bonnefont J-P, Colonna M et al. Infantile form of carnitine palmitoyltransferase II deficiency with hepatomuscular symptoms and sudden death: physiopathological approach to carnitine palmitoyltransferase deficiencies. J Clin Invest 1992; 87:859-864.
3. Finnochiaro G, Taroni F, Rochi M et al. cDNA cloning, sequence analysis, and chromosomal localization of the gene for human carnitine palmitoyltransferse. Proc Natl Acad Sci USA 1991; 88:661-665.
4. Bremer J. Carnitine. Metabolism and functions. Physiol Rev 1983; 1420-1480.
5. Feller AG, Rudman D. Role of carnitine in human nutrition. J Nutr 1988; 118:541-547.
6. Taroni F, Verderio E, Fiorucci S et al. Molecular characterization of inherited carnitine palmitoyltransferase II deficiency. Proc Natl Acad Sci USA 1992; 267:3758-8433.
7. Broderick TL, Quinney HA, Lopaschuck GD. Carnitine stimulation of glucose oxidation in the fatty acid perfused isolated working rat heart. J Biol Chem 1992; 267:3758-3763.
8. Pepine CJ. The therapeutic potential of carnitine in cardiovascular disorders. Clin Ther 1991; 13:2-21.
9. Siliprandi N, Di Lisa F, Menabio R. Clinical use of carnitine. Past, present, and future. Adv Exp Biol Med 1990; 272:175-181.
10. Kurahashi K, Andoh T, Sata K et al. Anesthesia in a patient with carnitine deficiency syndrome. Masui 1993; 42:1223-1226.
11. Schinetti ML, Mazzini A. Effect of L-carnitine on human neutrophil activity. Int J Tissue React 1986; 8:199-203.
12. Fattorossi A, Biselli R, Casciaro A et al. Regulation of normal human polymorphonuclear leucocytes by carnitine. Med Infamm 1993; 2:S37-S41.
13. Demirkol M, Sewell AC, Bohles H. The variation of carnitine content in human blood cells during disease: a study in bacterial infection and inflammatory bowel disease. Eur J Pediatr 1994; 153: 565-568.

14. Rook GAW, Attiyah RA, Foley N. The role of cytokines in the immunotherapy of tuberculosis and the regulation of agalactosyl IgG. Lymphokine Res 1989; 8:323-328.
15. Barnes PF, Fong SJ, Brennan PJ et al. Local production of tumor necrosis factor and IFNg in tuberculosis pleuritis. J Immunol 1990; 145:149-154.
16. Jirrillo E, Alatamura M, Munno I et al. Effects of acetyl-L-carnitine oral administration on lymphocyte antibacterial activity and TNF-a levels in patients with active pulmonary tuberculosis. A randomized double blind versus placebo study. Immunopharmacol Immunotoxicol 1991; 13:135-146.
17. Jirrillo E, Altamura M, Marcuccio C et al. Immunological responses in patients with tuberculosis and in vivo effects of acetyl-L-carnitine oral administration. Med Inflamm 1993; 2:S17-S20.
18. Youmans AS, Youmans GP. Effect of metabolic inhibitors on the formation of antibody to sheep erythrocytes on the development of delayed hypersensitivity, and on the immune response to infection with Mycobacterium tuberculosis in mice. Infect Immun 1978; 19:211-216.
19. Butler LD, Layman NK, Reidl PE et al. Neuroendocrine regulation of in vivo cytokine production and effects. I. In vivo regulatory networks involving the neuroendocrine system, intcrleukin-1 and tumor necrosis factor-alpha. J Neuroimmunol 1989; 24:143-153.
20. Matsuyama T, Kobayashi N, Yamamoto N. Cytokines and HIV infection: is AIDS a tumor necrosis factor disease? AIDS 1991; 5: 1405-1417.
21. Dezube BJ, Pardee AB, Beckett LA et al. Cytokine dysregulation in AIDS: in vivo overexpression of mRNA tumor necrosis factor-$\alpha$ and its correlation with that of the inflammatory cytokine GRO. J Acq Immun Defic Syndrome 1992; 1099-1104.
22. Mastroianni CM, Paoletti F, Valenti C et al. Tumor necrosis factor (TNF-$\alpha$) and neurological disorders in HIV infection. J Neurol Neurosurg Psychiat 1992; 55:219-221.
23. De Simone C, Calvani M, Catania S et al. Acetyl-L-catrnitine as a modulator of the neuroendocrine immune infection in HIV+ subjects. In: De Simone C, Martelli EA. eds. Stress, Immunity and Ageing. Amsterdam: Elsevier Publishers B.V. (Biomedical Division) 1989:125-138.
24. De Simone C, Tzantzoglou S, Jirrillo E et al. L-carnitine deficiency in AIDS patients. AIDS 1992; 6:203-205.
25. De Simone C, Tzantzoglou S, Famularo G et al. High-dose L-carnitine improves immunologic and metabolic parameters in AIDS patients. Immunopharmacol Immunotoxicol 1993; 15(1):1-12.
26. Glauser MP, Zanetti G, Baumgartner JD, Cohen J. Septic shock pathogenesis. Lancet 1991; 338:732-736.

27. Waage A, Halstensen A, Espevik T. Association between tumor necrosis factor in serum and fatal outcome in patients with meningococcal disease. Lancet 1987; I:355-357.

28. Vanderpoll T, Romijn JA, Endert E et al. Tumor necrosis factor mimics the metabolic response to acute infection in healthy humans. Am J Physiol 1991; 261:E457-E465.

29. Starnes HF, Warren RS, Jeevanandam H et al. Tumor necrosis factor and the acute metabolic response to tissue injury in man. J Clin Invest 1988; 82:1321-1325.

30. Suter E, Ullman GE, Hoffman RG. Sensitivity of mice to endotoxin after vaccination with BCG (bacillus Calmette-Guerin). Proc Soc Exp Bio Med 1958; 99:167-169.

31. Freudenberg MA, Galanos C. Tumor necrosis factor alpha mediates lethal activity of killed gram-negative and gram-positive bacteria in D-galactosamine-treated mice. Infect Immun 1991; 59:2110-2115.

32. Galanos C, Freudenberg MA, Krajewska D et al. Hypersensitivity to endotoxin. EOS J Immunol Immunopharmacol 1986; 6 (suppl. 3):78-81.

33. Galanos C, Freudenberg MA. Bacterial endotoxins: biological properties and mechanisms of action. Med Inflamm 1991; 2:S11-S16.

34. Takeyama N, Takagi D, Matsuo N et al. Altered hepatic fatty acid metabolism in endotoxicosis: effect of L-carnitine on survival. Am J Physiol 1989; 256:E31-E38.

35. Gallo LL, Tian Y, Orfalian Z et al. Amelioration of lipopolysaccharide-induced sepsis in rats by free and esterified carnitine. Med Inflamm 1993; 2:S51-S56.

36. Hulsmann WC, Dubelaar Ml, De Witt LEA, Persoon NLM. Cardiac lipoprotein lipase: effects of lipopolysaccharide and tumor necrosis factor. Mol Cell Biochem 1988; 79:137-145.

37. Hulsmann WC, Dubelaar ML. Carnitine requirement of vascular endothelial and smooth muscle cells in imminent ischemia. Mol Cell Biochem 1992; 116:125-129.

38. Hulsmann WC. Vulnerability of vascular endothelium in lipopolysaccharide toxicity: effect of (acyl) carnitine on endothelial stability. Med Inflamm 1993; 2:S21-S23.

39. Border JR, Burns GP, Rumph C, Shenk WG. Carnitine levels in severe infection and starvation: a possible key to the prolonged catabolic state. Surgery 1970; 68:175-179.

40. De Simone C, Delogu G, Fagioli A et al. Lipids and the immune system are influenced by L-carnitine. A study in elderly subjects with cardiovascular diseases. Int J Immunother 1985; 1:267-271.

41. De Simone C, Ferrari M, Lozzi A et al. Vitamins and immunity. II. influence of L-carnitine on the immune system. Acta Vitaminilogica et Enzymologica 1982; 4:135-140.

42. Carlsson M, Sundqvist MP. L-carnitine enhances lymphocyte mitogenesis in depleted traumatized and infected patients. Clin Nutr 1987; 6:39-44.

43. Monti D, Cossarizza A, Troiana L et al. Immunomodulatory properties of L-acetylcarnitine on lymphocytes from young and old humans. In: De Simone C, Martelli EA, eds. Stress, Immunity, and Ageing, a role for acetyl-L-carnitine. Amsterdam: Elsevier Science Publishers 1989; 83-96.

44. Kouttab N, De Simone C. Modulation of cytokine production by carnitine. Med Inflamm 1993; S25-S28.

45. Winter BK, Fiskum G, Gallo LL. Effects of L-carnitine on serum triglycerides and cytokine levels in rat models of cachexia and septic shock. Br J Cancer 1995; 72:1173-1179.

46. Elliott GR, Lauwen APM, Bonta IL. The effect of acute feeding of carnitine and propionyl carnitine on basal and A23187-stimulated eicosanoid release from rat carrageenin-elicited peritoneal macrophages. Br J Nutr 1990; 64:497-503.

47. Garrelds IM, Elliott GR, Pruimboom WM et al. Effects of carnitine and its congeners on eicosanoid discharge from rat cells: implications for release of TNFα. Med Inflamm 1993; S57-S62.

48. Renz H, Gong JH, Schmidt A et al. Release of tumour necrosis factor-alpha from macrophages: Enhancement and suppression are dose-dependent regulated by prostaglandin E2 and cyclic nucleotides. J Immunol 141:2388-2392.

49. Lehmmann V, Benninghoff B, Droge W. Tumour necrosis factor-induced activation of peritoneal macrophages is regulated by prostaglandin E2 and cAMP. J Immunol 1988; 141:957-959.

50. Flohe S, Heinrich PC, Schneider J et al. Time course of IL-6 and TNF-α release during endotoxin-induced endotoxin tolerance in rats. Biochem Pharmacol 1995; 41:1607-1614.

51. Rola-Pleszczynski M, Stankova J. Cytokine gene regulation by PGE2, LTB4 and PAF. Med Inflamm 1992; 1:5-8.

52. Tracey KJ, Fong Y, Hesse D et al. Anti-cachectin/TNF monoclonal antibodies prevent septic shock during lethal bacteremia. Nature 1987; 330:662-664.

53. Calandra T, Baumgartner JD, Grace CE et al. Prognostic values of tumor necrosis factor/cachectin, IL-1, IFNα and IFNγ in the serum of patients with septic shock. J Infec Dis 1990; 161:982-987.

54. Franks AK, Kujawa KI, Yaffe LJ. Experimental elimination of tumor necrosis factor in low-dose endotoxin models has variable effects on survival. Infec Immun 1991; 59:2609-2614.

55. Ruggiero V, D'Urso CM, Albertoni C et al. LPS-induced serum TNF production and lethality in mice: effect of L-carnitine and some acyl-derivatives. Med Inflamm 1993; 2:S43-S50.

56. Feuerstein G, Hallenbeck JM, Vanetta B et al. Effect of gram-negative endotoxin levels of serum corticosterone, TNF-α, circulating blood cells, and survival of rats. Circ Shock 1990; 30:265-278.

# CHAPTER 9

# Involvement of Carnitine in Reye's and Reye-Like Syndromes

Maria Teresa Tacconi

## DEFINITION OF REYE'S AND REYE-LIKE SYNDROMES

In 1963 Reye and colleagues described a new clinical pathological entity in childhood, called Reye's syndrome (RS),[1] characterized by non-inflammatory encephalopathy and fatty degeneration of the viscera. RS is a rare, acute, and often fatal metabolic disease affecting mostly 7- to 9-year old children after a few days of mild viral infection, treated with aspirin.[2,3] The link between viral infection and aspirin has been suggested by several epidemiological and clinical studies [4-7] and is further supported by the observed steep decline in RS cases since 1985, when professional and media warnings were issued against the use of aspirin during infections in children.[8-10] However, RS has reemerged in the last few years, suggesting that it has not vanished.[11]

The case definitions for RS epidemiological surveillance in the U.S. and the British Isles in the last decade (1981-1990)[12] and that of the Centers for Disease Control[13] group as RS all cases that present themselves with unexplained non-inflammatory encephalopathy and hepatopathy, characterized by alteration of one or more of the following laboratory parameters: serum hepatic transaminases more than three times the upper limit of normal, plasma ammonia concentration more than three times the upper limit of normal, or characteristic fatty infiltration of liver.

Both definitions are very general and can also be applied to illnesses whose causative agents are known; examples include valproic acid, an antiepileptic drug;[14] margosa oil, an extract from the neem tree, Azidichta indica A Juss, used as a traditional remedy in Hindu medicine,[15] hopantenate, a homolog of pantothenic acid used in Japan as a cerebral metabolic enhancer,[16] and toxins such as aflatoxin.[17] Some inherited metabolic diseases,

*Carnitine Today*, edited by Claudio De Simone and Giuseppe Famularo.
© 1997 Landes Bioscience.

too, like defects in ureagenesis, ketogenesis, branched-chain amino acid catabolism, carnitine transport, carbohydrate and pyruvate metabolism and fatty acid oxidation impairments[18,19] cause manifestations similar to those observed in RS. The term "Reye-like syndrome"(RLS) or "secondary RS" was introduced for these.

It is our opinion that RS and RLS comprise a class of multifactorial metabolic diseases with similar onset that can be grouped under the same pathogenetic pattern, principally involving derangement of liver mitochondria and then encephalopathy (for a review see ref. 20).

The pathogenesis of the disease can be summarized as follows: primary causative agents like fasting status and infections increase the catabolism and the subsequent flux of metabolites from peripheral tissues to the liver (fatty acids and amino acids); cytokines (TNF, IL-1 and IL-6) in particular mediate this effect during infection and experimental endotoxemia. Some drugs and other toxic compounds induce functional and morphological liver mitochondrial derangement. Oxidative metabolism is impaired, with subsequent stimulation of alternative pathways of oxidation (peroxisomal β-oxidation and microsomal ω-oxidation), producing unusual toxic acyl-CoA and dicarboxylic acids. Toxic compounds accumulate in the liver, affecting its functions and causing energy depletion (low ketone bodies and hypoglycemia).

Toxic products may be released into the circulation from which they reach other tissues, including the brain. Neurons and astrocytes in the brain may be affected differently: neurons suffer from the lack of energy and the toxic effects of dicarboxylic acids, the unusual acyl-CoA, ammonia and octanoic acid arriving from the bloodstream, and astrocytes may be directly affected by the β-oxidation derangement. Very important, though, may be the presence of a genetic predisposition which, by making the patient more sensitive to a particular causative agent, may facilitate the onset of RS and RLS.

## PATHOLOGICAL MANIFESTATION OF RS AND RLS

Clinical symptoms of RS are severe vomiting, progressive deterioration of consciousness, convulsions and coma. The metabolic alterations are high levels of hepatic transaminases, hypoglycemia, high levels of serum free fatty acids, low plasma ketone bodies, short- and medium-chain organic acidemia, increased excretion of carnitine and acylcarnitine in urine, and dicarboxylic aciduria.[1,21,22] Liver biopsies show alteration of mitochondrial morphology, with swelling, matrix expansion and reduction in number;[23] similar damage is present in the brain.[24] In patients who recover, mitochondrial morphology improves in parallel with recovery.[23] The activity of several mitochondrial enzymes is low in liver and brain of RS patients:

ornithine transcarbamylase, carbamylphosphate synthase, pyruvate carboxy-lase, succinate dehydrogenase, cytochrome c oxidase, citrate synthase, suc-cinate cytochrome c reductase, NADH rotenone-sensitive cytochrome c reductase, mitochondrial isoenzymes of fumarase and malate dehy-drogenases.[25-28]

It is generally believed that the mortality and morbidity of RS result from severe cerebral edema, which is the manifestation of a general insult to the mitochondrial structure and function[25,29] and in particular to the impairment of FA β-oxidation. This derangement may be involved in RS through multiple mechanisms. A general depletion of energy-giving prod-ucts may affect all tissues, but particularly neurons which depend on glu-cose and ketones as fuel. Accumulation of short, medium and long-chain acyl-CoA esters, as incomplete products of β-oxidation, may have toxic effects on some enzymatic systems.

Acyl-CoA derivatives could inhibit multiple enzymatic activities in-cluding key enzymes in gluconeogenesis, in the urea cycle and enzymes in-volved in ATP production.[30] Long-chain acyl-CoA derivatives, found in large amounts in RS serum,[31] can be oxidized in peroxisomes, which are increased in RS; but short and medium chain ones are only metabolized by ω-oxida-tion in microsomes, producing a number of unusual dicarboxylic acids, which are then excreted in plasma and urine.[32]

Agents associated with the development of RLS seem to act through an impairment of β-oxidation or of lipid metabolism. Uncoupling of oxi-dative/phosphorylative reactions, lowering of mitochondrial acetyl-CoA and free CoA levels and inhibition of β-oxidation by depletion of intra-mitochondrial ATP and free CoA were observed in rat mitochondria in vitro after margosa oil treatment.[33]

Alterations in plasma ketone bodies and FFA and in dicarboxylic ac-ids and medium-chain acyl carnitine in plasma and urine arise during valproic acid therapy.[34] In animals receiving valproic acid, hyper-ammonemia, hypocarnitinemia, mitochondrial swelling and microvesicular steatosis were observed in liver cells.[35,36] Excretion of dicarboxylic acids is abnormal during hopantenate-induced RLS.[37]

## INVOLVEMENT OF CARNITINE

Involvement of carnitine can be inferred, considering its key role in the transport of FA inside the mitochondria and in the metabolism of acetyl groups. β-oxidation inside the mitochondria depends on fatty acid trans-port from cytoplasm, in the form of acylcarnitine. Carnitine also regulates the transfer of acyl groups outside the mitochondria and exchanges acyl and acetyl groups with CoA, playing the well-known "buffer" role in preventing intracellular accumulation of acyl-CoA that may be toxic for many enzyme activities.

This observation is pertinent in RS and RLS. The disparity between extrahepatic mobilization, due to stimulated catabolic state, and the low hepatic clearance of metabolites leads to an accumulation of various fatty and organic acyl-CoA due to incomplete mitochondrial β-oxidation. In normal conditions the intracellular amount of these toxic compounds is kept low by transformation to the corresponding acylcarnitine which is used for oxidation or, if in excess, excreted into the urine.

In RS liver acyl-CoA derivatives may increase up to 4-fold and a large amount of free carnitine is needed to buffer them and release CoA. Muscle carnitine, which accounts for 98% of total body carnitine, is released, as evidenced by the low carnitine content of muscle during the acute phase of RS and the high levels of free carnitine and acylcarnitine in plasma in many but not all RS patients.[38,39] Urinary carnitine loss rises up to 40-fold,[30] with an excess of acyl carnitine over free carnitine. The acyl carnitine:free carnitine ratio is high in the livers of many RS patients.[39]

When no more free carnitine is available, toxic acyl-CoA esters accumulate, along with their adverse effects on enzyme functions. This condition can be considered a carnitine deficiency according to Stumpf: carnitine deficiency is present every time there is an accumulation of toxic acyl-CoA, whether or not depletion of carnitine from stores can be shown.[30] In valproate-induced RLS and in other disturbances involving damage in β-oxidation, a deficiency of carnitine could be demonstrated.[36,39] Prolonged fasting, often arising in RS and RLS, can be a cause of abnormal carnitine status.[40]

## CARNITINE TREATMENT IN RS AND RLS

Experimental models of RS in animals have been used to assess whether exogenous carnitine supplementation could be beneficial.

In mice with influenza virus-induced RLS, the inhibition of β-oxidation can be prevented by carnitine treatment.[41] In experimental RS induced by margosa oil, carnitine supplementation, particularly if associated with glucose, increases the rate of survival.[42] Carnitine prevents mitochondrial swelling induced by valproic acid.[36] Endotoxicosis in animals induces a syndrome resembling RS;[43] in this condition, too, carnitine increases the rate of survival and prevents alteration of hepatic fatty acid metabolism.

In a model of RS, rats were given low doses of endotoxin and aspirin, reproducing some of the hepatic metabolic alterations found in human RS such as low levels of ketone bodies, acetyl-CoA, low ATP/ADP ratio, and high levels of short and medium chain acyl-CoA intermediates.[44]

We used this model to investigate whether L-carnitine (LC) or acetyl-L-carnitine (ALC) helped to prevent hepatic alteration.[45] Fasted rats were treated with endotoxin (0.2 mg/kg i.p, 12 h before killing) plus aspirin (50 mg/kg i.p, 11 h before killing), and LC or ALC were given twice (500 mg/kg orally, 12 and 2 h before killing).

RLS rats showed a dramatic decrease of hepatic ketones and acetyl-CoA and an increase of isobutyryl-CoA and isovaleryl-CoA. Mitochondrial morphology was impaired with intracrystal swelling and increased electron density of the mitochondrial matrix. Determinants of mitochondrial membrane fluidity such as the microviscosity of mitochondrial lipids and the cholesterol-phospholipids ratio were decreased in both the inner and outer mitochondrial membrane fractions, suggesting a general increase in membrane fluidity.

LC and ALC reversed the decrease in ketone bodies and the toxic increase in short-chain acyl-CoA and the alteration in membrane morphology, whereas only ALC reversed the decrease in acetyl-CoA. LC and ALC prevented mitochondrial lipid alterations mainly in the inner membrane fraction.

These data suggest that carnitine, probably by keeping the endogenous pool large enough, protects the liver from toxic compounds which may impair various mitochondrial processes such as ATP production, lipid oxidation, gluconeogenesis and the urea cycle. Carnitine may act directly on ketone body levels, because supplementation of the endogenous pool, especially during catabolic-activated states like endotoxicosis or starving, stimulates hepatic fatty acid oxidation.

Few attempts have been made to treat RS or RLS patients with carnitine. One reason could be the difficulty of defining deficiency, since plasma levels of carnitine are often normal. However, plasma carnitine may be a misleading measurement, considering that plasma is the vector for transporting carnitine both from muscle to liver (to buffer toxic acyl-CoA) and from liver to kidney (where carnitine and acylcarnitine are excreted into the urine) and carnitine levels may fluctuate during the course of the disease. Instead, carnitine content may be inadequate at the sites where it is needed for its buffering activity.

To our knowledge there are only three studies of this nature. In 1983 Roe observed a slower clinical progression in six RS patients treated with carnitine.[38] Carnitine replacement led to clinical improvement of a three-year old child with repeated episodes of RLS.[46]

β-oxidation impairment was studied in 12 epileptic patients (3-19 years old) receiving valproate therapy, before and after carnitine supplementation (50 mg/kg).[34] A partial inhibition of β-oxidation in patients receiving valproate was corrected by carnitine administration.

On the basis of these findings and considering that carnitine is a relatively safe compound, it might be useful to run a controlled clinical trial to assess whether carnitine supplementation is beneficial in alleviating the severity of a pathology for which no real therapy is available. Of course, the intrinsic difficulties of such a trial cannot be denied, considering the low incidence of the disease.

REFERENCES

1. Reye RDK, Morgan G, Baral J. Encephalopathy and fatty degeneration of the viscera: A disease entity in childhood. Lancet 1963; 2:749-775.
2. Lee WM. Acute liver failure. New England J Med 1993; 329:1862-1872.
3. Linnemann CC, Shea L, Kauffman CA, Shiff GM, Partin JC, Schubert W. Association of Reye's syndrome with viral infection. Lancet 1974; 2:179-182.
4. Starko KM, Ray CG, Dominguez LB et al. Reye's syndrome and salicilate use. Pediatrics 1980; 66:859-864.
5. Halpin TJ, Holtzhauer FJ, Campbell RJ et al. Reye's syndrome and medication use. J Am Med Ass 1982; 248:687-691.
6. Waldman RJ, Hall WN, McGee H et al. Aspirin as a risk factor in Reye's syndrome. J Am Med Ass 1982; 247:3089-3094.
7. Hurwitz ES, Barrett MJ, Bregman D et al. Public health service study on Reye's syndrome and medication. New England J Med 1985; 313:849-857.
8. Soumerai SB, Ross-Degnan D, Spira Kahn J. Effects of professional and media warnings about the association between aspirin use in childhood and Reye's syndrome. The Milbank Quarterly 1992; 70 (1):154-182.
9. Porter JDH, Robinson PH, Glasgow JFT et al. Trends in the incidence of Reye's syndrome and the use of aspirin. Arch Dis Child 1990; 65:826-829.
10. Davis DL, Buffler P. Reduction of death after drug labeling for risk of Reye's syndrome. Lancet 1992; 340:1042.
11. Poss WB, Vernon DD, Dean JM. A reemergence of Reye's syndrome. Arch Pediatr Adolesc Med 1994; 148:879-882.
12. Green A, Hall SM. Investigation of metabolic disorders resembling Reye's syndrome. Arch Dis Child 1992; 67:1313-1617.
13. From the Centers for Disease Control. Reye syndrome surveillance. United States. J Am Med Ass 1991; 265:960.
14. Gerber N, Dickinson RG, Harland RC et al. Reye-like syndrome associated with valproic acid therapy. J Paediatr 1979 95:142-144.
15. Sinniah D, Baskaran G. Margosa oil poisoning as a cause of Reye's syndrome. Lancet 1981; 1:487-489.

16. Sugimoto T, Yasuhara Y, Nishida N et al. 3 cases of acute encephalopathy with calcium hopantenate administration. No To Hattatsu (Jpn) 1983; 15:258-259.

17. Hadidane R, Roger-Regnault C, Bouatour H et al. Correlation between alimentary mycotoxin contamination and specific diseases. Hum Toxicol 1985; 4:491-501.

18. Glasgow JFT, Moore R. Reye's syndrome 30 years on. Br Med J 1993; 307:950-951.

19. Rowe PC, Valle D, Brusilow SW. Inborn errors of metabolism in children referred with Reye's syndrome. J Am Med Ass 1988; 260: 3167-3170.

20. Visentin M, Salmona M, Tacconi MT. Reye's and Reye-like syndromes, drug related diseases? (Causative agents, etiology, pathogenesis and therapeutic approaches). Drug Metabolism Reviews 1995; 27:517-539.

21. Heubi JE, Partin JC, Partin JS et al. Reye's syndrome: current concepts. Hepatology 1987; 7:155-164.

22. Tonsgard JH. Urinary dicarboxylic acids in Reye syndrome. J Paediatr 1985; 107:79-84.

23. Dougherty CC, Gartside PS, Heubi JE et al. A morphometric study of Reye's syndrome. Am J Pathol 1987; 129:313-326.

24. Partin JC, Shubert WK, Partin JS. Mitochondrial ultrastructure in Reye's syndrome (encephalopathy and fatty degeneration of the viscera). New England J Med 1971; 285:1339-1341.

25. Van Coster RN, De Vivo DC, Blake D et al. Adult Reye's syndrome· A review with new evidence for a generalized defect in intra-mitochondrial enzyme processing. Neurology 1991; 41: 1815-1821.

26. De Vivo DC. Reye syndrome: a metabolic response to an acute mitochondrial insult? Neurology 1978; 28:105-108.

27. Sinatra F, Yoshida T, Applebaum M et al. Abnormalities of carbamylphosphate synthetase and ornithine transcarbamylase in liver of patients with Reye's syndrome. Pediatr Res 1975; 9: 829-833.

28. Snodgrass PJ, Delong GR. Urea-cycle enzyme deficiencies and an increase nitrogen load producing hyperammomemia in Reye's syndrome. New England J Med 1976; 294:855-860.

29. Brown JK, Imam H. Interrelationship of liver and brain with special reference to Reye's syndrome. J Inher Metab Dis 1991; 14:432-458.

30. Stumpf DA, Parker WD, Angelini C. Carnitine deficiency, organic acidemias and Reye's syndrome. Neurology 1985; 35:1041-1045.

31. Tonsgard JH. Serum dicarboxylic acids in patients with Reye's syndrome. J Paediatr 1986; 109:440-445.

32. Corkey BE, Hale DE, Glennon MC et al. Relationship between unusual hepatic acyl coezyme A profiles and the pathogenesis of Reye syndrome. J Clin Invest 1988; 82:782-788.

33. Koga Y, Yoshida I, Kimura A et al. Inhibition of mitochondrial functions by margosa oil: possible implications in the pathogenesis of Reye's syndrome. Paediatr Res 1987; 22:184-187.

34. Kossak BD, Schmidt-Sommerfeld E, Tonsgard GH et al. Fatty acid β-oxidation during valproic acid therapy and the role of carnitine. Ann Neurol 1991; 30:448-449.
35. Lewis JH, Zimmerman HJ, Garrett CT et al. Valproate-induced hepatic steatogenesis in rats. Hepatology 1982; 2:870-873.
36. Sugimoto T, Arak A, Nishida N et al. Hepatotoxicity in rats following administration of valproic acid: Effect of L-carnitine supplementation. Epilepsia 1987; 28:373-377.
37. Matsumoto M, Kuhara T, Inohue Y et al. Abnormal fatty acid metabolism in patients in hopantenate therapy during clinical episodes. J Chromatogr 1991; 562:139-145.
38. Roe CR, Millington DS, Maltby D et al. Status and function of L-carnitine in Reye's syndrome (RS) and related metabolic disorders. J Natl Reye's Syndrome Foundation 1983; 4:58-59.
39. Sugiyama N, Kidouchi K, Kobayashi M et al. Carnitine deficiency in inherited organic acid disorders and Reye syndrome. Acta Pediatr Jpn 1990; 32:410-416.
40. Matsuyuki M. Mitochondrial changes and carnitine status in fasting rats. Acta Paediatr Jpn 1990; 32:443-448.
41. Trauner DA, Horvith E, Davis LE. Inhibition of fatty acid beta- oxidation by influenza B virus and salicilic acid in mice: Implications for Reye's syndrome. Neurology 1988; 38:239-241.
42. Sinniah D, Sinniah R, Baskaran G et al. Evaluation of the possible role of glucose, carnitine, coenzyme Q10 and steroids in the treatment of Reye's syndrome using the margosa oil animal model. Acta Paediatr Jpn 1990; 32:462-468.
43. Takeyama N, Takagi D, Matsuo N et al. Altered hepatic fatty acid metabolism in endotoxicosis: Effect of L-carnitine on survival. Am J Physiol 1989; 256:E31-E38.
44. Kilpatrick LE, Polin RA, Douglas SD et al. Hepatic metabolic alterations in rats treated with low-dose endotoxin and aspirin: An animal model of Reye's syndrome. Metabolism 1989; 38:73-77.
45. Visentin M, Bellasio R, Tacconi MT. Reye syndrome model in rats: Protection against liver abnormalities by L-carnitine and acetyl-L-carnitine. J Pharm Exp Ther 1995; 275:1069-1075.
46. Matsubasa T, Ohtani Y, Miike T et al. Carnitine prevents Reye-like syndrome in atypical carnitine deficiency. Pediatric Neurol 1986; 2:80-84.

# CHAPTER 10

# Acylcarnitine and Chronic Fatigue Syndrome

Hirohiko Kuratsune, Kouzi Yamaguti, Yasuyoshi Watanabe, Mamoru
Takahashi, Ichiro Nakamoto, Takashi Machii, Gunilla B Jacobson,
Hirotaka Onoe, Kiyoshi Matsumura, Sven Valind, Bengt Långström and
Teruo Kitani

## SUMMARY

In 1992, we reported serum acylcarnitine (ACR) deficiency without free carnitine abnormality in the majority of 38 patients with chronic fatigue syndrome (CFS), which is characterized by prolonged general fatigue, myalgia and neuropsychiatric symptoms. There is a clear correlation between serum ACR concentration and performance status in patients with CFS. Up to the present, we have studied the serum carnitine concentrations of 146 patients with CFS, and confirmed that the vast majority of CFS patients have ACR deficiency. However, the physiological and biological roles of serum ACR are unclear.

Recently, we found an important feedback system in ACR metabolism. That is, the mammalian liver can supply a large amount of ACR at the time of danger in energy metabolism, and immediately salvage and conserve the unused ACR to provide for subsequent energy crises when the state of energy metabolism is improved. When the brain uptake of acetylcarnitine was investigated in normal Rhesus monkeys using different position labeled acetyl-L-carnitine and related molecules with $^{11}$C by positron emission tomography, the uptake values of radio-labeled acetyl-carnitine into the brain were quite different from the labeling positions of $^{11}$C, and the uptake value of [2-$^{11}$C]acetyl-L-carnitine was by far the highest among the $^{11}$C-labeled acetyl-L-carnitine and L-carnitine.

These findings indicate that endogenous serum ACR might be an important substance in mammals, and that it plays some role in conveying an acetyl moiety into the brain, especially in an energy crisis. There is a

*Carnitine Today,* edited by Claudio De Simone and Giuseppe Famularo.
© 1997 Landes Bioscience.

possibility that ACR deficiency in serum and/or cells might be related to the symptoms of patients with CFS. Indeed, we found that in patients with CFS who were supplemented with acetyl-carnitine, marked improvement of daily activity and reduction of the symptoms occurred.

## INTRODUCTION

Chronic fatigue syndrome (CFS) is currently an operational concept to clarify the unknown etiology of the syndrome characterized primarily by chronic fatigue.[1,2] The characteristic symptoms of CFS are prolonged generalized fatigue, muscle weakness, myalgia and postexertional malaise. However, the results of routine histological examination of muscles, assay of cytoplasmic enzymes of the skeletal muscle in venous blood and electromyography for patients with CFS are usually normal. Recently, several investigators have described the metabolic abnormalities in the muscle of patients with CFS, i.e. excessive intracellular acidosis of skeletal muscle,[3] impaired muscle protein synthesis and impediment of β-oxidation of palmitate in mitochondria,[4] but the pathogenic role of these findings remains to be determined.

Carnitine has important roles not only in the transport of long-chain fatty acids into the mitochondria as a long-chain fatty acid carnitine, but also in the modulation of the intramitochondrial CoA/acyl-CoA ratio (Fig. 10.1).[5,6] Deficiency of carnitine results in abnormal energy metabolism and/ or accumulation of toxic acyl-CoA compounds in the mitochondria. Therefore, we studied whether patients with CFS have carnitine abnormalities or not, and found a peculiar carnitine abnormality in CFS. That is, the majority of patients with CFS have an acylcarnitine (ACR) deficiency in serum, but their free carnitine (FCR) levels were within normal levels.[7,8] ACR means carnitine binding to fatty acid, and most investigators regard ACR as a transient substance of fatty acid metabolism in mitochondria at present. However, the vast majority of serum ACR are not the long-chain fatty acids carnitine, but the short-chain fatty acid carnitine, especially acetyl-carnitine.[9] The physiological and biological roles of serum ACR itself are not yet understood.

Recently, we found not only that mammals have a regulatory system of serum ACR,[10] but also the uptake values of serum ACR into the brain were extremely high.[11] There is a possibility that serum endogenous ACR might be an important substance for brain metabolism, and serum ACR deficiency in CFS might be associated with the signs and symptoms of patients with CFS. We describe here not only the ACR deficiency in CFS, but also ACR dynamics and physical roles in mammals.

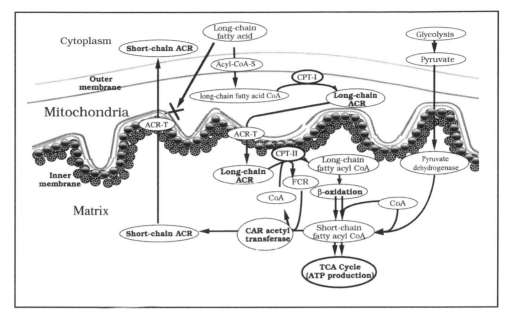

Fig. 10.1. Diagrammatic representation of the function of carnitine and acylcarnitine in mitochondria. FCR, free carnitine; ACR, acylcarnitine; CoA, coenzyme A; acyl-CoA-S, Acyl-CoA synthetase; CAT-I, carnitine acyltransferase 1; CAT-II, carnitine acyl-transferase 2; ACR-T, acylcarnitine translocase; TCA, tricarboxylic acid; CAR acetyl-T, carnitine acetyl transferase.

## ACYLCARNITINE (ACR) DEFICIENCY IN CFS

Serum ACR and free carnitine (FCR) concentrations were studied in 146 patients with CFS (64 males, 82 females) and 308 normal controls (177 males, 131 females). A diagnosis of CFS was made based on the clinical criterion proposed by Holmes GP et al.[2] Carnitine concentration was evaluated by the new enzymatic cycling method using NADH, thio-NAD+ and carnitine dehydrogenase, as previously reported.[12] Blood samples from patients with CFS and normal controls were taken before breakfast, and serum samples were stored at -80°C until measurement of carnitine concentration.

Since serum FCR concentration was higher in males than in females and serum ACR concentration was lower in males than in females,[7] we have compared the serum FCR and ACR levels in CFS patients with those of sex-matched normal controls.

In 1992, we reported that the majority of 38 patients with CFS had serum ACR deficiency without FCR abnormality.[13] Up to the present, we have studied 146 patients with CFS, and confirmed that the vast majority of CFS patients had ACR deficiency, but their FCR levels were normal. There

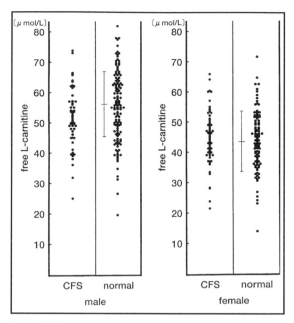

Fig. 10.2. Concentrations of free L-carnitine in the serum from patients with CFS and normal controls.

was no statistically significant difference in serum FCR concentration between CFS patients and normal controls (Fig. 10.2, Table 10.1). In contrast, the vast majority of patients with CFS had serum ACR deficiency, as indicated by a statistically significant difference in serum ACR concentration between CFS patients and normal controls (P < 0.001, Student's t test) (Fig. 10.3, Table 10.1). The serum ACR deficiency in patients with CFS was unrelated to the serum FCR concentration (Fig. 10.4).

Serum ACR concentration in our patients with CFS tended to increase during the period of improvement, while FCR concentration did not show such a tendency (Fig. 10.5).[7] There was a statistically significant difference in ACR concentrations at the initial examination phase of illness and that at the recovery phase of illness (P < 0.02, paired t test). When the performance levels of patients with CFS deteriorated, serum ACR concentrations declined again.[8] Since the bed-ridden patients with bone fractures did not have serum ACR deficiency, the reduced daily physical activity by itself did not cause a decrease of serum ACR.[8]

Recently, Plioplys et al studied serum ACR and FCR in 38 patients with CFS in the U.S., and reported that most of their CFS patients had both ACR and FCR deficiency in serum, when serum ACR and FCR levels of CFS patients in the U.S. were compared to those of Japanese normal controls.[14] The fact that the decrease in serum ACR was found in the majority of CFS patients in the U.S. suggests that serum ACR deficiency in patients with CFS may not be a local phenomenon particular to Japan. However, there is a significant difference in serum FCR and total carnitine (TCR)

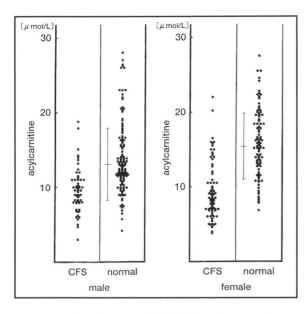

Fig. 10.3. Concentrations of acylcarnitine in the serum from patients with CFS and normal controls.

concentration between their CFS patients and Japanese CFS patients and/or Japanese normal controls. The weakness in their report is that they did not illustrate their data for normal controls in the U.S., despite using a different method for studying the concentration of ACR and FCR.

There is one more report from England[15] on serum carnitine levels. Recently, Majeed et al reported that serum ACR and FCR concentration levels of 27 patients with CFS were not different from those of 80 normal controls in England. However, they did not specify when the blood samples were taken from patients with CFS and normal controls. As described below, serum ACR concentration is significantly decreased after meals. Since in their report the levels of serum ACR in both normal controls and CFS patients were significantly lower than of Japanese normal controls, it seems

**Table 10.1. Serum FCR and ACR in CFS and normal controls**

|  | (n) | ACR (μM) | FCR(μM) |
|---|---|---|---|
| Normal Controls |  |  |  |
| Male | 177 | 13.4 +/– 4.6 | 56.1 +/– 10.7 |
| Female | 131 | 15.5 +/– 4.4 | 43.6 +/– 10.0 |
| CFS patients |  |  |  |
| Male | 64 | 9.7 +/– 2.9* | 52.2 +/– 8.8 |
| Female | 82 | 9.4 +/– 3.7* | 44.5 +/– 8.2 |

(n): number of cases, ACR: acylcarnitine,
FCR: free carnitine, *P < 0.001 vs normal controls

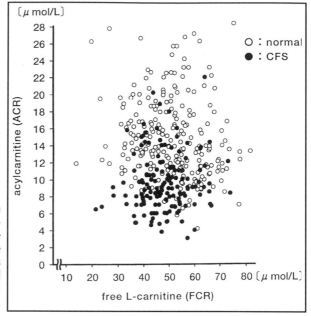

Fig. 10.4. Association between concentrations of free L-carnitine and acylcarnitine in the serum from patients with CFS (closed circles) and normal controls (open circles).

to be unclear whether the patients with CFS in England have serum ACR deficiency or not.

## ACR METABOLISM IN MAMMALS

Concerning the dynamics of ACR in serum, it is well known that serum ACR concentration increases during starvation. Since many investigators have reported increases in ACR and TCR concentration in the liver during starvation,[16-19] the increase of ACR in serum is thought to be associated with ACR production in the liver. However, there are conflicting reports in which the increase of ACR in the liver was suggested to be at least partly accounted for by the decrease in liver mass,[16] and perfused liver, whether from fed or fasted animals,[20] releases carnitine with the same ester content.

The increased concentration of ACR during starvation was reported to decrease to the basal level after 24 hours of refeeding in humans,[19] but no previous study has yet examined the immediate changes of ACR metabolism after refeeding. It is not known how and where most of this serum ACR is used and metabolized in the body. Therefore, we examined the concentrations of ACR, FCR and TCR in serum and livers of mice to clarify the changes in ACR metabolism during starvation and soon after refeeding.[10] Furthermore, we have studied the dynamics of ACR in several tissues in the Rhesus monkey and human using positron emission tomography (PET).

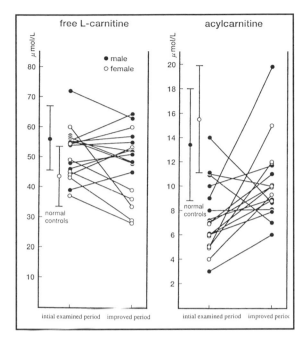

Fig. 10.5. Concentrations of free L-carnitine (left) and acylcarnitine (right) in the serum from patients with CFS at the period of initial examination (poor performance status phase) and at improving phase of illness. Reprinted from Kuratsune et al. Clin Infect Dis 1994; 18(Suppl 1):S62-67. © The University of Chicago Press.

THE EFFECT OF STARVATION AND REFEEDING ON ACR, FCR AND TOTAL CARNITINE (TCR) IN MICE[10]

Eight-week-old male C3H/He mice (20-25 g) were used in all experiments. The animals were divided into 4 groups as follows: in the first three groups, the mice were starved for 24 hours. In the first group, the mice were killed by decapitation after starvation without refeeding; in the second group, they were refed for 90 min before decapitation; and in the third group, they were refed for 180 min prior to decapitation. The fourth group was used as a control in which animals had free access to a balanced laboratory diet. This group (control) comprised 10 mice, while each of the other groups comprised 4 mice.

ACR concentration in the serum increased significantly after starvation ($68.8 \pm 2.6$ vs. $35.2 \pm 2.8$ µM). In contrast, FCR concentration in the serum fell from $41.7 \pm 0.4$ to $32.5 \pm 2.2$ µM after starvation. In the liver, acid-soluble ACR concentration (nmol/g wet tissue) increased significantly during starvation, and FCR concentration (nmol/g wet tissue) also increased slightly after starvation (from 227 to 246; +8% increased)(Fig. 10.6). After refeeding, the ACR concentration in serum quickly decreased below the basal levels (from $68.8 \pm 2.6$ to $21.9 \pm 1.1$ µM; after 90 min of refeeding). In contrast, FCR concentration in serum was increased slightly at 90 min after refeeding (from $32.5 \pm 2.2$ to $38.3 \pm 1.5$ µM). In the liver, acid-soluble FCR and TCR concentrations had significantly increased after 180 min of

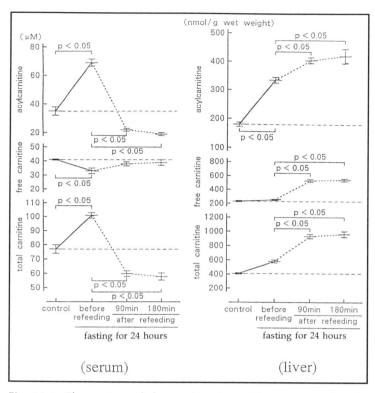

Fig. 10.6. Change in acyl, free and total carnitine concentrations in serum and liver during fasting and refeeding.

refeeding (from 246 to 536; +118% increase in FCR, and from 579 to 955; +64.9% increase in TCR), and acid-soluble ACR concentration was slightly increased (from 333 to 419; +26% increase) (Fig. 10.6).

The experiments with mice revealed that ACR concentration in serum increased after starvation, and promptly decreased below basal levels after refeeding. In addition, the fact that the decrease of ACR concentration in serum was accompanied by a significant increase of TCR in the liver after refeeding suggests the possibility that refeeding caused the uptake of serum ACR by the liver, because it is not likely that the increased level of TCR in the liver is immediately synthesized after refeeding.

## THE EFFECT OF ORAL ADMINISTRATION OF 75 GRAMS OF GLUCOSE ON ACR, FCR AND TCR IN NORMAL HUMAN VOLUNTEERS

When we studied the concentrations of FCR, ACR and TCR in serum before and after meals in normal human volunteers, an apparent decrease in serum ACR concentration was found, similar to the results in the mice experiments.[10] Furthermore, when we have studied the change of carnitine concentrations in 14 normal human volunteers using the glucose tolerance test, serum ACR concentration was clearly reduced at 120 min after glucose ingestion (from 14.1 to 10.2 $\mu$M; P < 0.001, Freadmann test), while FCR and TCR concentrations had not changed significantly (Table 10.2).[10] It is quite interesting to note that not only refeeding but also the ingestion of glucose alone during the fasting state causes a rapid decrease in serum ACR in normal human volunteers.

THE EFFECT OF INTRAVENOUS GLUCOSE ADMINISTRATION ON THE ACR UPTAKE
IN THE RHESUS MONKEY

To clarify the ACR dynamics before and after glucose administration, we studied ACR metabolism in the Rhesus monkey by positron emission tomography (PET) using [2-$^{11}$C] acetyl-L-carnitine. As shown in Fig. 10.7, most of the radio-labeled ACR gathered in the kidneys before glucose administration. However, a significant increase in ACR uptake by the liver was evoked immediately after glucose administration, accompanied by a decrease in serum ACR concentration (from 6.6 to 2.0 $\mu$M). Two hours after glucose administration, the changes of ACR uptake in the liver returned basal levels. Our mice experiments and PET studies in the Rhesus monkey using [2-$^{11}$C]acetyl-L-carnitine suggest that there is an important feedback system in which the mammalian liver can synthesize a large amount of ACR at times of danger to the energy metabolism, and immediately salvage and conserve the unused ACR to provide for subsequent energy crises when the state of energy metabolism is improved through meals.

It has been reported that ACR concentration in the human forearm artery blood during starvation was higher than that of the forearm vein blood,[9] and serum ACR has been thought to contribute to the flux of meta-

*Table 10.2. Changes in BS, IRI, ACR, FCR and TCR before and after oral admisnistration of glucose in normal human volunteers*

| | 75.0 grams of glucose administration | | | |
| | before | after 30 min. | after 60 min. | after 120 min. |
|---|---|---|---|---|
| BS (mg/dl) | 89.1±10.1 | 129.8±17.6 | 119.6±18.9 | 92.3±11.7 |
| IRI ($\mu$U/ml) | 5.9±3.1 | 39.9±13.4 | 40.1±15.5 | 15.7±7.1 |
| ACR ($\mu$M) | 14.1±4.6 | 13.2±3.7 | 11.5±2.8* | 10.2±2.9** |
| FCR($\mu$M) | 70.2±14.5 | 71.3±14.9 | 69.3±13.8 | 69.3±13.8 |

BS: plasma glucose level, IRI: immunoreactive insulin
ACR:acylcarnitine, FCR: free carnitine, TCR total carnitine,
*P < 0.05; **P < 0.001, after glucose administration
Reprinted with permission from Yamaguti K, Kuratsune H et al. Biochem Biophys Res Commun 1996; 225:740-746.

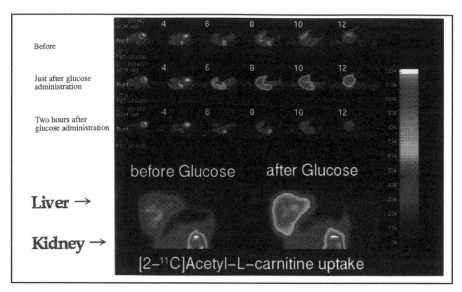

Fig. 10.7. [2-¹¹C]acetyl-L-carnitine uptake in the liver and kidney of rhesus monkey before and after glucose administration. Reprinted with permission from Yamaguti K, Kuratsune H et al. Biochem Biophys Res Commun 1996; 225:740-746. See color figure in insert.

bolic fuel, such as ketone bodies. However, there is a clear difference in concentration between ketone bodies and ACR during starvation. Judging from blood concentrations, the contribution of serum ACR as fuel is only one hundredth that of ketone bodies. There is a possibility that serum ACR might be used for providing acetyl units to some biosynthetic process in the tissues.

By studying the metabolism of acetyl-L-carnitine in mice at a fasting or feeding state using [1-¹⁴C]acetyl-L-carnitine, most of the [1-¹⁴C]acetyl-L-carnitine was stated to have changed to ¹⁴CO2, but some of the ¹⁴C in the liver was located in the fatty acids of phospholipid and triacylglycerols.[21] It was suggested that the acetyl moiety of acetyl-L-carnitine entered a biosynthetic pathway. This raises the possibility that acetyl-carnitine might provide acetyl units for some biosynthetic processes which require acetyl CoA. Since Farrell et al did not study the change of ACR metabolism soon after refeeding, a significant increase in ACR uptake by the liver evoked by refeeding was not noted. However, judging by our results and their observations, the acetyl moiety of ACR taken up by the liver after refeeding might enter the lipid biosynthetic pools to provide for subsequent periods of starvation. Since the mammalian liver is not capable of changing ketone bodies to acetyl CoA, ketone bodies produced by the liver during fasting are never taken up by the liver after refeeding and have to be used in the peripheral tissues. In this respect, there is a clear difference between ACR and ketone bodies.

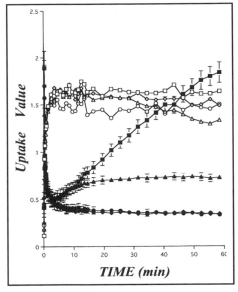

Fig. 10.8. Time courses of the uptake value of ACM, ACN, ACC and CRN into the whole brain (closed symbols) and temporal muscle (open symbols) of rhesus monkeys. ACM, [2-[11]C]acetyl-L-carnitine (■, □); ACN, [1-[11]C]acetyl-L-carnitine (▲, △); ACC, acetyl-L-[methyl-[11]C]carnitine (◆, ◇); CRN, L-[methyl-[11]C]carnitine (●, ○). Each symbol represents the mean uptake value for a given time and bars represent standard errors (n = 6 in ACM, 5 in ACN, 5 in ACC, 4 in CRN). When bars are not shown the errors were smaller than the symbols.

*TIME (min)*

## THE UPTAKE OF ACR IN THE BRAIN OF RHESUS MONKEYS AND HUMANS

When the brain uptake was studied in Rhesus monkeys using several [11]C-labeled acetyl-L-carnitine and related molecules with PET, the uptake value of [11]C-labeled acetyl-L-carnitine varied depending on the positions of [11]C-radiolabel.[11] Figure 10.8 shows the time courses of the uptake value of [2-[11]C]acetyl-L-carnitine (ACM), [1-[11]C]-acetyl-L-carnitine (ACN), acetyl-L-[methyl-[11]C]carnitine (ACC), L-[methyl-[11]C]carnitine (CRN) into the whole brain. The uptake values of CRN and ACC were almost identical and extremely low, while the brain uptake of ACN was slightly higher in comparison. When ACM was used as the tracer, we found that the uptake value of ACM was farther elevated. Previous studies of the brain uptake of acetyl-carnitine investigated the use of acetyl-L-[[3]H]carnitine, and as a result the brain uptake of acetyl-carnitine had been regarded as extremely low.[21] It is of notable interest that the uptake value of [11]C-labeled acetyl-L-carnitine varied depending on the positions of [11]C-radiolabel, and that the uptake value of ACM was by far the highest among [11]C-labeled acetyl-L-carnitine and L-carnitine. Surprisingly, the uptake value of ACM in the brain was higher than that in the temporal muscle after 120 min of the initial injection. Since there was no significant difference in the disappearance rate from whole blood among these four radioactive tracers (data not shown), the reason why the uptake value of ACM was noticeably high in the brain is not due to the difference of its concentration in the blood.

There is a clear difference in the brain uptake between carnitine labeled acetyl-carnitine (ACC) and acetyl moiety labeled acetyl-carnitine (ACM and ACN), suggesting that the acetyl moiety may be separated from acetyl-carnitine before the uptake into the brain parenchyma and only a part of acetyl moiety is taken up into the brain, or that the acetyl moiety may be separated from acetyl-carnitine immediately after uptake into the brain, and carnitine moiety is quickly discharged from the brain.

Furthermore, the fact that there is a significant difference between the uptake values of ACN and ACM (Fig. 10.1) suggests that endogenous serum acetyl-L-carnitine has some role in conveying an acetyl moiety into the brain and that an unknown metabolic pathway of the $[2\text{-}^{11}C]$acetyl moiety might be rather active in the brain. If the acetyl moieties of acetyl-carnitine enters the tricarboxylic acid (TCA) cycle only for synthesis of ATP, the $^{11}C$ of both acetyl moiety of acetyl-L-carnitine will be expired as $^{11}CO_2$, and so this big difference of uptake value between ACN and ACM could not be established.

Judging from these findings, there is a possibility that the acetyl moiety of acetyl-carnitine taken up into the brain may enter the TCA cycle at least once, and then the $^{11}C$ of the $[1\text{-}^{11}C]$acetyl moiety may be expired as $^{11}CO2$, but the $^{11}C$ of the $[2\text{-}^{11}C]$acetyl moiety may not. It is known that the $^{11}C$ of the $[2\text{-}^{11}C]$acetyl-moiety is not expired as $^{11}CO_2$ at the first cycle. Therefore, the $[2\text{-}^{11}C]$acetyl moiety may slip out of TCA cycle and enter the GABA shunt as an $\alpha$-keto-$[^{11}C]$glutaric acid. It may be used for biosynthesis of an important neurometabolic substance like glutamic acid and GABA.

Figure 10.9 shows the PET images showing the distribution of CRN and ACM in a horizontal section and sagittal section of the head of Rhesus monkeys. There is a significant difference in uptake into the brain between CAR and ACM.

Figure 10.10 shows the uptake of ACM in the human brain. A high uptake of acetyl-carnitine was found in the human brain cortex, analogous to the uptake in Rhesus monkeys. The uptake of ACM was higher in gray matter than in white matter.

## HYPOTHESIS: THE ROLE OF ACR IN THE ETIOLOGY OF CFS

The increase of glycolysis that occurs through exercise produces a great deal of acetyl CoA in the mitochondria. In such a situation, numerous enzymes are inhibited by a low CoA/acyl-CoA ratio in muscle cell. To modulate the intramitochondrial CoA/acyl-CoA ratio, carnitine is bound to short-chain fatty acid CoAs, and it changes to acylcarnitine. The majority of these short-chain acylcarnitines discharge into the blood (Fig. 10.1). The regulatory system of serum ACR is also useful for maintaining the acyl radical produced by muscle cells through exercise (Fig. 10.11).

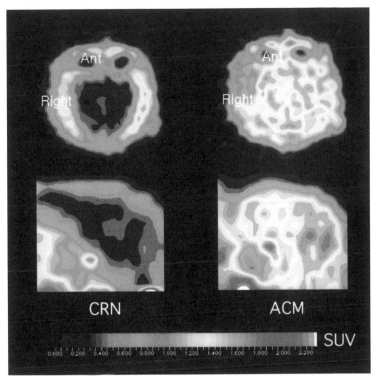

Fig. 10.9. PET scans showing the distribution of CRN (left images) and ACM (right images) in a horizontal section (upper images) and sagittal section (lower images) of the head of rhesus monkeys. These images were constructed from 30 min to 45 min after injection of the radioactive tracer. CRN, L-[methyl-$^{11}$C]carnitine; ACM, [2-$^{11}$C]acetyl-L-carnitine. See color figure in insert.

As mentioned above, the vast majority of radio-labeled acetyl-carnitine gathered in the kidneys, but less than 1.0% of the radio-labeled acetyl-carnitine was excreted in urine after two hours of intravenous injection. These findings indicate that serum ACR is not unused, but rather a necessary substance in mammals. It is regulated by the liver, kidneys and muscles (Fig. 10.11).

Recently, much attention has been paid to the pharmaceutical effects of acetyl-carnitine on the central nervous system.[22-27] Many investigators have tried to seek a role for acetyl-carnitine, and found improvement of performance in spatial learning tasks in aged rats,[22] enhancement of rat brain energy and phospholipid metabolism,[23] prolongation of survival of adult rat sensory neurons,[24] activation of protein kinase C and an anti-amnesic effect[25] and an inhibitory effect on apoptosis.[26] Furthermore, the progression of Alzheimer's disease has been reported to be significantly reduced in patients who had received acetyl-carnitine for one year in a double-blind, randomized and controlled clinical trial.[27]

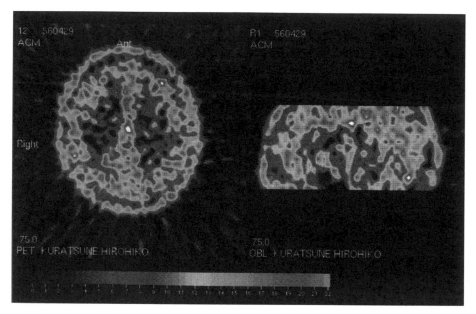

Fig. 10.10. PET scans showing the distribution of ACM in a horizontal section (left image) and sagittal section (right image) of the human brain. These images were constructed from 30 min to 45 min after injection of the radioactive tracer. ACM, [2-$^{11}$C]acetyl-L-carnitine. See color figure in insert.

These findings and our data suggest that serum endogenous ACR might be an important substance for brain metabolism, and that serum ACR deficiency in CFS might be related to the neuro-psychiatric symptoms of CFS.

Many investigators have suggested that patients with CFS have various abnormalities, such as reactivation of latent viruses, immune system dysfunctions, abnormal regulation of the hypothalamo-pituitary-adrenal axis, abnormal production of cytokines and neuro-muscular dysfunction. Recently, we discovered a possible link between CFS and infection with Borna disease virus, which is a neurotropic RVA virus.[28,29] However, judging from these diverse and sometimes conflicting abnormalities found in CFS, it seems difficult to explain the cause of CFS from a single pathogenesis.

Figure 10.12 illustrates our hypothesis concerning the etiology of CFS.[8] Our hypothesis is the following: regardless of whether the trigger is stress, viral infections or unknown factors, which may lead to abnormalities of cytokine production and immune system dysfunction and/or abnormal regulation of the hypothalamo-pituitary adrenal axis, the final result is invariably acylcarnitine metabolic dysfunction. There is a possibility that a deficiency of serum and cellular endogenous acylcarnitine in CFS might be related to cellular dysfunction in the brain, resulting in general fatigue and neuro-psychological symptoms.

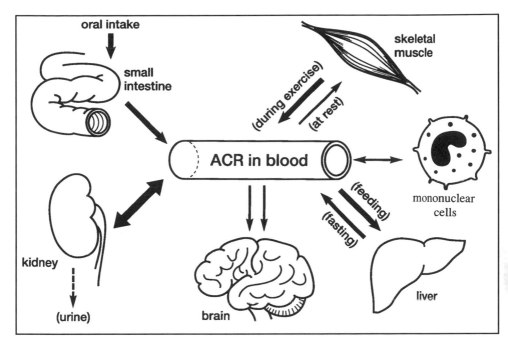

Fig. 10.11. The dynamics of acylcarnitine (ACR) in mammals.

It has been reported that ACR represents more than 90% of the total carnitine pool in inactivated mononuclear phagocytes, but that ACR quickly decreases by 50% after phorbol-estel activation.[30] In 1995, Majeed et al reported that ACR and FCR concentrations in peripheral mononuclear cells were low in their CFS patients.[15] If ACR in cells was associated with the cellular activation process or cellular functions, the deficiency of ACR in serum and/or cells might be related to the abnormality of the immune system found in CFS patients.

## ACETYL-L-CARNITINE TREATMENT FOR PATIENTS WITH CFS

A 21-year-old woman was admitted to our hospital because of severe fatigue. Before acetyl-carnitine administration, she had received several treatments: administration of anti-inflammatory drugs, minor tranquilizers and Chinese drugs. However, she was unable to carry on normal activity, even unable to perform light tasks. Since her serum acylcarnitine concentration was extremely low (7.2 μM), she requested supplementary therapy of acylcarnitine. We administered 4.0 grams of acetyl-carnitine per day for 2 weeks. Table 10.3 summarizes her symptoms, signs of natural killer (NK) activities and serum ACR before and after acetyl-carnitine treatment. Before acetyl-carnitine treatment, she had severe general fatigue, low grade fever, sore throat, myalgia etc., but after 5 days of treatment, her symptoms

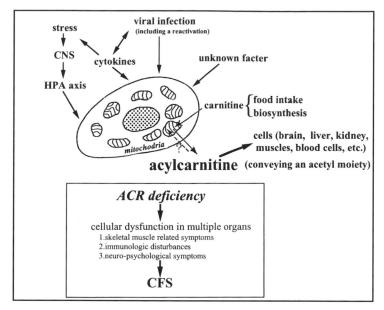

Fig. 10.12. Hypothesis: the role of acylcarnitine in the etiology of CFS. CFS, central nervous system; HPA axis, hypothalamo-pituitary-adrenal axis, – – →, hypothetical pathway.

gradually decreased, and after just 2 weeks of administration, she was able to go shopping. Her NK activity had also improved from 9.0% to 15.7%. However, 2 months after treatment was terminated, her general fatigue gradually deteriorated, and finally she often stayed in bed for over half a day.

In this case, there was a recurrence of most of her symptoms 2 months after termination of acetyl-carnitine treatment. Since the supplement of acetyl-carnitine is not a treatment for the cause of ACR deficiency itself, it is reasonable to assume that the recurrence of most of her symptoms was due to the discontinuation of acetyl-carnitine supplementation. However, the fact that supplementation of acetyl-carnitine caused marked improvement in her daily activities and reduction of her symptoms during treatment suggests the possibility that the supplementation of acetyl-carnitine may become a useful new treatment for CFS patients with acylcarnitine deficiency. Acetylcarnitine treatment is now in progress in several patients with CFS who have a deficiency of serum ACR. When the effectiveness of a therapy is estimated in the treatment of a disease, the placebo effects should be considered, and thus a double-blind controlled study should be implemented as a matter of course.

**Table 10.3. The changes of symptoms, NK activities and acylcarnitine concentrations before and after acetyl-L-carnitine administration**

| symptoms | Acetyl-L-carnitine administration (4.0g/day, 14 days, oral administration) | | |
|---|---|---|---|
| | before | just after treatment | 2 months after treatment |
| *General fatigue | +++ | + | ++ |
| *Low grade fever | +++ | + | +++ |
| *Prolonged fatigue after exercise | +++ | – | +++ |
| *Neuropsychologic complaints | +++ | – | +++ |
| *Hypersomnia | ++ | – | ++ |
| *Insomnia | ++ | – | – |
| Myalgia | +++ | ++ | ++ |
| Sore throat | +++ | ++ | + |
| Headache | + | + | – |
| Painful lymph nodes | – | – | – |
| Muscle weakness | – | – | – |
| Arthralgia | – | – | – |
| | | | |
| NK activities, (E:T ratio) | | | |
| (10:1) | 9.0 | 15.7 | 15.5 (%) |
| (20:1) | 14.7 | 22.2 | 30.9 |
| Serum acylcarnitine | 7.2 | 9.6 | 8.9 (µM) |
| Serum free carnitine | 39.3 | 39.7 | 29.8 |

\* symptoms which were improved markedly during ACR administration
+++ severe symptoms, ++ moderate symptoms, + light symptoms, - no symptoms

REFERENCES

1. Shafran SD. The chronic fatigue syndrome. Am J Med 1991; 90:730-739.
2. Holmes GP, Kaplan JE, Gantz NM et al. Chronic fatigue syndrome: a working case definition. Ann Intern Med 1988; 108:387-389.
3. Arnold DL, Bore PJ, Radda GK et al. Excessive intracellular acidosis of skeletal muscle on exercise in a patient with a post-viral exhaustion/fatigue syndrome. A 31P nuclear magnetic resonance study. Lancet 1984; 1:1367-1369.
4. Edwards RHT, Newham DJ, Peters TJ. Muscle biochemistry and pathophysiology in post-viral fatigue syndrome. Br Med Bull 1991; 47:826-837.
5. Rebouche CJ. Carnitine metabolism and human nutrition. J Appl Nutr 1988; 40:99-111.

6. Breningstall GN. Carnitine deficiency syndrome. Pediat Neurol 1990; 6:75-81.
7. Kuratsune H, Yamaguti K, Takahashi M et al. Acylcarnitine deficiency in chronic fatigue syndrome. Clin Infect Dis 1994: 18(Suppl 1):S62-67.
8. Kuratsune H, Yamaguti K, Takahashi M et al. Abnormal cellular carnitine metabolism in chronic fatigue syndrome. EOS-J Immunol Immunopharmacol 1995; (1-2):40-44.
9. Bartlett K, Bhuiyan AKMJ, Aynsley-Green A et al. Human forearm arteriovenous differences of carnitine, short-chain acylcarnitine and long-chain acylcarnitine. Clinical Science 1989; 77:413-416.
10. Yamaguti K, Kuratsune H, Watanabe Y et al. Acylcarnitine metabolism during fasting and after refeeding. Biochem Biophys Res Commun 1996; 225:740-746.
11. Kuratsune H, Yamaguti K, Watanabe Y et al. High uptake of [2-$^{11}$C]acetyl-L-carnitine into the brain: a PET study. Biochem Biophys Res Commun 1997; 231:488-493.
12. Takahashi M, Ueda S, Misaki H et al. Carnitine; A new enzymatic cycling method using dehydrogenase. Clin Chem 1994; 40/5:817-821.
13. Kuratsune H, Yamaguti K, Takahashi M et al. Acylcarnitine deficiency in chronic fatigue syndrome. First international CFS/ME clinical and research conference. N.Y. October, 1992.
14. Plioplys AV, Plioplys S. Serum levels of carnitine in chronic fatigue syndrome: clinical correlates. Biol Psychiatry 1995; 32:132-138.
15. Majeed T, DeSimone C, Famularo G et al. Abnormalities of carnitine metabolism in chronic fatigue syndrome. Eur J Neurology 1995; 2:425-428.
16. Brass EP, Hoppel CL. Carnitine metabolism in the fasting rat. J Biol Chem 1978; 253:2688-2693.
17. Seccombe DW, Hahn P, Novak M. The effect of diet and development on blood levels of free and esterified carnitine in the rat. Biochim Biophys Acta 1978; 528:483-489.
18. Frohlich J, Seccombe DW, Hahn P et al. Effect of fasting and esterified carnitine levels in human serum and urine: Correlation with serum levels of free fatty acid and β-hydroxybutyrate. Metabolism 1978; 27:555-561.
19. Hoppel CL, Genuth SM. Carnitine metabolism in normal-weight and obese human subjects during fasting. Am J Physiol 1980; 238: E409-415.
20. Sandor A, Cseko J, Kispal G, Alkonyi I. Surplus acylcarnitine in the plasma of starved rats derive from the liver. J Biol Chem 1990; 265:22313-22316.
21. Farrell S, Vogel J, Bieber LL. Entry of acetyl-L-carnitine into the biosynthetic pathways. Biochim Biophys Acta 1986; 876:175-177.

22. Ghirardi O, Milana S, Ramacci MT, Abgelucci L. Effect of acetyl-L-carnitine chronic treatment on discrimination models in aged rats. Physiol Behav 1988; 44:769-773.
23. Aureli T, Miccheli A, Ricciolini R et al. Aging brain: effect of acetyl-L-carnitine treatment on rat brain energy and phospholipid metabolism. A study by 31P and 1H NMR spectroscopy. Brain Res 1990; 526:108-112.
24. Formenti A, Arrigoni E, Sansone V. Effects of acetyl-L-carnitine on the survival of adult rat sensory neurons in primary cultures. Int J Devl Neuroscience 1992; 10:207-214.
25. Pascale A, Milano S, Corsico N. Protein kinase C activation and anti-amnesic effect of acetyl-L-carnitine: in vitro and in vivo studies. Eur J Pharmacol 1994; 265:1-7.
26. Galli G, Fratelli M. Activation of apoptosis by serum deprivation in a teratocarcinoma cell line: Inhibition by L-acetyl-carnitine. Exp Cell Res 1993; 204:54-60.
27. Bowman BAB. Acetyl-carnitine and Alzheimer's disease. Nutr Rev 1992; 50:142-144.
28. Nakaya T, Takahashi H, Nakamura Y, et al. Demonstration of Borna disease virus RNA in peripheral blood mononuclear cells derived from Japanese patients with chronic fatigue syndrome. FEBS Lett 1996; 378:145-149.
29. Kitani T, Kuratsune H, Fuke I, et al. Possible correlation between Borna disease virus infection and Japanese patients with chronic fatigue syndrome. Microbiol Immunol 1996; 40:459-462.
30. Kurth L, Fraker P, Bieber L. Utilization of intracellular acylcarnitine pools by mononuclear phagocytes. Biochim Biophys Acta 1994; 1201:321-327.

# CHAPTER 11

# L-Carnitine, a Modulator of Immunometabolic Homeostasis in Subjects Infected with the Human Immunodeficiency Virus

Claudio De Simone, Sonia Moretti, Sonia Marcellini,
Vito Trinchieri, Antonio Boschini and Giuseppe Famularo

## INTRODUCTION

The inexorable decline in the numbers of CD4 T lymphocytes, which have a central role in the immune response to pathogens, and their association with the loss of cell-mediated immunity are major hallmarks of advancing acquired immunodeficiency syndrome (AIDS).

Theories about the causes of this loss of CD4 cells range from their destruction or dysfunction directly caused by infection with the human immunodeficiency virus (HIV) to accelerated apoptosis resulting from unregulated cytokine production, abnormal expression of Fas or endogenous antioxidant deficiency and oxidant stress.[1,2]

The observation that many patients with AIDS manifest multiorgan failure, including central and peripheral nervous system disease, cardiac dysfunction, and a wasting syndrome, has suggested the view that HIV-associated syndromes may possess metabolic or nutritional components. It is conceivable that the metabolic toxicity of drugs commonly used in the management of HIV-infected patients, including approved antiretroviral drugs, and the nutritional deficiency usually recognized in these subjects, further impair the cellular metabolism and substantially contribute to apoptosis.[2,3]

We have focused our recent work on the investigation of carnitine metabolism in HIV-infected patients. We report here data which

Carnitine Today, edited by Claudio De Simone and Giuseppe Famularo.
© 1997 Landes Bioscience.

convincingly demonstrate that carnitine deficiency may be found in this population. This strongly points to a potential role for L-carnitine supplementation in the therapy of HIV infection. Work in progress in our laboratory has demonstrated that L-carnitine therapy has a strong favorable impact on lymphocyte apoptosis as well as on CD4 cell counts and HIV load, the two best independent predictors of developing AIDS-related complications. Taking all these data into account, it appears that L-carnitine therapy could contribute to slowing down the clinical and immunological progression of the infection.

## IMMUNOMODULATING PROPERTIES OF L-CARNITINE

The observation that leukocytes, including peripheral blood mononuclear cells (PBMCs), are enriched in carnitines[4] first suggested that L-carnitine and its congeners may regulate the immune networks.

The influence of the pool of carnitines on lymphocyte functions predominantly or exclusively relies on carnitine-dependent energy production from fatty acids. The PBMC carnitine content can be regarded under a pharmacokinetic standpoint as an independent compartment, but under several conditions PBMCs can either lose carnitines or have an increased but unmet carnitine demand. This results in reduced energy production and impaired functional capability.

Previous reports have demonstrated the enhancement of immune responses by L-carnitine supplementation.[5-7] In addition, L-carnitine has been shown to protect cells against toxicity of reactive oxygen intermediates[8] and this correlates with the anti-apoptotic activity exerted by L-carnitine and its congeners under in vitro conditions.[9]

A reduced pool of carnitines has been recently found in either serum or tissues, or both, in disorders with unregulated immune responses such as the chronic fatigue syndrome[10,11] and septic shock.[12] This further supports the view that a normal endogenous pool of carnitines is crucial to the maintenance of normal immune networks.

## SERUM AND CELLULAR CARNITINE DEFICIENCY IN HIV-INFECTED SUBJECTS

HIV-infected subjects, both adults and children, can have impaired nutritional profiles secondary to HIV-associated complications. Micronutrient deficiencies are common in this population, and it can be expected that there may exist concomitant L-carnitine deficiency. However, only a few studies directed at investigating the extent of L-carnitine deficiency, either primary or secondary, in HIV-infected patients have been reported.

We investigated 29 adult patients with AIDS, adequate profiles of nutrition, and no evidence of myopathy or cardiac dysfunction. Most of them (72%) had reduced serum levels of both total and free L-carnitine compared to healthy controls. Furthermore, we observed that even the serum levels of short-chain carnitine were frequently reduced.[13,14] By contrast, a minority of patients (14%) had levels of carnitines in the normal or even the high range.[13,14] In yet another study carried out on a series of 30 adult patients, 37% of patients were found to have levels of total L-carnitine above the upper limit of the normal range.[15] In the study of Tomaka et al, no L-carnitine deficiency was noted in screening HIV-infected subjects from a private practice for various vitamins and minerals but no correlation with zidovudine or other nucleoside analog status was reported.[16] In very preliminary findings, Mintz and coworkers have found deficiencies of total and free L-carnitine in 25% of children with HIV infection who have received zidovudine for longer than 6 months.[17]

An important issue in investigating carnitine metabolism in HIV-infected people is to assess whether carnitine deficiency in serum is associated with deficiency in tissues since there is evidence that the serum concentrations of carnitines do not closely mirror the pool within cells.[18,19] In other words, even significant differences may be found between serum and cellular levels, pointing out that serum concentrations of carnitines should not be regarded as reliable indicators of the whole-body pool of carnitines. Thus, even in patients with AIDS the measurement of serum levels may be a fallacious index.

This background prompted us to investigate the levels of carnitine in PBMCs in AIDS patients, which are most likely to closely reflect the levels in tissues. As expected, patients with AIDS had reduced carnitine concentrations in PBMCs, whether or not serum levels were reduced.[14,20] Therefore, patients with AIDS may have carnitine deficiency at the level of PBMCs, and probably in most tissues, irrespective of whether concentrations in their sera are normal or reduced. No data are available about the cellular levels of free and short-chain carnitine because of the difficulty in obtaining an adequate number of cells from these subjects.[14,20]

In addition, in this study we found a strong relationship between the frequency of mitogen-driven PBMCs entering the S and G2-M phases of the cell cycle and the intracellular concentration of carnitine.[14,20] We previously observed that the pool of PBMCs from AIDS patients that are hyporesponsive to mitogen stimulation, as shown by a frequency of less than 20% cells in the S and G2-M phases, can be significantly augmented if the culture is pretreated with L-carnitine in doses ranging from 100 to 200 pg/ml.[14] By contrast, L-carnitine addition did not enhance proliferative responses in subjects who possessed normoresponsive PBMCs (more than 20% of cells in the S and G2-M phases) to mitogens.[14] These data are in agreement with the hypothesis discussed above that an adequate intracellular pool of carnitines might contribute to maintain the integrity of immune responses. Remarkably, an optimal lipid milieu is required for lymphocyte proliferation and cytokine production[21] and L-carnitine supplementation of patients with unregulated lipid metabolism has been shown to enhance immune functions, probably by correcting the impaired lipid metabolism at the lymphocyte level.[5-7] If we assume that disturbances in lipid metabolism[22-24] caused by either HIV per se[25-30] or the unregulated production of cytokines, such as tumor necrosis factor (TNF)-alpha, associated with the infection[31,32] are crucial to the progressive impairment of immune functions during the course of HIV infection, then the carnitine depletion observed in AIDS patients can be considered a contributing factor.

## CARNITINE DEFICIENCY AND MITOCHONDRIAL TOXICITY OF NUCLEOSIDE ANALOGS

### Skeletal Myopathy

There is evidence that zidovudine (AZT) causes severe mitochondrial myopathy, with generalized weakness, myalgia, raised creatinkinase and transaminase levels, muscle softening and atrophy.[33]

Microscopically, "ragged red fibers," a characteristic marker of mitochondrial myopathies, are found as a consequence of the subsarcolemmal accumulation of mitochondria.[33] By transmission electron microscopy the mitochondria are enlarged and swollen and contain disrupted cristae and paracrystalline inclusions, and biochemical assays performed on muscle homogenates reveal abnormal mitochondrial respiratory function.[33]

The depletion of mitochondrial DNA is crucial to the pathogenesis of AZT-myopathy.[33] However, recent studies have reported that the pool of carnitines is reduced in the skeletal muscles of subjects with AZT-myopathy.[34,35] Furthermore, a markedly elevated ratio of esterified/free carnitine is found in the plasma from these subjects,[35] and this probably reflects a disturbance of fat oxidation.

Although the reasons for the decreased pool of muscle carnitines in AZT-myopathy are unclear, this reduction is likely to play a pathogenic role. Carnitine is essential for the transport of long-chain fatty acids into the mitochondria and for their subsequent beta-oxidation. The muscle carnitine deficiency in patients with AZT-myopathy can therefore substantially contribute to the defect of beta-oxidation that causes the typical lipid accumulation within skeletal muscles.

It is reasonable that the low carnitine levels in skeletal muscles of subjects taking AZT are the consequence of impaired carnitine uptake by the dysfunctioning mitochondria. The subsequent shift toward the glycolytic pathway can lead to an excess of cytoplasmic acetyl-CoA and the esterification of free carnitine, which is then exported.

The hypothesis has been tested that as long as an adequate amount of carnitines is present in the muscle, energy production can be maintained and AZT-myopathy prevented. Under in vitro conditions, L-carnitine has been shown to prevent and improve both the morphological abnormalities of mitochondria and the accumulation of fat droplets induced by AZT in normal human myotubes.[36,37] Thus, it is conceivable that L-carnitine supplementation could be a useful tool for preventing and/or treating the mitochondrial toxicity of AZT. Studies are currently in progress to test this hypothesis.

A derangement in carnitine metabolism may take place in even other tissues, in addition to the skeletal muscles, in subjects treated with AZT or other nucleoside analogs. For example, macrovesicular and microvesicular hepatic steatosis has been observed in association with AIDS and with the use of AZT.[38-41] A similar syndrome of hepatic failure and fatty liver has been reported after treatment with didanosine (ddI)[42,42] and zalcitabine (ddC).[38] These reports are of particular interest in the light of the recent tragic outcome with fialuridine (FIAU), a new nucleoside analog for the treatment of hepatitis B, since several patients treated with FIAU had severe or fatal lactic acidosis in association with microvesicular steatosis after eight weeks of therapy.[44] These changes were assumed to be due to a gradual uncoupling of mitochondrial oxidative metabolism. Unfortunately, so far no data are available about the carnitine metabolism in the liver of these subjects. Nevertheless, it is intriguing to note that the clinical picture of lactic acidosis and hepatic failure induced by nucleoside analogs closely resembles that of subjects with Reye's syndrome or toxic reactions produced by valproic acid.[45] Decreased levels of carnitines are found in these two disorders and carnitine supplementation has been shown to improve their course.[46,47] Taken together, these data indirectly add weight to the view that carnitine deficiency can be a factor contributing to the mitochondrial toxicity of nucleoside analogs.

## NEUROTOXICITY

The use of such nucleoside analogs as ddI, ddC, and stavudine (d4T) may be burdened by the onset of severe dose-limiting peripheral neuropathy.[48-51] ddI, ddC and d4T inhibit mitochondrial DNA polymerase and reduce the mitochondrial DNA content and this is considered responsible for their neurotoxicity.[33,52] Nevertheless, other, as yet unknown, factors may intervene in the pathogenesis of the neurotoxicity.

Acetyl-carnitine regulates the metabolism and function of peripheral nerves[53-55] and contributes to their regeneration following injury[53,56-58] by enhancing both the levels and binding of nerve growth factor to its receptor.[59-63] Additional properties of acetylcarnitine are the ability to correct the age-dependent impairment of mitochondrial DNA transcription[64] and sustain the oxidative metabolism of mitochondria.[65,66]

We have recently shown that patients with clinically manifest, painful, peripheral neuropathy that developed during treatment with different regimens of ddI, ddC, and d4T had reduced levels of acetylcarnitine in their sera but the levels of total carnitine were normal.[67] Thus, the acetylation of carnitine to acetylcarnitine appears impaired in these subjects, probably as a result of the mitochondrial toxicity of nucleoside analogs. By contrast, subjects who did not experience peripheral neuropathy while taking AZT or ddI as the only antiretroviral regimen had normal levels of acetylcarnitine.[67] Thus, the finding of overtly low levels of acetyl-carnitine appeared associated with the development of peripheral neuropathy during treatment with the nucleoside analogs ddI, ddC and d4T.

In our opinion, these data support the view that acetylcarnitine deficiency has a role in the pathogenesis of nucleoside analog-related peripheral neurotoxicity. Furthermore, this is in agreement with most studies demonstrating that neurotoxicity is common during treatment with such nucleoside analogs as ddI, ddC and d4T, whereas AZT mainly accumulates in the skeletal muscle and is rarely neurotoxic.[33]

Even though the metabolic pathways linking acetyl-carnitine deficiency to the neurotoxic effects of nucleoside analogs require further investigation, the exogenous supplementation of acetyl-carnitine in patients taking ddI, ddC or d4T appears a reasonable hypothesis.

## ETIOLOGY OF CARNITINE DEFICIENCY IN AIDS

HIV infection is a high-risk condition for developing carnitine deficiency. Many mechanisms producing carnitine deficiency may be involved (Table 11.1), but the effect of AZT on mitochondrial function is probably a predominant mechanism. Furthermore, HIV-infected patients are prone to nutritional problems associated with malabsorption due to an inadequate diet or chronic diarrhea because of HIV-related enteropathy, multiple opportunistic infections and malignancies, which may lead to a considerable degree of malabsorption, thus creating a secondary carnitine deficiency. HIV-related kidney abnormalities, which result in a strong increase of urinary carnitine excretion, and a shift toward glycolytic pathways with breakdown of fats to form fatty acids and their subsequent rebuilding, which utilizes energy and could account for the unregulated carnitine consumption, are additional mechanisms contributing to the pathogenesis of carnitine deficiency in these subjects. Even the use of pivaloyl antibiotics, cephalosporines, and sulfadiazine and pyrimethamine[68] may contribute to the pathogenesis of carnitine deficiency in HIV-infected subjects. Since L-carnitine is a safe compound and freely available in the drugstore at a low cost, many HIV-infected subjects supplement their drug regimen with L-carnitine, in combination or not with standardized antiretroviral regimens. This could obscure the true extent of the carnitine deficiency. Furthermore, the majority of these patients do not report this to the physicians taking care of them. This is a relevant issue since the unclear extent of L-carnitine supplementation could represent a significant bias for the interpretation of the results of trials designed to investigate the efficacy of antiretroviral regimens. Likewise, the overwhelming use of nucleoside analogs and antibiotics in HIV-infected people makes it very difficult to distinguish the natural history of carnitine deficiency from the effects of drug toxicity. Additionally, the investigation of carnitine metabolism in HIV-infected patients has been regarded as trivial by many researchers and only a small number of laboratories and investigators have reported data concerning this issue, and reproducible findings in additional centers would be desirable. Consequently, the pathogenesis of carnitine deficiency in HIV-infected subjects and the therapeutic potential of L-carnitine supplementation have not been so far fully elucidated.

## IMPACT OF L-CARNITINE THERAPY ON LYMPHOCYTE MITOGEN RESPONSIVENESS AND CARNITINE CELLULAR CONTENT

Pilot trials have demonstrated that L-carnitine supplementation improves several immunologic and metabolic parameters in patients with AIDS.

High-dose L-carnitine (6 g per day for two weeks) resulted in amelioration of the mitogen-driven proliferative responses of PBMCs.[14,20,69] When PBMCs were isolated from patients exposed to high-dosed L-carnitine supplementation, there was an enhancement of in vitro mitogenic responses to phytohemagglutinin, again measured as a function of the percent of lymphocytes entering the S and G2-M phases.[14,20,69] This was paralleled by a significant trend towards restoration of PBMC carnitine content, accompanied by an increase in serum levels.[14,20,69]

The enhancement of mitogen-driven proliferative PBMC responses raised the concern of increased HIV replication, but p24 antigen levels, a marker of HIV replication, did not rise in L-carnitine-treated in patients with detectable p24 at base-line, and no conversion to detectable p24 occurred patients with undetectable levels at base-line.[14,20,69]

At the end of the study period, serum triglycerides were decreased with respect to pretreatment values, and the decline was associated with a reduction of serum TNF-alpha levels.[14,69] Furthermore, the elevated baseline serum levels of beta-2-microglobulin, a surrogate marker for survival in HIV-infected subjects and a potential marker for HIV encephalitis, were also reduced following treatment with L-carnitine.[14,69] However, these early reports failed to show any increase in CD4 counts.[14,20,69] This suggested that the enhanced mitogen responsiveness of PBMCs following L-carnitine treatment was the result of the effects of L-carnitine at the single cell level. Although no clinical correlation was investigated, there were a number of

---

**Table 11.1. Causes of carnitine deficiency in HIV-infected persons**

---

Malabsorption (opportunistic infections and cancer of small intestine)
HIV-related enteropathy
HIV-related kidney abnormalities
Unregulated carnitine consumption associated with derangements in
lipid metabolism
Drugs
    Antiretroviral nucleoside analogs (AZT,ddI,ddC,d4T)
    Pivaloyl-antibiotics (pivampicillin, pivmecillinam)
    Cephalosporines
    Sulfadiazine
    Pyrimethamine

---

participants who reported subjective improvements in "energy levels," "well-being," and weight gain.

## IMPACT OF L-CARNITINE THERAPY ON LYMPHOCYTE APOPTOSIS, CD4 CELL DECLINE AND HIV VIREMIA

Lymphocytes from HIV-infected individuals undergo inappropriate apoptosis, a major mechanism for the decline in CD4 and CD8 cells that drives the disease progression toward AIDS. Indeed, lymphocyte apoptosis correlates with disease progression and lower CD4 counts and a high degree of apoptosis has been detected in HIV-infected progressors in comparison to long-term nonprogressors,[70] a unique population of subjects who remain clinically healthy and immunocompetent over an extended period of time despite chronic infection with HIV. In general, more rapid declines in CD4 counts and more rapid disease progression correlate with lower CD4 counts and higher HIV load. In turn, an increase in CD4 counts along with a decrease in viral load explain a significant part of the treatment effect observed with antiretroviral therapy.

Recent studies have demonstrated that the activation of the sphingomyelin pathway and the generation of ceramide, an endogenous mediator of apoptosis and HIV replication, are involved in the pathogenesis of HIV infection. Ceramide is generated from sphingomyelin hydrolysis via the action of a sphingomyelin-specific form of phospholipase C, a sphingomyelinase, which might initiate signalling leading to programmed cell death in response to several mechanisms implicated in the inappropriate apoptosis seen in HIV-infected subjects, such as the chronic expression of Fas and the unregulated activation of the receptor for TNF.[71-73] In addition, ceramide has been shown to increase following HIV infection[74] and potently induce the virus replication.[75,76] Patients with AIDS have significantly higher lymphocyte-associated ceramide levels in comparison to long-term nonprogressors, but both AIDS patients and long-term nonprogressors have elevated levels compared to healthy individuals.[77,78] As expected, the frequency of lymphocytes undergoing apoptosis differs between AIDS patients and long-term nonprogressors since a higher frequency of apoptotic CD4 and CD8 cells has been measured in AIDS patients than in long-term nonprogressors.[78] These differences in the levels of ceramide appear associated with differences in lymphocyte counts and HIV viremia. In fact, higher CD4 and CD8 counts have been found in long-term nonprogressors than in AIDS patients, whereas the viral load is more elevated in the AIDS group.[78] In addition, a moderate inverse relationship links ceramide levels and CD4 counts in long-term nonprogressors and a slight tendency towards a positive association between HIV plasma load and ceramide levels has been recognized in patients with AIDS.[78]

These data strongly add weight to the in vitro observations suggesting a critical role for ceramide in both HIV replication and apoptotic loss of T lymphocytes. It is conceivable that fluctuations in lymphocyte-associated ceramide content may accompany or precede an accelerated rate of lymphocyte apoptosis and viral replication. In turn, strategies directed at down-modulating lymphocyte-associated ceramide could slow the clinical progression of the infection.

Early reports have suggested the potential of L-carnitine and its congeners to act as anti-apoptotic compounds.[9] More recently, L-carnitine has been shown to interfere with the Fas-triggered apoptotic signalling through down-modulating ceramide.[79,80] The inhibition of ceramide generation by L-carnitine appears to involve the inhibition of the acidic sphingomyelinase; by contrast, the Fas-activated neutral sphingomyelinase, which has not been implicated in generating ceramide relevant to Fas-induced apoptosis, is not significantly influenced by L-carnitine treatment.[79,80]

Taken all into account, this background prompted us to investigate whether L-carnitine supplementation of HIV-infected patients could impact on lymphocyte apoptosis, ceramide generation, CD4 counts and viral load.

In the first study, we investigated the effects of short-term L-carnitine therapy on the apoptosis of CD4 and CD8 cells as well as on ceramide generation.[81] Briefly, ten male patients with AIDS received via the intravenous route L-carnitine (6 grams) in normal saline over a two-hour period each day for five days. Blood samples for measuring CD4 and CD8 counts, the frequency of cells undergoing apoptosis, and the levels of PBMC-associated ceramide were taken at base-line, at day 3 (T1), and at day 6 (T2).

Apoptotic CD4 cells significantly decreased at both T1 and T2 measurements compared to the base-line and a trend towards declining counts of apoptotic CD8 was also observed.[81] These changes in the frequency of apoptotic cells were associated with a trend towards increasing counts of total lymphocytes as well as CD4 and CD8 cells.[81] Remarkably, when L-carnitine therapy was interrupted the counts of apoptotic CD4 and CD8 cells returned to base-line levels within one week.[81]

Even the levels of PBMC-associated ceramide were decreased by L-carnitine therapy with respect to base-line and the decrease was statistically significant at both T1 and T2 measurements. Furthermore, the ceramide levels were well correlated with the frequency of apoptotic CD4 cells and moderately with the frequency of apoptotic CD8 cells.[81]

We are currently investigating the impact of long-term L-carnitine treatment on CD4 counts and HIV viremia, the two best independent predictors of the risk of developing AIDS-related complications (De Simone et al, manuscript in preparation). It should be noted that we recruited into this study a unique population of HIV-infected subjects: 1) all individuals lived in a community devoted to the rescue of drug addicts; 2) none of them had carnitine deficiency; 3) all subjects had progressively declining CD4 counts during the pre-treatment follow-up period; 4) all subjects rejected treatment with antiretroviral drugs.

The patients were administered L-carnitine (6 grams) in normal saline through the intravenous route over a two-hour period each day for 4 months. Then, L-carnitine was administered at the same dosage by the oral route each day for 2 months, in order to improve patients' compliance. Blood samples were taken at base-line (T0), at day 15 (T1), at day 30 (T2), at day 60 (T3), at day 120 (T4) and at day 180 (T5).

Preliminary analysis of the results has shown that the decline in CD4 counts during the pre-treatment follow-up period was reverted by L-carnitine therapy. Indeed comparing the change in CD4 counts (pre-treatment to T0) vs (T3-T0) and vs (T4-T0) we observed a significant improvement in the CD4 rate. While CD4 counts declined an average of 0.08 cells per day from an early date until L-carnitine treatment was started, the interval from T0 until T3 had an increase of 0.73 cells per day and the net effect was an overall gain of 0.81 cells per day compared to the rate of pre-treatment decline (P 0.024). Similarly, the interval from T0 until T4 had an increase of 0.64 CD4 cells per day and the net effect was an overall gain of 0.72 cells per day compared to the rate of pre-treatment decline (P 0.024). Even on the remaining time points there was a trend towards improvement in the CD4 rate, but the differences did not reach statistical significance. An overall daily gain of even CD8 cells was recognized, but the impact of L-carnitine therapy did not reach statistical significance.

The possibility that this effect of L-carnitine therapy may reflect a response to the drug itself and not a drug-induced protection from CD4 cell death has not been tested in this study. However, the reversal in CD4 cell decline we observed appeared associated with a strong reduction in the frequency of apoptotic CD4 and CD8 lymphocytes and this seems to rule out a margination effect or redistribution of already formed cells.

HIV viremia, expressed as serum RNA levels, was measured at base-line and after 6 months of L-carnitine therapy (T5). Viral load was on average reduced at T5 compared to base-line. HIV RNA levels were markedly reduced in 8/11 subjects; of the remaining three, two had no significant changes whereas one had a 5-fold increase in the viral load. Of note, L-carnitine has no direct antiretroviral activity (H. Mitsuya, personal communication).

The levels of PBMC-associated ceramide were reduced by L-carnitine therapy with respect to base-line as well. We measured decreased levels of ceramide throughout the study period at each time point, and the changes were statistically significant compared to base-line on T4 and T5. Remarkably, at each time point the levels of ceramide correlated weakly to moderately with the frequency of apoptotic CD4 and CD8 cells and HIV viremia.

The results of this study are very encouraging. The relevant finding was that long-term L-carnitine therapy reverted the decline of CD4 cells, and a net gain was obtained, through decreasing apoptosis and controlled HIV replication. The improvement in these parameters appears mediated by the down-modulation of ceramide. The favorable impact of L-carnitine therapy on CD4 cell counts and HIV load, the two best independent predictors of disease progression, suggests an important potential for L-carnitine administration in the management of HIV-infected people. In addition, no toxicity of L-carnitine therapy was recognized and a significant improvement in the Karnofsky score and in the ability to perform regular daily activities was observed in treated subjects.

It is clear that HIV-infected subjects receiving only L-carnitine therapy are not likely to experience an indefinite stabilization in their disease course. In turn, treatment with approved antiretroviral drugs is frequently hampered by their relatively weak antiviral activity, toxicity, the emergence of resistant viral strains and cross-resistance. In addition, access and cost of antiretroviral therapy are major obstacles to inadequately served populations throughout the world. In our opinion, L-carnitine should be considered for the treatment of people infected with HIV but not in imminent danger of progression or with a slow decay. This is a reasonable alternative to the option to wait for another six or twelve months while the medical and economic issues concerning the new antiretroviral regimens are sorted so that they could be regarded as an effective alternative to currently approved regimens that are too difficult or costly to sustain. The safety and low cost of L-carnitine therapy further support this view.

## CONCLUDING REMARKS

There is a growing body of evidence in the literature that HIV-infected subjects, particularly those receiving treatment with nucleoside analogs, may possess a carnitine deficiency syndrome. Such a deficiency can be measured in serum, PBMCs, or skeletal muscle and, possibly, other tissues. Taken together, available data indicate that HIV-infected subjects require exogenous L-carnitine. The results of ongoing clinical trials of L-carnitine therapy involving the correlation with parameters of disease progression are encouraging. Furthermore, L-carnitine has a low toxicity profile and, in turn, an improvement in global well-being and in the ability to participate in daily activities is frequently recognized in L-carnitine-receiving subjects. In addition, to address issues of the efficacy of L-carnitine therapy, further studies are warranted with the pursuit of providing guidelines for dosing and the timing of starting L-carnitine therapy.

REFERENCES

1. Fauci AS, Pantaleo G, Stanley S, Weissman D. Immunopathogenetic mechanisms of HIV infection. Ann Intern Med 1996; 124:654-663.
2. De Simone C, Famularo G, Cifone G, Mitsuya H. HIV-1 infection and cellular metabolism. Immunol Today 1996; 17:256-258.
3. Famularo G, Moretti S, Marcellini S, Alesse E, De Simone C. Cellular dysmetabolism:the dark side of HIV-1 infection. J Clin Lab Immunol 1996 48:123-132.
4. Deufel T. Determination of L-carnitine in biological fluids and tissues. J Clin Chem Clin Biochem 1990; 28:307-311.
5. Monti D, Cossarizza A, Troiano L, Arrigoni Martelli E, Franceschi C. Immunomodulatory properties of L-acetylcarnitine on lymphocytes from young and old humans. In: De Simone C, Arrigoni Martelli E, eds. Stress, Immunity and Ageing. A Role for L-acetylcarnitine. Amsterdam: Elsevier, 1989:83-96.
6. De Simone C, Delogu G, Fagiola A et al. Lipids and the immune system are influenced by L-carnitine. A study in elderly subjects with cardiovascular diseases. Int J Immunother 1:267-271, 1985.
7. De Simone C, Ferrari M, Meli D, Midiri G, Sorice F. Reversibility by L-carnitine of immunosuppression induced by emulsion of soya bean oil, glycerol and egg lecithin. Drug Res 1982; 32:1485-1485.
8. Monti D, Troiano L, Tropea F et al. Apoptosis - programmed cell death: a role in the aging process? Am J Clin Nutr 1992; 55: 1208S-1214S.
9. Famularo G, De Simone C, Tzantzoglou S, Trinchieri V. Apoptosis, anti-apoptotic compounds and TNF-alpha release. Immunol Today 1994; 15:495-496.
10. Kuratsune H, Yamaguti K, Takahashi M, Misaki H, Tagawa S, Kitani T. Acylcarnitine deficiency in chronic fatigue syndrome. Clin Infect Dis 1994; 18:S62-S67.

11. Majeed T, De Simone C, Famularo G, Marcellini S, Behan PO. Abnormalities of carnitine metabolism in chronic fatigue syndrome. Eur J Neurol 1995; 2:425-428.
12. Famularo G, De Simone C, Arrigoni Martelli E, Jirillo E. Carnitine and septic shock: a review. J Endotoxin Res 1995; 2:141-147.
13. De Simone C, Tzantzoglou S, Jirillo E et al. Carnitine deficiency in AIDS patients. AIDS 1992; 6:203-205.
14. Famularo G, De Simone C. A new era for carnitine? Immunol Today 1995; 16:211-213.
15. Bogden JD, Baker H, Frank O et al. Micronutrient status and human immunodeficiency virus (HIV) infection. Ann NY Acad Sci 1990; 587:189-195.
16. Tomaka FL, Cimoch PJ, Reiter WM et al. Prevalence of nutritional deficiencies in patients with HIV-1 infection. Int Conf AIDS 1994 (Abs. PB 0898).
17. Mintz M. Carnitine in human immunodeficiency virus type I/Acquired Immune Deficiency Syndrome. J Child Neurol 1995; 10:2S40-2S44.
18. Bohmer T, Rydning A, Solberg HE. Carnitine levels in human serum in health and disease. Clin Chem Acta 1974; 57:55-61.
19. Tripp ME, Shug AL. Plasma carnitine concentrations in cardiomyopathy patients. Biochem Med 1984; 32:199-206.
20. De Simone C, Famularo G, Tzantzoglou S, Trinchieri V, Moretti S, Sorice F. Carnitine depletion in peripheral blood mononuclear cells from patients with AIDS: effect of oral L carnitine. AIDS 1994, 8:655-660.
21. Herzberg VL. Human T lymphocytes require lipid as either lipoprotein or nonesterified fatty acid for in vitro activation. Immunol Invest 1991; 20:507-513.
22. Hommes MJT, Romijn JA, Endert E et al. Basal fuel homeostasis in symptomatic human immunodeficiency virus infection. Clin Sci 1991; 80:359-365.
23. Stein TP, Nutinsky C, Condolucci D et al. Protein and energy substrate metabolism in AIDS patients. Metabolism 1990; 39:876-881.
24. Grunfeld C, Feingold RK. Metabolic disturbances and wasting in the acquired immunodeficiency syndrome. N Engl J Med 1992; 327: 329-337.
25. Aguilar JJ, Anel A, Torres JM et al. Changes in lipid composition of human peripheral blood lymphocytes infected by HIV. AIDS Res Hum Retroviruses 1991; 7:761-765.
26. Apostolov K, Barker W, Wood CB et al. Fatty acid saturation index in peripheral blood cell membranes in AIDS patients. Lancet 1987; i:695-697.
27. Apostolov K, Barker W, Galpin SA. Syncytia formation in HIV-1-infected cells is associated with an increase in cellular oleic acid. FEBS Lett 1989; 250:241-244.

28. Klein A, Mercure L, Gordon P et al. The effect of HIV-1 infection on the lipid fatty acid content in the membrane of cultured lymphocytes. AIDS 1990; 4:865-867.
29. Marchalonis J. Structure and Role of Phospholipids in the Lymphocyte Plasma Membrane. New York: Marcel Dekker Inc., 1987: 171-222.
30. Lynn WS, Tweedale A, Cloyd MW. Human immunodeficiency virus (HIV-1) cytotoxicity: perturbation of the cell membrane and depression of phospholipid synthesis. Virology 1988; 163:43-51.
31. Matsuyama T, Kobayashi N, Yamamoto N. Cytokines and HIV infection: is AIDS a tumor necrosis factor disease? AIDS 1991; 5:1405-1417.
32. Memon RA, Feingold KR, Moser AH, Doerller W, Grunfeld C. In vivo effects of interferon-alpha and interferon-gamma on lipolysis and ketogenesis. Endocrinology 1992; 131:1695-1702.
33. Lewis W, Dalakas MC. Mitochondrial toxicity of antiviral drugs. Nature Med 1995; 1:417-422.
34. Dalakas MC, Leon-Monzon ME, Bernardini I, Gahl WA. Zidovudine-induced mitochondrial myopathy is associated with muscle carnitine deficiency and lipid storage. Ann Neurol 1994; 35:482-487.
35. Campos Y, Arenas J. Muscle carnitine deficiency associated with zidovudine-induced mitochondrial myopathy. Ann Neurol 1994; 36:680-681.
36. Semino-Mora C, Leon-Monzon ME, Dalakas MC. Effect of L-carnitine on the zidovudine-induced destruction of human myotubes. Part I: L-carnitine prevents the myotoxicity of AZT in vitro. Lab Invest 1994; 71: 102-112.
37. Semino-Mora MC, Leon-Monzon ME, Dalakas MC. Effect of L-carnitine on the zidovudine-induced destruction of human myotubes. Part II: treatment with L-carnitine improves the AZT-induced changes and prevents further destruction. Lab Invest 1994; 71: 773-781.
38. Chattha G, Arieff AI, Cummings C, Tierney LM Jr. Lactic acidosis complicating the acquired immunodeficiency syndrome. Ann Intern Med 1993; 118:37-39.
39. Freiman JP, Helfert KE, Hamrell MR, Stein DS. Hepatomegaly with severe steatosis in HIV-seropositive patients. AIDS 1993; 7:379-385.
40. Gopinath R, Hutcheon M, Cheema-Dhadli, Halperin M. Chronic lactc acidosis in a patient with acquired immunodeficiency syndrome and mitochondrial myopathy: biochemical studies. J Am Soc Nephrol 1992; 3:1212-1219.
41. Gradon JD, Chapnick EK, Sepkowitz DV. Zidovudine-induced hepatitis. J Intern Med 1992; 231:317-318.
42. Lai KK, Gang DL, Zavacki JK, Cooley TP. Fulminant hepatic failure associated with 2',3'-dideoxyinosine (ddI). Ann Intern Med 1991; 115:283-284.

43. Bissuel F, Bruneel F, Habersetzer F et al. Fulminant hepatitis with severe lactic acidosis in HIV-infected patients on didanosine therapy. J Intern Med 1994; 235:367-371.
44. McKenzie R, Fried MW, Sallie R et al. Hepatic failure and lactic acidosis due to fialuridine (FIAU), an investigational nucleoside analogue for chronic hepatitis B. N Engl J Med 1995; 333:1099-1105.
45. Balistreri WF. Reye's syndrome and its metabolic mimickers. In: Balistreri WF, Stocker JT, eds. Pediatric Hepatology. New York: Hemisphere, 1990; 183-202.
46. Matsuda I, Ohtani Y. Carnitine status in Reye's and Reye-like syndrome. Pediatr Neurol 1986; 2:90-94.
47. Castro-Gago M, Novo I, Rodriguez-Segade S. Effects of valproic acid on the urea cycle and carnitine metabolism. Int Pediatr 1990; 5:54-57.
48. Simpson DM, Maltagliati M. Neurologic manifestations of HIV infection. Ann Intern Med 1994; 121:769-785.
49. Faulds D, Brogden RN. Didanosine. A review of its antiviral activity, pharmacokinetic properties and therapeutic potential in human immunodeficiency virus infection. Drugs 1992; 44:94-116.
50. Whittington R, Brogden RN. Zalcitabine. A review of its pharmacology and clinical potential in acquired immunodeficiency syndrome (AIDS). Drugs 1992; 44:656-683.
51. Browne MJ, Mayer KN, Chapee SB et al. 2',3'-didehydro-3'deoxythymidine (d4T) in patients with AIDS or AIDS related complex: a phase I trial. J Infect Dis 1993; 167:21-29.
52. Chen CH, Vasquez-Padua M, Cheng YC. Effect of anti-human immunodeficiency virus nucleoside analogs on mitochondrial DNA and its implication for delayed toxicity. Mol Pharmacol 1991; 39:625-628.
53. Pettorossi VE, Brunetti V, Carrobi L, Della Torre G, Grassi S. L-acetylcarnitine enhances functional muscle reinnervation. Drugs Exp Clin Res 1991; 17:119-125.
54. Rampello L, Giammona G, Aleppo G, Favit A, Fiore L. Trophic action of acetyl-L-carnitine in neuronal cultures. Acta Neurol 1992; 14:15-21.
55. Forloni G, Angeretti N, Smiroldo S. Neuroprotective activity of acetyl-L-carnitine: studies in vitro. J Neurosci Res 1994; 37:92-96.
56. Rosenthal RE, Williams R, Bogaert YE, Getson PR, Fiskum G. Prevention of postischemic canine neurological injury through potentiation of brain energy metabolism by acetylcarnitine. Stroke 1992; 23:1312-1317.
57. De Angelis C, Scarfo C, Falcinelli M, Reda E, Ramacci MT, Angelucci L. Levocarnitine acetyl stimulates peripheral nerve regeneration and neuromuscular junction remodelling following sciatic nerve injury. Int J Clin Pharmacol Res 1992; 12:269-279.
58. Tenconi B, Donadoni L, Germani E et al. Intraspinal degenerative atrophy caused by sciatic nerve lesions prevented by acetyl-L-carnitine. Int J Clin Pharmacol Res 1992; 12:263-267.

59. Piovesan P, Pacifici L, Taglialatela G, Ramacci MT, Angelucci L. Acetylcarnitine treatment increases choline acetyltransferase activity and NGF levels in the CNS of adult rats following total fimbria fornix transection. Brain Res 1994; 633:77-82.

60. De Simone R, Ramacci MT, Aloe L. Effect of acetyl-L-carnitine on forebrain cholinergic neurons of developing rats. Int J Dev Neurosci 1991; 9:39-46.

61. Taglialatela G, Angelucci L, Ramacci MT, Werrbach Perez K, Jackson GR, Perez Polo JR. Stimulation of nerve growth factor receptors in PC12 cells by acetyl-L-carnitine. Biochem Pharmacol 1992; 44:577-585.

62. Taglialatela G, Navarra G, Cruciani R, Ramacci MT, Alema GS, Angelucci L. Acetyl-L-carnitine increases nerve growth factor levels and choline acetyltransferase activity in the central nervous system of aged rats. Exp Gerontol 1994; 29:55-66.

63. Castorina M, Ferraris L. Acetyl-L-carnitine affects aged brain receptorial system in rodents. Life Sci 1994; 54:1205-1214.

64. Gadaleta MN, Petruzzella V, Renis M et al. Reduced transcription of mitochondrial DNA in the senescent rat: tissue dependence and effect of L-carnitine. Eur J Biochem 1990; 187:501-506.

65. Villa RF, Turpenoja L, Benzi G et al. Action of L-acetylcarnitine on age-dependent modifications of mitochondrial membrane proteins from rat cerebellum. Neurochem Res 1988; 13:509-516.

66. Villa RF, Gorrini A. Action of L-acetylcarnitine on different cerebral mitochondrial populations from hippocampus and striatum during aging. Neurochem Res 1991; 16:1125-1132.

67. Famularo G, Moretti S, Marcellini S et al. Acetyl-carnitine deficiency in AIDS patients with neurotoxicity on treatment with antiretroviral nucleoside analogs. AIDS 1997 (in press).

68. Famularo G, Matricardi F, De Simone C. Carnitine deficiency: primary and secondary syndromes. In: De Simone C, Famularo G, eds. Carnitine Today. Austin: RG Landes 1997; 119-172.

69. De Simone C, Tzantzoglou S, Famularo G et al. High-dose L-carnitine improves immunologic and metabolic parameters in AIDS patients. Immunopharmacol Immunotoxicol 1993; 15:1-12.

70. Gougeon ML, Lecoeur H, Dulioust A et al. Programmed cell death in peripheral lymphocytes from HIV-infected persons. J Immunol 1996; 156:3509-3520.

71. Spiegel S, Foster D, Kolesnick R. Signal transduction through lipid second messengers. Curr Op Biol 1996; 8:159-167.

72. Cifone MG, De Maria R, Roncaioli P et al. Apoptotic signaling through CD95 (Fas/APO-1) activates an acidic sphingomyelinase. J Exp Med 1994; 177:1547-1552.

73. Cifone MG, Roncaioli P, De Maria R et al. Multiple pathways originate at the Fas/APO-1 (CD95) receptor: sequential involvement of

phosphatidylcholine-specific phospholipase C and acidic sphingomyelinase in the propagation of the apoptotic signal. EMBO J 1995;
14:5859-5868.

74. Van Veldhoven PP, Matthews JJ, Bolognesi DP, Bell RM. Changes
in bioactive lipids alkylacylglycerol and ceramide occur in HIV-infected cells. Biochem Biophys Res Commun 1992; 187:209-216.

75. Rivas CI, Golde DW, Vera JC, Kolesnick RN. Involvement of the
sphingomyelin pathway in TNF signaling for HIV production in
chronically infected HL-60 cells. Blood 1993; 83:2191-2197.

76. Papp B, Zhang D, Groopman JE, Byrn RA. Stimulation of human
immunodeficiency virus type I expression by ceramide. AIDS Res
Hum Retroviruses 1994; 10:775-780.

77. De Simone C, Cifone MG, Roncaioli P et al. Ceramide, AIDS and
long-term survivors. Immunol Today 1996; 17:48-49.

78. De Simone C, Cifone MG, Di Marzio L et al. Cell-associated ceramide
in HIV-1-infected subjects. AIDS 1996; 10:675-676.

79. Di Marzio L, Alesse E, Roncaioli P et al. Influence of L-carnitine on
Fas crosslinking-induced apoptosis and ceramide generation in T cell
lines: Correlation with its effects on purified acidic and neutral
sphingomyelinase in vitro. Proceedings of The American Association of Physicians (in press).

80. Alesse E, Di Marzio L, Roncaioli P et al. Effect of L-carnitine on
Fas-induced apoptosis and sphingomyelinase activity in human T cell
lines. In: De Simone C, Famularo G, eds. Carnitine Today. Austin:RG
Landes 1997; 259-270.

81. Cifone MG, Alesse E, Di Marzio L et al. Effect of L-carnitine treatment in vivo on apoptosis and ceramide generation in peripheral
blood lymphocytes from AIDS patients. Proceedings of The American Association of Physicians (in press).

# CHAPTER 12

# Effect of L-Carnitine on AZT-Induced Mitochondrial Toxicity: Studies on Human Muscle Cultures

Cristina Semino-Mora and Marta E. Leon-Monzon

## INTRODUCTION

Mitochondrial myopathy in zidovudine-treated patients was initially reported in 1990 by Dalakas.[1] Zidovudine (AZT) is one of the nucleotide analogs, the antiretroviral drugs, provided to patients infected with human immunodeficiency virus (HIV) to control the amount of virus present in those individuals and avoid the full development of the disease (AIDS).[2] The first treatment consisted of a high dose of AZT for prolonged periods; in some of the HIV-patients treated with this regimen, it was observed that AZT caused a myopathic disease that was called "AZT myopathy."[1,3,4,5] Muscle biopsy studies from those patients revealed that this myopathy was histologically characterized by an increased number of a unique type of muscle fiber described as ragged red fibers.[1,6] When the muscle biopsies were studied by electron microscopy, a proliferation of mitochondria with enlarged size and abnormal cristae was observed.[1,6,7] Molecular analysis has also determined a severe reduction of the mitochondrial DNA in the muscle of HIV patients treated with AZT.[6] We and others have reported on the mechanism by which AZT damages the muscle.[8-11] Our studies were performed in vitro, using human muscle cultures,[8,12,13] and in vivo, using rats treated with daily intraperitoneal injections of AZT.[8] In an effort toward preventing this disease, our laboratory has also found that L-carnitine (3-hydroxy-4-methyl-ammoniobutanoate) in our model systems prevents and improves the pathological alterations caused by AZT.[12,13]

L-carnitine regulates the substrate flux and energy balance across cell membranes by modulating the transport of long-chain fatty acids into

*Carnitine Today,* edited by Claudio De Simone and Giuseppe Famularo.

mitochondria and their β-oxidation.[14-18] Moreover, L-carnitine exerts in vitro a protective effect on the ammonium sulfate-induced structural changes of mitochondria and it can stimulate state 4 of the respiration chain, exerting a protective effect against the oxidative damage of calcium-loaded mitochondria.[19] L-carnitine is currently being utilized for the treatment of ischemic heart disease due to its immunological properties.[20] Recent studies analyzed its role in disorders with unregulated responses, such as AIDS,[20-22] septic shock[20,23] and chronic fatigue syndrome (CFS).[24]

## IN VITRO STUDIES

### EXPERIMENTAL DESIGNS

Muscle cultures were established from human skeletal muscle removed from patients undergoing routine diagnostic muscle biopsies.[8,12,13,25] Five different concentrations of AZT from 0.01 μM (0.0027 μg/ml) to 500 μM (135 μg/ml) were used for a period of 1 to 3 weeks to determine the optimal concentration that would reproduce the morphological alterations observed in the muscle biopsy specimens.[12] We found that AZT at a dose of 250 μM (67.5 μg/ml) for 3 weeks induced important quantitative changes in various organelles of the myotubes;[12,13] at lower concentrations (100 μM) AZT induced a substantial increase in the absolute number of mitochondria (Fig.12.1). The dose of 250 μM was used to assess whether or not L-carnitine could have a beneficial effect on the AZT-treated cultures. The study of the potential effect of L-carnitine was carried out in three sets of cultures. In the first set, the muscle cultures were exposed to both AZT (250 μM) and L-carnitine (5 mM) for 3 weeks; in the second set, muscle cultures received AZT for 3 weeks, followed by another 3 weeks in the presence of 5 mM L-carnitine alone; in the third set, human cultures were treated with 250 μM AZT for a total of 6 weeks, but after the third week L-carnitine was also added. Human muscle cultures without any treatment were used as controls in each set. At the end of the three or six weeks all cultures were examined by: a) light microscopy; b) enzyme histochemistry using oil-red O stain to detect accumulation of lipid droplets; c) immunocytochemistry using the monoclonal antibody Leu-19, that specifically immunostains N-CAM expressing myotubes but not fibroblasts;[12,13,26] and d) electron microscopy. By electron microscopy we examined the morphology and counted the number and the volume occupied by each organelle/unit volume of tissue volumetric density (Vvi),[12,13,27] The mean number of Vvi for each organelle within the myotubes (including mitochondria, nuclei, endoplasmic reticulum, lysosomes, lipid droplets, myofibrils, Golgi apparatus, vacuoles and glycogen) treated with both AZT and L-carnitine was compared to the mean number of organelles within the myotubes treated only with AZT and to the mean number of organelles in the untreated, control, cultures.

EFFECT OF AZT (250 μM) ON HUMAN MUSCLE CULTURES

By the third week, the 250 μM dose of AZT inflicted significant damage to the myotubes. The number of myotubes/field, detected by immunocytochemistry, decreased by the end of the third week from $24.89 \pm 0.96$ to $3.43 \pm 0.62$ ($p < 0.001$) (Fig. 12.2B). Histochemical staining with oil-red-O showed an accumulation of lipid droplets in the cytoplasm of the myotubes (Fig. 12.3B). By electron microscopy, morphological abnormalities were seen in the mitochondria consisting of swelling, increased size, bizarre shape, vesiculation, lamellar inclusions and multiple concentric cristae (Fig. 12.4B-D). An increment in the Vvi of the lipid droplets was also noted from $0.70 \pm 0.34$ to $12.22 \pm 4.91$ ($p < 0.05$) (Fig. 12.5B) as well as an increment in the lysosomes from $1.23 \pm 0.32$ to $15.60 \pm 3.66$ ($p < 0.05$).

EFFECTS OF L-CARNITINE ON THE AZT/L-CARNITINE-TREATED MYOTUBE CULTURES

By the third week, the muscle cultures treated with both 250 μM of AZT and 5 mM of L-carnitine were better preserved than the parallel cultures treated only with AZT, described in the previous paragraph. An increase number of Leu-19-positive-myotubes from $3.43\pm0.62$ in the AZT alone, to $9.44\pm1.23$ ($p < 0.001$) in the AZT/L-carnitine (Fig. 12.2C), and $24.88\pm0.86$ in the untreated control cultures were observed. The accumulations of lipid droplets dramatically diminished in the AZT/L-carnitine-treated cultures from $12.22\pm4.91$ to $1.37\pm0.69$ (Fig. 12.3C and 5C). The Vvi of the lysosomes decreased from $15.60\pm3.66$ to $3.97\pm1.45$ ($p < 0.001$). The ultrastructural morphology of the mitochondria and the rough endoplasmic reticulum was preserved (Fig. 12.4 E). The Vvi of the myofibrils, however,

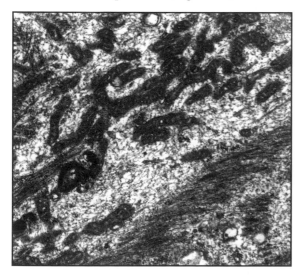

Fig. 12.1. Electron micrographs of human muscle in tissue cultures treated with 100 μM AZT. Observe significant proliferation of mitochondria (X 32,000).

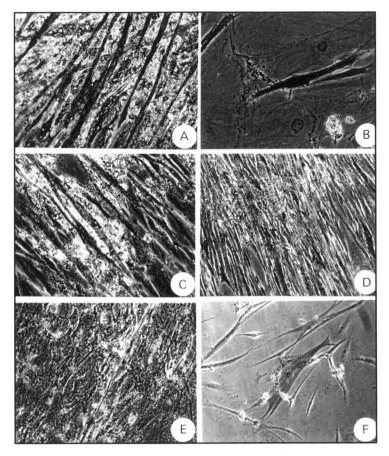

Fig. 12.2 A-F. Effect of AZT on human myotubes in culture. Representative flasks from each of cultures were immunoreacted with N-CAM antibodies. Cultures treated with 250 µM AZT, (B) show a reduction of myotubes compared with the untreated control cultures (A). C: cultures treated simultaneously with 5 mM L-carnitine and 250 µM AZT demonstrate significant prevention of the myotoxic effect of AZT, as shown by the increase in the number of myotubes. D: cultures treated for 3 weeks with 250 µM AZT followed by 3 weeks with L-carnitine also show an increment in the number of myotubes when compared to cultures treated only with AZT (B). E: cultures treated with AZT for 3 weeks, followed by no drugs (only medium) for 3 more weeks note a decreased number of myotubes when compared to cultures which received L-carnitine (D). F: cultures treated with AZT (for 6 weeks) and L-carnitine (from 3rd to 6th week) also show an increased number of the myotubes (X 200). See color figure in insert.

did not change with the carnitine treatment since it remains low (5.60 ± 1.59) in the AZT/L-carnitine-treated cultures compared to 18.03 ± 2.17 in the untreated control cultures (p < 0.001). According to our morphological data L-carnitine had a beneficial effect on the human myotubes when is administered simultaneously with AZT.

EFFECT OF L-CARNITINE ON CULTURES AFTER 3 WEEKS OF AZT TREATMENT

By the sixth week (AZT for 3 weeks and L-carnitine for 3 weeks), the muscle cultures showed an increased number of Leu-19-positive myotubes, from 3.43 ± 0.62 (AZT, 3 weeks) to 23.00 ± 1.56 (6 weeks, 3 weeks AZT alone followed by 3 weeks L-carnitine), compared to 3.83 ± 1.23 (6 weeks, 3 weeks AZT followed by 3 weeks without treatment) (p < 0.001) (Fig. 12.2D,E). The accumulation of lipid droplets dramatically diminished from 12.22 ± 4.91 to 0.03 ± 0.02 (p < 0.001) compared to 0.18 ± 0.07 in the untreated cultures and 1.26 ± 0.51 in the cultures treated with medium alone after AZT-treatment. (Figs. 12.3D, 3E, 5D, 5E). We found by electron microscopy in the third week that the mitochondria in the L-carnitine-treated cultures were morphologically normal (Fig. 12.4F), in contrast to the mitochondria in the medium-treated cultures, which continued to show lamellar inclusions, vesiculations, and undefined cristae (Fig. 12.4G). The Vvi of the myofibrils had increased approaching the range of the chrono-logical control cultures to 9.80 ± 1.85 from 2.18 ± 1.25. Our data show that L-carnitine reverted the damage caused by the AZT treatment on human myotubes.

EFFECT OF L-CARNITINE ON CULTURES TREATED ONLY WITH AZT FOR THREE WEEKS AND WITH A MIXTURE OF AZT/L-CARNITINE FOR AN ADDITIONAL THREE WEEKS

After 6 weeks, the number of Leu-19-positive myotubes in the AZT-treated cultures that received L-carnitine was 6.87 ± 1.35/field compared to 3.3 ± 0.74 in the cultures treated with AZT alone (p < 0.0025) and 10.1 ± 1.56 in the untreated control cultures (Fig. 12.2F). Electron microscopy, after 6 weeks of AZT-treatment, showed 57.89 ± 5.64% of abnormal mito-chondria with high densities, vacuolation and lamellar inclusions (Fig. 12.4H). In contrast, only a few changes were noted in the mitochon-dria of the L-carnitine-treated cultures (Fig. 12.4I). The Vvi of the lipid droplets in the carnitine-treated cultures was reduced compared with AZT-treated cultures, from 5.06 ± 1.44 to 2.72±0.72 (p < 0.05) (Fig. 12.3F). No significant differences were noted in the Vvi of the lysosomes. The Vvi of the myofibrils in the L-carnitine-treated cultures increased compared with AZT-treated cultures that did not receive L-carnitine, from 2.5 ± 0.52 to 5.37 ± 0.76 (p < 0.05). Our results indicate that L-carnitine had a protective effect on the human myotubes even when the AZT-treatment is continued.

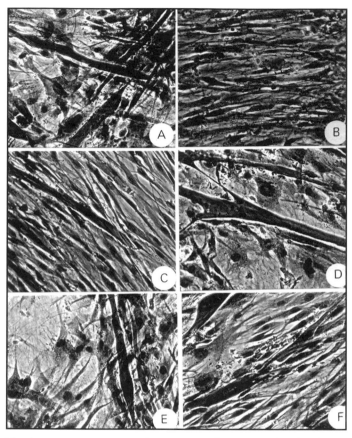

Fig. 12.3 A-F. Human muscle in tissue culture stained with oil-red-
O. Cultures treated with 250 μM demonstrate a remarkable increase
of lipid droplets (B) compared to the untreated control cultures (A).
C: cultures treated with 5 mM L-carnitine together with 250 μM
AZT resulted in substantial reduction of lipid droplets. Observe the
significant reduction in the lipid droplets in cultures treated with
carnitine (3 weeks) after AZT treatment (3 weeks) (D) and in cultures treated with complete medium after AZT treatment (3 weeks)
(E). F: cultures treated with AZT for 6 weeks and carnitine (from
3rd to 6th week) demonstrate also a reduction in the lipid droplets
(X 200). See color figure in insert.

These data may provide an indication for the use of a combined therapy in
the treatment of HIV-infected individuals.

## IN VIVO STUDIES

### EXPERIMENTAL DESIGNS

Two concentrations of AZT, low dose: 20mg/kg/day and high dose:
40 mg/kg/day, were used for each arm of the cohort; these concentrations

were based on the daily therapeutic doses. One group of 2 rats received only the different doses of AZT (1 animal per dose) intraperitoneally daily for 116 days. A second group of 3 animals each received L-carnitine (100 mg/kg/day) together with each dose of AZT during 116 days. A third group of 2 animals each received a first dose of AZT (55 days) followed by L-carnitine alone (61 days). A fourth group of 2 animals each received first AZT (either low or high) for 55 days followed by AZT/L-carnitine for 61 days. A fifth group of 1 animal each received first AZT (low or high dose) for 86 days followed without AZT treatment for 61 additional days, to assess the reversibility of the morphological changes. Animal controls only received i.p. saline solution (2 rats) or L-carnitine (2 rats) for the same periods. Muscle biopsies were performed in one animal from each group at day 55, day 86, and at the end of the treatments. They were evaluated with: modified Gomori's thrichrome, oil-red-O, cytochrome c oxidase (COX), ATPase, NADH and SDH,[28] quantification of the COX(-) fibers and ragged-red fibers (RRF), electron microscopy and morphometric studies calculating the volumetric density of mitochondria/per unit volume of tissue.[27]

EFFECT OF AZT IN RATS

The AZT-treated rats lost up to 22.5% of their weight, but regained 77% of it three months after the drug was withdrawn. The histological study of the muscle biopsies revealed: a) ragged-red fibers increased after AZT-therapy from 13.06 + 1.89% to 27.89 ± 2.89% in rats treated with low-AZT-dose (p < 0.05), and 36.91 ± 2.03% in rats treated with high-AZT-dose (p < 0.001); and b) COX(-) fibers increased from 66.97 ± 3.80% in control rats to 80.96 ± 4.19% in rats treated with low-dose-AZT (p < 0.001) and to 77.93 ± 3.26% in rats treated with high-dose-AZT (p < 0.05). After discontinuting AZT in the recovered animals, the percentage of RRF and COX(-) also decreased.

Electron microscopy revealed an increase in the absolute number of mitochondria per area from 8.13 ± 0.99 in the controls to 21.50±3.29 in the rats treated with low-AZT-dose (p < 0.001). An increment in the abnormal mitochondria was observed in rats treated with high-AZT-dose, 47.65 ± 4.04% vs 1.98 ± 1.33% in control rats (p < 0.001). However this number decreased after AZT withdrawal [47.65 ± 4.04% vs 26.56 ± 3.27% respectively (p < 0.001)]. Mitochondrial abnormalities consisted of myelin membranes, electron-dense inclusions, and vacuolization with disrupted cristae.

PRELIMINARY RESULTS OF L-CARNITINE IN AZT-TREATED RATS

a) Rats treated for 116 days with AZT and carnitine together

In the muscle of animals treated with 20 mg/kg/day AZT and L-carnitine, the percentage of RRF decreased from 27.89 ± 2.89 in animals treated

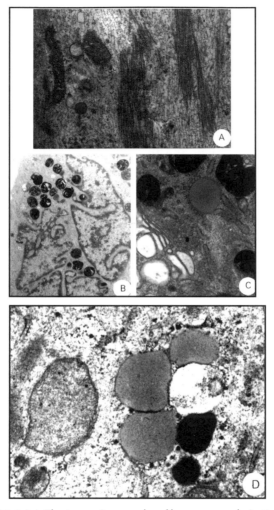

Fig. 12.4 A-I. Electron micrographs of human muscle in tissue culture treated with 250 μM AZT (B-D) show abnormal mitochondria with swelling, increased size (D), vacuolization and lamellar inclusions (B,C) compared to control untreated cultures (A). Cultures treated with 5 mM L-carnitine together with 250 μM AZT (E) and carnitine alone (3 weeks) after AZT treatment (3 weeks) (F) demonstrate rescue of the mitochondria structure. G: cultures treated with medium alone for 3 weeks post-AZT treatment; there are still abnormal mitochondria with swelling, vesiculation and myelin figures. H: cultures treated with 250 μM AZT for 6 weeks, observe abnormal mitochondria with loss of cristae, vesiculation and lamellar inclusions. I: Cultures treated with AZT (for 6 weeks) and carnitine (from 3rd to 6th week), cells show remarkable recovery and the mitochondria have normalized.(A,C,D,E,F,H,I: X 32,000 and B,G: X 12,000).

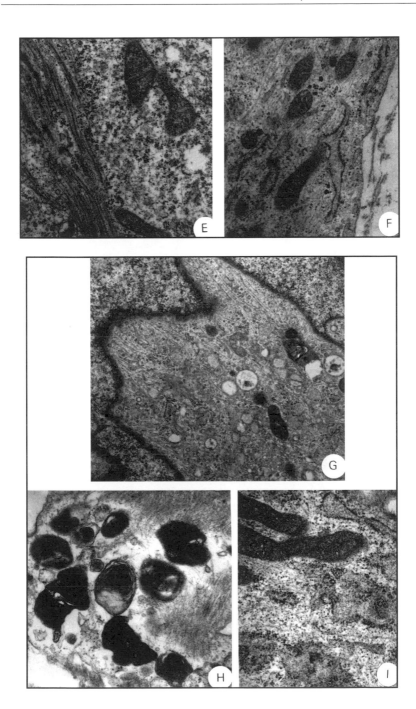

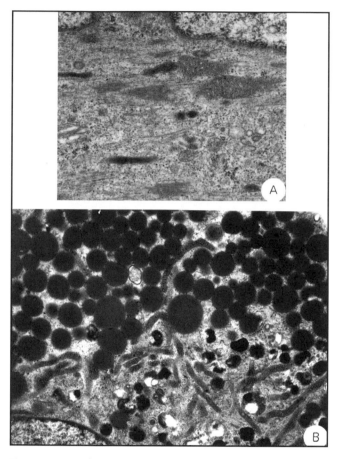

Fig. 12.5 A-E. Electron micrographs of human muscle in tissue culture treated with AZT for 3 weeks (B); note the dramatic increase of the lipid droplets, compared to control (A). C: cultures treated with carnitine together with AZT show significant reduction in the lipid droplets. In cultures treated with carnitine (3 weeks) after AZT-treatment (3 weeks) (D) and culture treated with medium (3 weeks) after AZT-treatment (3 weeks), an accumulation of lipids is not observed. (A,C,D,E: X 32,000 and B: X 12,000).

only with AZT to $15.56 \pm 1.70\%$ ($p < 0.001$), approaching the value of the control animals ($13.06 \pm 1.89$). The effect of L-carnitine was also seen in the number of COX(-) fibers, which decreased significantly from $80.96 \pm 4.19$ to $63.05 \pm 4.03$ ($p < 0.05$), compared to control at $66.97 \pm 3.80$. Ultrastructural morphometric studies showed that the number of mitochondria decreased from $24.20 \pm 1.57$ to $10.83 \pm 0.63$ in those animals treated concurrently with L-carnitine ($p < 0.001$). The percentage of abnormal mitochondria decreased from $47.65 \pm 4.04\%$ in high-AZT dose treatment to

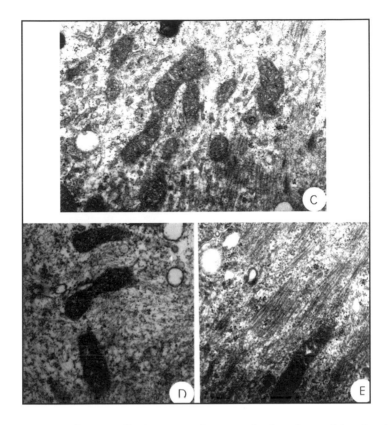

20.20±4.83%. These preliminary results, namely that L-carnitine in vivo has an effect on the AZT-treated muscles, need to be confirmed with additional counting before reaching a final conclusion. Furthermore, even if confirmed, the functional significance of these changes in rats is unclear.

**b) Rats treated for 55 days with AZT, followed by carnitine for 61 days**

Preliminary results in animals treated first with low-AZT dose and then with L-carnitine showed a decrease in the percentage of RRF, from 36.91 ± 2.03% to 26.69 ± 2.41%, and of the COX(-) fibers from 80.96 ± 4.19% to 59.32 ± 2.73% (p < 0.001). The percentage of abnormal mitochondria observed with high-AZT-dose decreased from 47.65 ± 4.04% to 38.49 ± 3.74%. No effect of carnitine was noted in the high-AZT-dose treatment animals.

The significance of these findings is unknown and needs further confirmation and correlation with functional studies.

# CONCLUSIONS

The present results established that L-carnitine in vitro applied concurrently with AZT 1) prevented the destructive effect of AZT on the myotubes and their mitochondria; 2) can enhance the recovery of the myotubes and their mitochondria when AZT is withdrawn; and 3) can restore the integrity and function of the myotubes while AZT treatment continues. Whether similar effects occur in vivo in animals can not be determined until additional counting is performed.

The mechanism by which L-carnitine exerts such a protective effect on the mitochondria is unknown. L-carnitine, in vitro, interacts with the mitochondrial membrane's cardiolipin, modifying the permeability of the membrane and protecting the physical mechanism of the mitochondria.[29] This mechanism has been proposed for the protective effect of L-carnitine on the ammonium acetate-induced swelling,[19] and may be also proposed for its protective effect on the AZT-induced mitochondrial toxicity.[12,13,19,29-31] AZT causes not only structural, but also functional, abnormalities in the mitochondria by uncoupling their oxidative phosphorylation and decreasing the enzymatic activity of the respiratory chain complex I and III.[8,32,33] Consequently, the long chain fatty acids cannot be effectively utilized, resulting in the accumulation of the lipid droplets.[12,13,34,35] L-carnitine facilitates $\beta$-oxidation of fatty acids and the concentration of acetyl-CoA in the cytosol.[14-18] Additionally, AZT inhibits state 4 of respiration,[8,30,32,33] and carnitine stimulates state 4 and removes fatty acids.[12,13,36]

REFERENCES

1. Dalakas MC, Illa I, Pezeshkpour GH et al. Mitochondrial myopathy caused by long-term zidovudine therapy. N Eng J Med 1990; 322: 1098-1105.
2. Fischl MA, Richman DD, Grieco MH and the AZT Collaborative Working group. The efficacy of azidothymidine (AZT) in the treatment of patients with AIDS and AIDS-related complex: a double-blind, placebo-controlled trial. N Engl J Med 1987; 317:185-191.
3. Gertner E, Thun JR, William DN et al. Zidovudine-associated myopathy. Am J Med 1988; 86:814-818.
4. Gorard DA, Henry K, Guiloff RJ. Necrotising myopathy and zidovudine. Lancet 1988; 1:1050.
5. Helbert M, Fletcher T, Peddle B, Harris JRW, Pinching AJ. Zidovudine-associated myopathy. Lancet 1988; 2:689-690.
6. Arnaudo D, Dalakas M, Shanske S et al. Depletion of muscle mitochondrial DNA in AIDS patients with zidovudine-induced myopathy. Lancet 1991; 337:508-510.
7. Cupler EJ, Danon MJ, Jay C et al. Early features of zidovudine-associated myopathy: histopathological findings and clinical correlations. Acta Neuropathol 1995; 90:1-6.
8. Lamperth L, Dalakas MC, Dagani F et al. Abnormal skeletal and car-

diac muscle mitochondria induced by zidovudine (AZT) in human muscle in vitro and in animal model. Lab Invest 1991; 65:742-751

9. Lewis W, Papoian T, Gonzalez B et al. Mitochondrial ultrastructural and molecular changes induced by zidovudine in rats hearts. Lab Invest 1991; 65:228-236.

10. Lewis W, Gonzalez B, Chomyn A, Papoian T. Zidovudine induces molecular, biochemical, and ultrastructural changes in rat skeletal muscle mitochondria. J Clin Invest 1992; 89:1354-1360.

11. Lewis W, Dalakas MC. Mitochondrial toxicity of antiviral drugs. Nature Medicine 1995; 1:417-422.

12. Semino-Mora MC, Leon-Monzon ME, Dalakas MC. The effect of L-carnitine on the zidovudine-induced destruction of human myotubes. Part I: L-carnitine prevents the myotoxicity of AZT in vitro. Lab Invest 1994; 71:102-112.

13. Semino-Mora MC, Leon-Monzon ME, Dalakas MC. The effect of L-carnitine on the AZT-induced destruction of human myotubes. Part II: Treatment with L-carnitine improves the AZT-induced changes and prevents further destruction. Lab Invest 1994; 71:773-781.

14. Bieber LL. Carnitine. Ann Rev Biochem 1988; 57:261-283.

15. Bremer J. Carnitine-metabolism and functions. Physiol Rev 1983; 63:1420-1480.

16. Carpenter S, Karpati G. Pathology of Skeletal Muscle. New York: Churchill Livingstone, 1984.

17. Di Mauro S, Bonilla E, Zeviani M et al. Mitochondrial myopathies. Ann Neurol 1985; 17:521-538.

18. Engel AG. Carnitine deficiency syndromes and lipid storage myopathies. In: Engel AG, editor. Myology. New York: McGraw-Hill, 1986;1663-1696.

19. Bellei M, Batelli D, Guarriero DM et al. Changes in mitochondrial activity caused by ammonium salts and the protective effect of carnitine. Biochem Biophys Res Commun 1989; 158:181-188.

20. Famularo G, De Simone C. A new era for carnitine. Immunol Today 1995; 16: 211-213

21. De Simone C, Famularo G, Tzantzoglou S et al. Carnitine depletion in peripheral blood mononuclear cells from patients with AIDS: effect of oral L-carnitine. AIDS 1994; 8:655-660.

22. De Simone C, Tzantzoglou S, Famularo G et al. High dose L-carnitine improves immunologic and metabolic parameters in AIDS patients. Immunopharmacol Immnunotoxicol 1993; 15:1-12.

23. Foresta P, Ruggiero V, D'Urso C et al. Protective effect of ST 899, a new PAF receptor antagonist, in endotoxin-induced shock in mice. Intensive Care Med 1994; 20:S156.

24. Kuratsune H, Yamaguti K, Takahashi M, et al. Acylcarnitine deficiency in chronic fatigue syndrome. Clin Infect Dis 1994; 18:S62-S67.

25. Askanas V, Engel WK. A new program for investigating adult skeletal muscle grown aneurally in tissue culture. Neurology 1975; 25:58-67.

26. Illa I, Leon-Monzon M, Dalakas MC. Regenerating and denervated human muscle fibers and satellite cells express N-CAM recognized by monoclonal antibodies to NK cells. Ann Neurol 1992; 31:46-52.

27. Weibel ER. Stereological principles for morphometry in electron microscopy cytology. Int Rev Cytol 1969; 26:235-302.

28. Dalakas MC. Morphological changes in the muscles of patients with postpoliomyelitis neuromuscular symptoms. Neurology 1988; 38:99-104.

29. Batelli D, Bellei M, Arrigoni-Martelli E, Muscatello U, Bobyleva V. Interaction of carnitine with mitochondria cardiolipin. Biochim Biophys Acta 1992; 1117:33-36.

30. Kim CS, Roe CR, Ambrose WW. L-carnitine prevents mitochondrial damage induced by octanoic acid in the rat choroid plexus. Brain Res 1990; 536:335-338.

31. Mokhova E, Arrigoni-Martelli E, Bellei M et al. The protecting effect of L-carnitine on $Ca^2$ -loaded rat liver mitochondria. FEBS 1991, 289: 187-189.

32. Mhiri C, Baudrimont M, Bonne G et al. Zidovudine myopathy: a distinctive disorder associated with mitochondrial dysfunction. Ann Neurol 1991; 29:606-614.

33. Chariot P, Gherardi R. Partial cytochrome C oxidase deficiency and cytoplasmic bodies in patients with zidovudine myopathy. Neuromuscul Disord 1991; 5:357-363.

34. Dalakas MC, Leon-Monzon M, Bernardini I et al. The AZT-induced mitochondrial myopathy is associated with muscle carnitine deficiency and lipid-storage. Ann Neurol 1994; 35:482-487.

35. d'Amati G, Lewis W. Zidovudine azidothymidine causes early increases in mitochondrial ribonucleic acid abundance and induced ultrastructural changes in cultured mouse muscle cells. Lab Invest 1994; 71:879-884.

36. Modica-Napolitano JS. AZT causes tissue-specific inhibition of mitochondrial bioenergetic function. Biochem Biophys Res Commun 1993; 194:170-177.

# Possible Anti-Apoptotic Activity of Carnitines on Excitatory Amino Acid-Induced Neurotoxicity

Edoardo Alesse, Grazia Cifone, Adriano Angelucci,
Francesca Zazzeroni and Claudio De Simone

## INTRODUCTION

Glutamate is the primary excitatory neurotransmitter in the brain. At the neuronal synapse, it interacts with a variety of receptors that specify neurotransmitter interactions and transmit information into target cells. The vast majority of synapses in the central nervous system use glutamate as a neurotransmitter to produce rapid neuronal excitation.[1,2] Glutamate neurotransmission also participates in neuronal plasticity and neurotoxicity. Neuronal plasticity elicited by glutamate is exemplified by long-term potentiation (LTP) in the hippocampus[3] and long term depression in the cerebellum.[4] However, at supraphysiological concentrations, it is a potent excitotoxin that causes neuronal death through a cascade of cationic and second messenger events.[5,6] In fact, in many neurologic disorders, injury to neurons may be partly caused by overstimulation of receptors for excitatory amino acids, including glutamate and aspartate. These neurologic conditions range from acute insults such as stroke, hypoglycemia and epilepsy to chronic neurodegenerative diseases such as Hungtington's disease, AIDS-dementia complex, amyotrophic lateral sclerosis, and perhaps Alzheimer's disease. Furthermore, a plethora of unrelated molecules including HIV gp120, HIV-Tat, tumor necrosis factor (TNF)-α, platelet-activating factor (PAF), interleukin-6 (IL-6), arachidonic acid metabolites, reactive oxygen species and nitric oxide (NO)[7-15] can trigger neuronal cell death by converging their actions into a common pathway that involves ionotropic glutamate receptors (glutamate-activated ion channels that regulate intracellular $Ca^{2+}$).

*Carnitine Today*, edited by Claudio De Simone and Giuseppe Famularo.

Thus, specific blockers of the NMDA subtype of glutamate receptors, such as MK801 or nemantine, effectively block in vitro the toxic effects of several candidate neurotoxins. These findings suggest that glutamate, besides constituting the direct toxic stimulus in some neurodegenerative diseases, may be a key contributor in some situations, such as HIV-induced neurodegeneration.[16]

## GLUTAMATE AND CANCER

Glutamate has been found to inhibit the membrane transport of cystine and to impair the function of macrophages and lymphocytes in vitro.[17,18] In patients with advanced colon carcinoma, elevated plasma glutamate concentrations have also been found to quantitatively correlate with reduced lymphocyte reactivity in these persons. After tumor resection, plasma glutamate levels returned to the normal range levels within 1 week of surgery. Concomitantly, a rapid recovery of lymphocyte reactivity toward concanavalin A was observed. Lymphocyte responses against pokeweed mitogen and phytohemoagglutinin, in contrast, remained impaired for at least 6 months, indicating that elevated glutamate levels in patients with colorectal carcinoma are associated with a long-lasting defect in the immune system.[13]

## GLUTAMATE MAY MEDIATE SOME NEUROLOGICAL DISORDERS

That glutamate and other amino acids act as neurotoxins was first described in the 1970s, when these agents were given orally to immature animals. Acute neurodegeneration was observed in those areas not well protected by the blood-brain barrier, notably the arcuate nucleus of the hypothalamus. The mechanisms of glutamate-induced neurodegeneration are divergent and activation of all the classes of ionotropic glutamate receptors has been implicated.[20]

### ISCHEMIC CELL DAMAGE

Prolonged periods of neuronal tissue anoxia (cardiac arrest, thrombosis) result in ischemic damage and neurotoxicity. Oxygen deprivation leads to a depletion of energy stores, with concomitant acidosis and release of free radicals. Subsequently, the inability of neurons to maintain their resting potential causes membrane depolarization with release of glutamate from presynaptic terminals. The postsynaptic AMPA ($\alpha$-amino-3-hydroxy-5-methyl-4-isoxazolepropionate) and NMDA (N-methyl-D-aspartate) receptors are then activated by the released glutamate and the $Ca^{2+}$ concentration increased intracellularly by its entry through the NMDA receptor complex and voltage-sensitive $Ca^{2+}$ channels.[21,22] The intracellular increase of $Ca^{2+}$ will trigger a cascade of second messengers, many of which remain activated long after the initial stimulus is removed. If the cell is unable to recover its resting potential, a positive feedback loop is triggered, leading to neuronal cell injury or death. The type of cell death undergone by neurons may depend on the intensity of the exposure to the excitatory amino acid and may involve two temporally distinct phases: necrosis, associated with extreme energy failure in mitochondria; and apoptosis, cell recovery of mitochondrial function after a moderate or mild insult followed by a default program of programmed cell death.

NEURODEGENERATIVE DISORDERS

Disorders of excitatory amino acid transmission have been implicated in different chronic neurodegenerative diseases. For some of them, there is good evidence of glutamate receptor involvement (Hungtington's disease, AIDS dementia complex, neuropathic pain syndrome), whereas for others the evidence is only suggestive (Alzheimer's disease, amyotrophic lateral sclerosis, Parkinsonism). As discussed below, a large number of in vitro studies have suggested that apoptosis may play an important role in these pathologies. This is supported by in vivo studies reporting the detection of in situ DNA fragmentation in epileptic brain damage,[23] and in brain specimens from patients with Alzheimer's disease.[24] Remarkably, αβ peptide has been shown to induce neurodegeneration and apoptosis in transgenic mice.[25] A serin-protease inhibitor, nexin I, which is present at decreased concentrations in brain regions affected by Alzheimer's disease, including the hippocampus, has been shown to rescue motor neurons from both naturally occurring and axotomy-induced cell death.[26] Probably, necrosis may also participate in the pathogenesis of neurodegeneration.

AMYOTROPHIC LATERAL SCLEROSIS (ALS)

A systemic defect in glutamate metabolism has been documented in patients with ALS, in whom the glutamate plasma concentration was 100% higher than in matched controls; these patients also showed abnormal glutamate clearance following oral glutamate administration.[27] Elevated glutamate levels have also been detected in the cerebrospinal fluid of ALS patients.[28] Furthermore, post-mortem examination of neuronal tissue has revealed selective depletion of glutamate in the central nervous system (CNS).[29] At the cellular level, glutamate is rapidly eliminated from the synapse by an energy-dependent high-affinity transport system present in both astrocytes and nerve terminals.[30-32] In ALS patients, glutamate transport velocity was found to be significantly impaired in the spinal cord, neocortex and cortex. This transport defect was due to a decrease in the relative abundance of the transport protein (e.g., astroglial specific transporter).[33-34] Defects in the clearance of extracellular glutamate, due to faulty transport, could lead to neurotoxic levels of extracellular glutamate and thus be pathogenic in ALS.

## ALZHEIMER'S DISEASE

Alzheimer's disease is a neurological disease that affects about one out of six individuals past the age of sixty.[35-36] Clinically, patients present with memory loss, personality changes and symptoms of cortical disconnection. Pathological brain changes include the presence of senile plaques, neurofibrillary tangles and granulovacuolar degeneration in the cerebral cortex, amygdala, olfactory tubercle and hippocampus.[37] Neurochemical studies of this pathology indicate the presence of several, altered transmission systems, including the glutaminergic system. A recent in vitro study suggests that β-amyloid protein can lead to apoptotic cell death by means of a nitric oxide-mediated process, triggered by $Ca^{2+}$ entry-activated NMDA-gated channels.[38] Furthermore, there is evidence that MPTP-induced destruction of nigrostriatal dopaminergic neurons can be attenuated by NMDA antagonists and that β-amyloid protein, which accumulates in Alzheimer's disease, can potentiate excitotoxic degeneration. The β-amyloid protein can form calcium channels in bilayer membranes, which may contribute to its neurotoxic effects.[39]

## AIDS AND AIDS DEMENTIA COMPLEX

Apoptosis is likely to be an important mechanism in HIV-associated lymphocyte depletion and also in HIV encephalitis. In both cases, glutamate alterations may play a relevant role. A large body of evidence indicates that AIDS may be the consequence of a virus-induced cysteine deficiency. HIV-infected persons, at all stages of the disease, have markedly decreased plasma cystine and cysteine concentrations, decreased intracellular glutathione and elevated plasma glutamate levels. High extracellular glutamate levels worsen the cysteine deficiency since glutamate competitively inhibits the membrane transport of cystine. In vitro lymphocyte functions are augmented by even slight elevations of extracellular cysteine deficiency and are inhibited by the elevation of the extracellular glutamate concentrations. In view of the decreased levels of the bona fide anti-oxidants, cysteine and glutathione, one may expect to find manifestations of oxidative damage, but the contribution of the oxidative damage to the immunopathology of HIV infection remains to be determined.[40] With regard to the AIDS dementia complex, the HIV-associated neurological manifestations, it affects 40-60% of the AIDS population and the virally induced cytopathology can be identified at autopsy in over 90% of cases. Since the burden of HIV infection within the CNS correlates with the severity of clinical dementia, it is likely that viral infection is crucial for the induction of neurological disease.[41] Nonetheless, the degree of neuropathological damage detected in the brain of individuals affected by HIV dementia is often less than what might be expected in light of the severity of the clinical presentation. It is particularly striking that relatively few cells in the CNS are productively infected by HIV-1 and that these cells are almost exclusively cells of the monocyte lineage. Three major hypotheses have been proposed to explain the observation that HIV severely compromises the CNS despite infecting relatively few cells: 1) secretion of neurotoxic viral products by infected microglial and brain macrophages; 2) aberration in the production of neurotoxic cytokines or other cellular factors caused by HIV-1 induced immune activation; and 3) disruption of intercellular communication and astrocyte function caused by non-productive infection of astrocytes. Candidate neurotoxins are viral and cellular gene products, such as the Tat protein and gp120, that may use a direct or indirect mechanism of action. In fact, gp120 partially exerts its neurotoxic action indirectly by triggering the release of secreted factors from monocytic cells, including TNF-α and nitric oxide.[8,42] These observations imply that immune activation may be crucial in the pathogenesis of HIV dementia. Indeed, the intracerebral expression of TNF-α mRNA has been found to be upregulated in this situation.[43] Furthermore, intracerebral levels of arachidonic acid metabolites, including prostaglandins, are also elevated in the CNS of individuals with HIV dementia.[44] These observations are in agreement with the in vitro findings that TNF-α, arachidonic acid metabolites, and PAF are produced at high levels by activated HIV-infected monocytes. In addition, PAF and TNF-α are toxic to cultured human fetal neurons. Moreover, intracranial administration of the TNF-α inhibitor, pentoxifylline, blocks the neurotoxic effect of the Tat protein.[10] Elevated levels of quinolinic acid, a glutamate agonist, are also observed in the CSF of patients with AIDS dementia complex.[45] Hence, a series of different molecules, (including HIV gp120, HIV-Tat, TNF-α, PGs, NO, etc.) can trigger or participate in neuronal cell death, both in vivo and in vitro. To hypothesize any potential therapeutic approach, it is important to analyze the mechanism through which these factors act. One possible answer is that these neurotoxins may converge upon a common pathway that involves ionotropic glutamate receptors. In fact, NMDA antagonists block the toxic effect of gp120 and PAF[46,15] while antagonists of non-NMDA glutamate receptors inhibit the neurotoxic effects of Tat and TNF-α.[11,13] Thus, glutamate may be a crucial contributor to HIV-induced neurological damage, via an excitotoxic mechanism (increase of the intracellular $Ca^{2+}$). If this hypothesis is true, astrocytes may play an important role in the neuropathogenesis of AIDS, due to their role in regulating extracellular glutamate concentrations in the CNS, while several candidate neurotoxins (e.g.,TNF-α) are able to alter glutamate transport in astrocytes.[47] Inhibition of glutamate receptors by TNF-α negatively influences neuronal uptake of cysteine, which is the limiting precursor for glutathione, thereby sensitizing the neuron to oxidative injury. Besides the NMDA receptor, four subtypes of the AMPA-glutamate receptor (A, B, C and D) are present in the CNS. Analysis of the AMPA receptor network, showed a strong decrease in both gene and protein expression for the Glu-R A receptor in patients who died of AIDS.

The altered host gene expression observed may compromise cell viability and function. There are many AMPAergic neurons throughout the brain, in which an alteration in the AMPA gene and receptor protein expression could not only impair transmission but also render those cells more vulnerable to further insult or death.[48] Interestingly, besides being the final pathway toward which different neurotoxic stimuli such as TNF-α and arachidonate metabolites converge, the glutaminergic system may also participate in generating, at least in vitro, some of these toxic molecules. In fact glutamate stably enhances the activity of phospholipase A2 in brain cortex cultures probably by a mechanism involving $Ca^{2+}$ and PKC. This phenomenon could partly explain the glutamate cytotoxicity.[49]

## PHARMACOTHERAPY FOR EXCITATORY AMINO ACID-INDUCED NEUROTOXICITY

There are several sites at which glutamate-mediated damage might be attenuated. For example, the synthesis and release of glutamate could be reduced or its uptake increased. The effect of glutamate could also be antagonized. Moreover, at the receptor level, certain drugs may be used to inhibit distal neurotoxic events triggered by receptor overstimulation. Several agents are available for these purposes, but the clinical side effects greatly restrict the range of these useful molecules.

Carnitine could be a useful molecule in the managment of different pathological conditions related to glutamate dysmetabolism. First, carnitine and acethylcarnitine are cheap, reliable and safe molecules. In fact, no major side effects are observed even during long term treatment. Second, different potential targets are present in the pathogenesis of several bona fide glutamate-induced diseases. Indeed, we previously described the anti-apoptotic action of carnitine on the lymphocytes of HIV-infected patients and we showed a clear correlation with the decreased levels of ceramide, a potential apoptotic messenger, in peripheral blood lymphocytes.[50,51] In this context, in addition to a direct effect of carnitine on sphingomyelinase activity, which generates ceramide,[52] a potential antioxidant action of this molecule has been postulated.[53] Furthermore, preliminary experiments in our laboratory indicate the possibility that carnitines may correct unbalanced glutamate metabolism (unpublished results). This latter finding prompted us to carnitines as useful molecules for the treatment of immunodeficiency as well as for the AIDS dementia complex. The following additional experimental evidence encourages the use of carnitine in different neurological disorders involving apoptosis:

1) Cytokines, such as TNF-α, are likely to play an important role in the development of AIDS dementia complex and other neurological disorders. In studies on inflammation, there is evidence that carnitine may downmodulate TNF-α production, thus acting on a possible pathogenetic element.[54,55]

2) Recently, it has been reported that L-carnitine was able to increase the affinity of glutamate for metabotropic receptors of the quisqualate type, thereby preventing the neurotoxicicity mediated by NMDA receptors.[56]

3) The neurotransmitter activity of glutamate released into synaptic terminals is terminated by its reuptake into pre- and post-synaptic neurons and into astrocytes.[57] The high affinity transport system is operated by an energy-dependent mechanism.[58] Several lines of evidence have indicated that sodium-dependent high affinity uptake of glutamate is inhibited in acute, as well as chronic, models of hyperammoniemia.[59] The uptake of glutamate by astrocytes is also inhibited in vitro by TNF-α.[47] The role of L-acetyl-carnitine in reestablishing the decreased reuptake in hyperammoniemia conditions could be predicted in terms of reversal. The altered synaptic membrane properties improve the energy supply for the normal function of $Na^+/K^+$ ATPase activity. Furthermore, the reduction of cytokine levels, such as TNF α, could contribute to the normalization of glutamate reuptake in all neurodegenerations involving an abnormal immune response.

Altogether, these observations suggest that the interesting properties of carnitines should be considered for the treatment of some neurological or general diseases related to apoptosis and glutamate dysfunction.

REFERENCES

1. Sommer B, Seeburg PH. Glutamate receptor channels: novel properties and new clones. Trends Biol Sci 1992; 13:291-296.
2. Monaghan DT, Bridges RJ, Cotman CW. The excitatory amino acid receptors: their classes, pharmacology, and distinct properties in the function of the central nervous system. Annu Rev Pharmacol Toxicol 1989; 29:365-402.
3. Collingridge GL, Bliss TVP. NMDA receptors - their role in long-term potentiation. Trends Neurosci 1987; 10:288-293.
4. Ito M. Long-term depression. Annu Rev Neurosci 1989; 12:85-102.
5. Choi DW. Glutamate neurotoxicity and diseases of the nervous system. Neuron 1989; 1:623-634.
6. Manev H, Costa E, Wroblewski ST, Guidotti A. Abusive stimulation of excitatory amino acid receptors: a strategy to limit neurotoxicity. Faseb J 1989; 4:2789-2797.

7. Toggas SM, Masliam E, Rockenstein EM et al. Central nervous system damage produced by expression of the HIV-1 coat protein gp120 in transgenic mice. Nature 1994; 367:188-193.

8. Koka P, He K, Zack JA. Human immunodeficiency virus 1 envelope proteins induce interleukin 1, tumor necrosis factor $\alpha$, nitric oxide in glial cultures derived from fetal, neonatal, and adult human brain. J Exp Med 1995; 182:941-952.

9. Benos DJ, Hann BH, Bubien JK. Envelope glycoprotein gp120 of human immunodeficiency virus type 1 alters ion transport in astrocytes: implications for AIDS dementia complex. Proc Natl Acad Sci USA 1994; 91:494-498.

10. Philippon V, Vellutini C, Gambarelli D et al. The basic domain of the lentiviral Tat protein is responsible for damages in mouse brain: involvement of cytokines. Virology 1994; 205:494-498.

11. Magnuson DSK, Kundensen BE, Geiger JD. Human immunodeficiency virus type I Tat activates non-N-methyl-D-aspartate excitatory amino acid receptors and causes neurotoxicity. Ann Neurol 1995; 37:373-380.

12. Wesselingh SL, Power C, Glass JD. Intracerebral cytokine messenger RNA expression in acquired immunodeficiency syndrome dementia. Ann Neurol 1993; 33:576-582.

13. Gelhard HA, Dzenko KA, DiLoreto D et al. Neurotoxic effects of tumor necrosis factor in primary human neuronal cultures are mediated by activation of the gltamate AMPA receptor subtype: implications for AIDS neuropathogenesis. Dev Neurosci 1993; 15:417-422.

14. Young MC, Pulliam L, Lau A. The HIV envelope protein gp120 is toxic to human brain-cell cultures through the induction of interleukin-6 and tumor necrosis factor-$\alpha$. AIDS 1995; 9:137-143.

15. Gelbard HA, Nottet HSLM, Swindells S. Platelet activating factor: a candidate HIV-1-induced neurotoxin. J Virol 68:4829-4836.

16. Dewhurst S, Gelbard HA, Fine SM, Neuropathogenesis of AIDS. Mol Med Today, 1996; 16-23.

17. Watanabe H, Bannai S. Induction of cystine transport activity in mouse peritoneal macrophages. J Exp Med 1987; 165:628-640.

18. Eck HP, Droge W. Influence of the extracellular glutamate concentration on the intracellular cysteine contentration in macrophages and on the capacity to release cystine. Biol Chem Hoppe-Seyler 1989; 370:109-113.

19. Eck HP, Betzler M, Schlag P, Droge W. Partial recovery of lymphocyte activity in patients with colorectal carcinoma after curative surgical treatment and return of plasma glutamate concentrations to normal levels. J Cancer Res Clin Oncol 1990; 116:648-650.

20. Dingledina R, McBain CJ. Excitatory amino acid transmitters. In: Siegel, GJ ed. Basic Neurochemistry Molecular, Cellular, and Medical Aspects. Raven Press, Ltd New York, 5:367-387.

21. Sommer B, Keynanen K, Verdoorn TA et al. Flip and flop: A cell specific functional switch in glutamate-operated channels of the C.N.S. Scienze 1990; 249:1580-1585.

22. Hume RI, Dingledine R, Heinemman SF. Identification of a site in glutamate receptor subunits that controls calcium permeability. Science 1991; 253:1028-1032.

23. Pollard HB, Cantagrel S, Charriant-Marlangue C, Moreau J, Ben Ar, Y. Apoptosis associated DNA fragmentation in epileptic brain damage. NeuroReport 1994; 5:1053-1055.

24. Lassmann H, Bancher C, Breitschopf H et al. Cell death in Alzheimer's disease evaluated by DNA fragmentation in situ. Acta Neuropathol 1995; 89:35-41.

25. LaFerla FM, Tinkle BT, Bierberich CJ et al. The Alzheimer's Aβ peptide induces neurodegeneration and apoptotic cell death in transgenic mice. Nature Genetics 1995; 9:21-30.

26. Houenou LJ, Turner PL, Li L et al. A serine protease inhibitor, protease nexin I, rescues motoneurons from naturally occurring and axotomy-induced cell death. Proc Natl Acad Sci USA 1995; 92:895-899.

27. Ptaitakis A, Caroscio JT. Abnormal glutamate metabolism in amyotrophic lateral sclerosis. Ann Neurol 1987; 22:575-579.

28. Rothstain JD, Tsai G, Kuncl RW. Abnormal excitatory amino acid metabolism in amyotrophic lateral sclerosis. Ann Neurol 1990; 28:18-25.

29. Plaitakis A. Altered glutaminergic mechanism selective motor neuron degeneration in amyotrophic lateral sclerosis: possible role of glycine. Adv Neurol 1991; 56:319-328.

30. Fonnum F. Glutamine and Glutamate in Mammals. Kvamme E, ed. Boca Raton, FL. CRC Press Inc, 1988; 2:57-69.

31. Shank RP, Aprison MH. Glutamine and Glutamate in Mammals. Kvamme E, ed. Boca Raton:FL, CRC Press Inc, 1988; 2:3-19.

32. Hertz L, Schousboe A. Glutamine and Glutamate in Mammals, Kvamme E, ed. Boca Raton:FL, CRC Press Inc, 1988; 2:39-55.

33. Shaw PJ, Chinnry RM, Ince PG. D-aspartate binding sites in the normal human spinal cord and changes in motor neuron disease: A quantitative autoradiographic study. Brain Res 1994; 655:195-201.

34. Rohstein JD, Van Kammen M, Levey AI et al. Selective loss of glial glutamate transporter GLT-1 in amyotrophic lateral sclerosis. Ann Neurol 1995; 38:73-84.

35. Khachaturian ZS. Diagnosis of Alzheimer's Disease. Arch Neurol 1985; 42:1097-1105.

36. Terry RD, Peck A, Deteresa R et al. Some morphometric aspects of the brain in senile dementia of the Alzheimer type. Annal Neurol 1981; 10:184-192.

37. Hyman BT, Van Hoesen GW, Damasio AR et al. Alzheimer's disease: cell-specific pathology isolates the hippocampal formation. Science, 1984; 225:1168-1170.

38. Le W, Colom LV, Xie WJ et al. Cell death induced by β-amyloid 1-40 in MES 23.5 hybrid clone: the role of nitric oxide and NMDA-gated channel activation leading to apoptosis. Brain Res 1995; 686:49-60.

39. Arispe N, Rojas E, Pollard HB. Alzeimer disease amyloid β protein forms calcium channels in bilayer membranes: blockade by tro methamine and aluminium. Proc Natl Acad Sci USA 1993; 90: 567-571.

40. Droge W, Eck H-P, Mihm S, Galter D. Abnormal redox regulation in HIV infection and other immunodeficiency diseases. In: Pasquier C et al. Oxidative Stress, Cell Activation, and Viral Infection. Birkhauser Verlag Basel/Switzerland, 1994; 285-298.

41. Wiley CA, Chim C. Human immunodeficiency virus encephalitis is the pathological correlate of dementia in acquired immunodeficiency syndrome. Ann Neurol 1994; 36:674-676.

42. Dawson VL, Dawson TM, Uhl GR, Snyder SH. Human immunode-ficiency virus type I coat protein neurotoxicity mediated by nitric oxide in primary cortical cultures. Proc Natl Acad Sci USA 1993; 90:3256-3259.

43. Wesseling HSL, Power C, Glass JD. Intracerebral cytokine messen-ger RNA expression in acquired immunodeficiency syndrome dementia. Ann Neurol 1993; 33:576-582.

44. Griffin DE, Wesselingh SL, McArthur JC. Elevated central nervous system prostaglandins in human immunodeficiency virus-associated dementia. Ann Neurol 1994; 35:592-597.

45. Heyes MP, Brew BJ, Martin A et al. Quinolinic acid in cerebrospi-nal fluid and serum in HIV-1 infection: Relationship to clinical and neurological status. Ann Neurol 1991; 29:202-209.

46. Lipton SA, Gendelma HE. Dementia associated with the acquired immunodeficiency syndrome. New Engl J Med 1995; 332:934-940.

47. Fine SM, Angel RA, Perry SW et al. Tumor necrosis factor α inhib-its glutamate uptake by primary human astrocytes. J Biol Chem 1994; 15303-15306.

48. Everall IP, Hudso L, Al-Sarraj S et al. Decreased expression of AMPA receptor messenger RNA and protein in AIDS: A model for HIV-associated neurotoxicity. Nature Med 1995; 1:1174-1178.

49. Kim DK, Rordorf G, Nemenoff RA et al. Glutamate stably enhances the activity of two cytosolic forms of phospholipase A2 in brain cor-tical cultures. Biochem J 1995; 310:83-90.

50. De Simone C, Cifone MG, Roncaioli P et al. Ceramide, AIDS, and long-term survivors. Immunol Today 1996; 17:48.

51. De Simone C, Cifone MG, Di Marzio L et al. Cell-associated ceramide in HIV-1-infected subjects. AIDS 1996; 10:675-688.

52. Cifone G, Alesse E, Di Marzio L et al. Effect of L-carnitine treat-ment in vivo on apoptosis and ceramide generation in peripheral

blood lymphocytes from AIDS patients. Proc Ass Am Phys, accepted for publication, 1996.
53. Buttke TM, Sandstrom PA. Oxidative stress as a mediator of apoptosis. Immunol Today 1994; 15:7-10.
54. De Simone C, Famularo G, Tzantzoglou S et al. Carnitine depletion in peripheral blood mononuclear cells from patients with AIDS: Effects of oral L-carnitine. AIDS 1994; 8:655-660.
55. Famularo G, De Simone C, Tzantzoglou S, Trinchieri V. Apoptosis, anti-apoptotic compounds and TNF-α release. Immunol Today 15:495-496.
56. Felipo V, Minana MD, Cabedo H, Grisolia S. L-carnitine increases the affinity of glutamate for quisqualate receptors and prevents glutamate neurotoxicity. Neurochemical Res 1994; 19:373-377.
57. Shank RP, Campbell GL. Amino acid uptake, content, and metabolism by neuronal and glial enriched cellular fractions from mouse cerebellum. J Neurosci 1984; 4:58-60.
58. Erecinska M. The neurotransmitter amino acid transport systems. A fresh outlook on an old problem. Biochem Pharmacol 1987; 36:3547-3555.
59. Mena EE, Cotman CW. Pathologic concentrations of ammonium ions block L-glutamate uptake. Exp Neurol 1985; 89:259-263.

# INDEX